Animal Nutrition Made Easy

(A Unique blend of MCQs and questions for competitive exams, NET, ICAR-ARS, etc.)

Animal Nutrition Made Easy

(A Unique blend of MCQs and questions for competitive exams, NET, ICAR-ARS, etc.)

Authors :

Jaswinder Singh, Ph.D. Animal Nutrition

Department of Veterinary and Animal Husbandry Extension Education

Jaspal Singh Hundal, Ph.D. Animal Nutrition

Department of Animal Nutrition

Guru Angad Dev Veterinary and Animal Sciences University, Ludhiana, Punjab

SSPH

SATISH SERIAL PUBLISHING HOUSE

403, Express Tower, Commercial Complex

Azadpur, Delhi-110033 (India)

Phone : 011-27672852, Fax : 91-11-27672046

e-mail : info@satishserial.com, hkjain1975@yahoo.com

Website : www.satishserial.com

Published by :

SATISH SERIAL PUBLISHING HOUSE
403, Express Tower, Commercial Complex, Azadpur, Delhi-110033 (INDIA)
Phone : 011-27672852 Fax : 91-11-27672046
E-mail : info@satishserial.com, hkjain1975@yahoo.com

ISBN 978-93-86200-94-5

Composed, Designed & Printed in India

I dedicate this book to my daughters
"Ekam " and "Amrit"

— Jaswinder

I dedicate this book to my son " Sukhanwar"

— Jaspal

Preface

Animal feeding is very vital aspect of livestock farming so does the science related with this subject i.e. Animal Nutrition. This subject is much applied essential and a must for all veterinary students. The whole profitability of farming revolve around this subject. But Veterinary students consider it as one of the most difficult subject. In our opinion it may be due to that this subject was taught them during the early years of graduation when they are not mature enough to understand the importance of this subject. Moreover as a whole, subject was taught to cover the topic of syllabus rather than to teach its practical relevance.

Attempt was made through this book to provide the animal nutrition in a question forms so that students and competitive exam aspirants go through the subject in a easy way. This book has been divided into 30 chapters.

As per our knowledge, it will be first exclusive book in India which covers the animal nutrition subject in multiple choice questions and other common questions which an animal nutritionist must know. Though written with Indian context, but we are sure that this will find wider application in other countries.

We are highly indebted to our better half's Manpreet Kaur and Ranjit Kaur for the understanding, they have shown along with shouldering the responsibilities which would otherwise vested on us.

Jaswinder Singh
Jaspal Singh Hundal

Contents

C. Nutrients Requirements and Feeding of Different Animals
(by Dr Jaspal Singh Hundal)

D. Others (by Dr Jaswinder Singh)

BASIC OF ANIMAL NUTRITION

by Dr Jaswinder Singh

Chapter 1

History of Animal Nutrition

Definition of Animal Nutrition

Animal nutrition is made up of two words i.e. animal and nutrition. Dictionary means of animal is any living thing, other than a human being, that can feel and move or a creature with four legs, as distinct from a bird, a reptile, a fish or an insect. Examples are cattle, sheep, goat, horse, dogs and cat, etc.

It can be defined as science of dietary food for animals providing bases on which to formulate a complete and balanced feed intake in accordance with the animal need.

It is sum of/series of process involved intake, assimilation utilization, waste production involving chemical and physiological activities.

It is integration of soil, plant, animal science, biochemistry, engineering, biotechnology, etc..

It is the study of nutrition process as well as the components of food, their action, interaction and balance in relation to health and disease in animals.

In dictionary terms, nutrition is "The series of processes by which an organism takes in and assimilates food for promoting growth and replacing worn or injured tissues". Therefore, nutrition involves various chemical reactions and physiological processes, which transform foods into body tissues and activities. It involves the ingestion, digestion, and absorption of the various nutrients, their transport to all body cells, and the removal of unusable elements and waste products of metabolism. So, animal nutrition is the science of nourishment of animals.

Relationship with other branches of sciences: Animal nutrition has a direct relationship with Physics, Chemistry, Biochemistry, Physiology, Genetics and Breeding, Anatomy and Histology, Biology, Mathematics and Microbiology without which complete study of animal nutrition is impossible. So, relative study of other sciences are also necessary and helpful for the animal nutritionists.

History of Animal Nutrition

Milestones in the development of Animal Nutrition

S.No.	Scientists/Year	Contribution/Discovery
1.	A. Lavosier (1762)	Founder of Animal Nutrition, Nature of respiration calorimeter. He also introduces balance and thermometer in nutritional studies.
2.	Menghini (1746)	Iron present in blood
3.	James Lind (1753)	Treatise of the scruvy
4.	Lavosier and Laplace (1780)	Devised the first animal Calorimeter
5.	Albrecht Thaer (1810)	Hay Equivalent
6.	Friedrich Tiedemann and Leopold Gmelin (1827)	First isolated the "taurine" in the bile of cattle (*Bos taurus*), hence its name
7.	William Prout (1834)	Nature of food
8.	G.J. Mulder (1838)	Gave the name protein
9.	Gruby and Delafond (1843)	Rumen protozoa
10.	G. Haubner (1855)	First to conduct digestion trial
11.	Henneberg and Stohman (1861)	Proximate analysis of feed stuffs
12.	W.O. Atwater (1892)	First human respiration calorimeter
13.	J.B.F. Magendie (1783-1855)	Essentiality of food nitrogen
14.	Lawes and J.H. Gilbert (1855)	Slaughter experiment in farm animals
15.	Oscar Kellner (1851-1911)	Starch equivalent system of energy evaluation
16.	Mikhail Tswett (1903)	Chromatogarphy
17.	Armsby (1903)	First respiration Calorimeter to study cattle

18.	AAFCO (1990)	Association of American Feed Control Official (AAFCO) establishment
19.	J.L. Hills (1910)	Used the term TDN
20.	Casimir Funk (1912)	Coined the term vitamine
21.	Leonard A. Maynard (1942)	Chairman of the NRC committee on animal nutrition
22.	Max Kleiber (1893-1976)	Use of weight to the 0.75 power instead of surface are for energy metabolism
23.	E.J. Underwood (1905-1980)	Mineral nutrition in livestock
24.	McCollum and Davis (1915)	Distinguish between "Fat soluble vitamin A" and Water soluble B nomenclature
25.	Moore (1929)	Reported that animal body converts carotene into Vitamin A
26.	George B Dantzig (1946-1947)	Liner Programme
27.	CLFMA-1967	Compound Livestock Feed Manufacturer Association (CLFMA) establishment
28.	P.J. Van Soest (1960)	Fibre estimation in feed stuffs
29.	Orpin (1975)	Anaerobic fungi in sheep rumen
30.	A. Bhattacharya (1980)	Study of recycling poultry waste as feed stuffs
31.	Indian Veterinary Research Institute, Izatnagar (1939)	Various research in animal nutrition
32.	National Dairy Research Institute, Karnal (1952)	Various research in animal nutrition
33.	N.D. Kehar (1950)	Nutritive value of non-conventional feeds. Wet alkali treatment to straw
34.	K.C. Sen (1954)	Nutritive value of Indian cattle feeds and feeding of farm animals
35.	S.K. Talapatra (1964)	Methods to estimate minerals in feeds and fodders
36.	Indian Council of Agricultural Research (1985)	Feeding standard for various categories of livestock

37.	K. Pradhan	Chairman of National Committee to develop ICAR feeding standards
38.	NRC (National Research Council, USA) 1942	Nutrient requirements for livestock
39.	ARC (Agriculture Research Council U.K.) 1959	Nutrient requirements for livestock
40.	Hungate (1966)	Rumen microbiology
41.	Lander and Dharmani (1923)	Started proximate analysis in India at Lalaypur, Faislabad (now in Pakistan)
42.	Animal Nutrition Division, IVRI (1928)	Animal Nutrition Division, IVRI was established
43.	J.E. Sirllow (1930)	Given the name "Degnalla disease"
44.	INRA-The French National Agriculture Research Institute (1950)	Formalin treatment of vegetable protein for protein protection
45.	Dairy Cattle Nutrition, NDRI (1956)	Dairy Cattle Nutrition Division, NDRI was established
46.	Tilley & Terry (1963)	*In vitro* method
47.	Mitchell (1964)	Ideal protein concept
48.	Burrough and Coworker (1975)	Concept of metabolisable protein
49.	Czerkawski & Breckenridge (1977)	Rumen simulation technique (rusitec)
50.	Mehraj and Orskov (1977)	*In sacco* method
51.	Menke *et al* (1979)	*In vitro* gas production method
52.	Czerkawski (1986)	Devised the "Rusitec" an artificial rumen system
53.	Sinffen *et al* (1992)/Chalupa and Sniffen	Cornell Net Carbohydrate and Protein (CNCP) of analysis
54.	National Institute of Animal Nutrition and Physiology, Bangalore (1995)	National Institute of Animal Nutrition and Physiology, Bangalore was established
55.	William C Rose	Discovered amino acid "Threonine"

❑❑❑

Chapter 2

Classification of Feedstuffs

Nutrition	In dictionary meaning it is defined as series process by which an organism takes in and assimilates feed for promoting growth and replacing worn or injured tissue.
Feed	Any material fed to the animal or eaten by the animal as a part of its daily ration. Or in simple words food for human beings and feed for animals.
Forage	Vegetable feed for domestic animals. It is a broader term generally refers to feed fresh or preserved, gathered and used as feed for animals, such as pasturage hay, silage and green feed.
Fodder	Synonymous with forage Or the cultivated forages are known as fodder.
Roughage	Feeds of a bulky and fibrous nature like cereal straw fodders, etc. with a CF content more than 18 % and TDN contents less than 60 %.
Concentrate	Feed which are low in fibre and high in TDN. All such feed which have CF content less than 18% and TDN more than 60 % and supply all the primary nutrients are called concentrate.

But there is exception to this roughage and concentrate concept, we cannot divide all the feedstuff into two categories, for example corn silage which has more than 18 % CF but it also has about 70 % TDN, similarly lush green grasses are high in fibre but their digestibility is also very high.

Nutrient	The chemical substances found in feed materials, which are necessary for maintenance, production and health of the animal. They are six in number carbohydrate, fat, protein, minerals, vitamin and water.
Diet	Mixture of ingredients including water which is consumed by animal on a particular time or on prescribed schedule of the day is known as diet.
Ration	The amount of feed consumed by the animal in 24 hours is known as ration.

Classification of feedstuff

Why we need the classification?

1. Feeds with similar nutritive characteristics are grouped together.
2. Such grouping helps in the selection of feedstuffs for formulation of ration to cater the need of the animal.
3. This also helps in the substitutions of one feed with another feed from the same group, no two feedstuffs are alike in chemical composition and characteristics, so we can substitute the one feedstuff with other from the same group depending upon availability of price of other feedstuff.

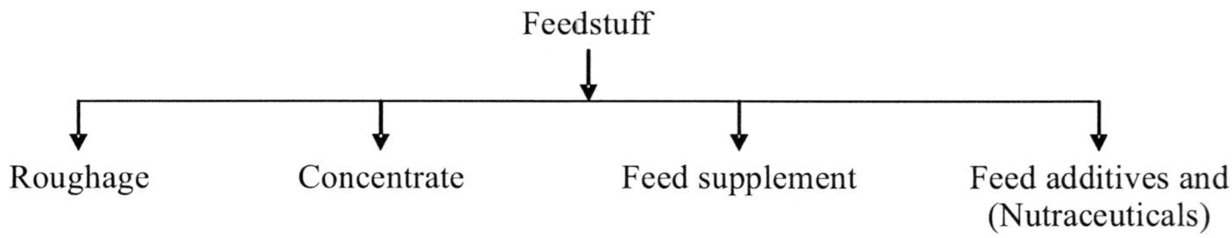

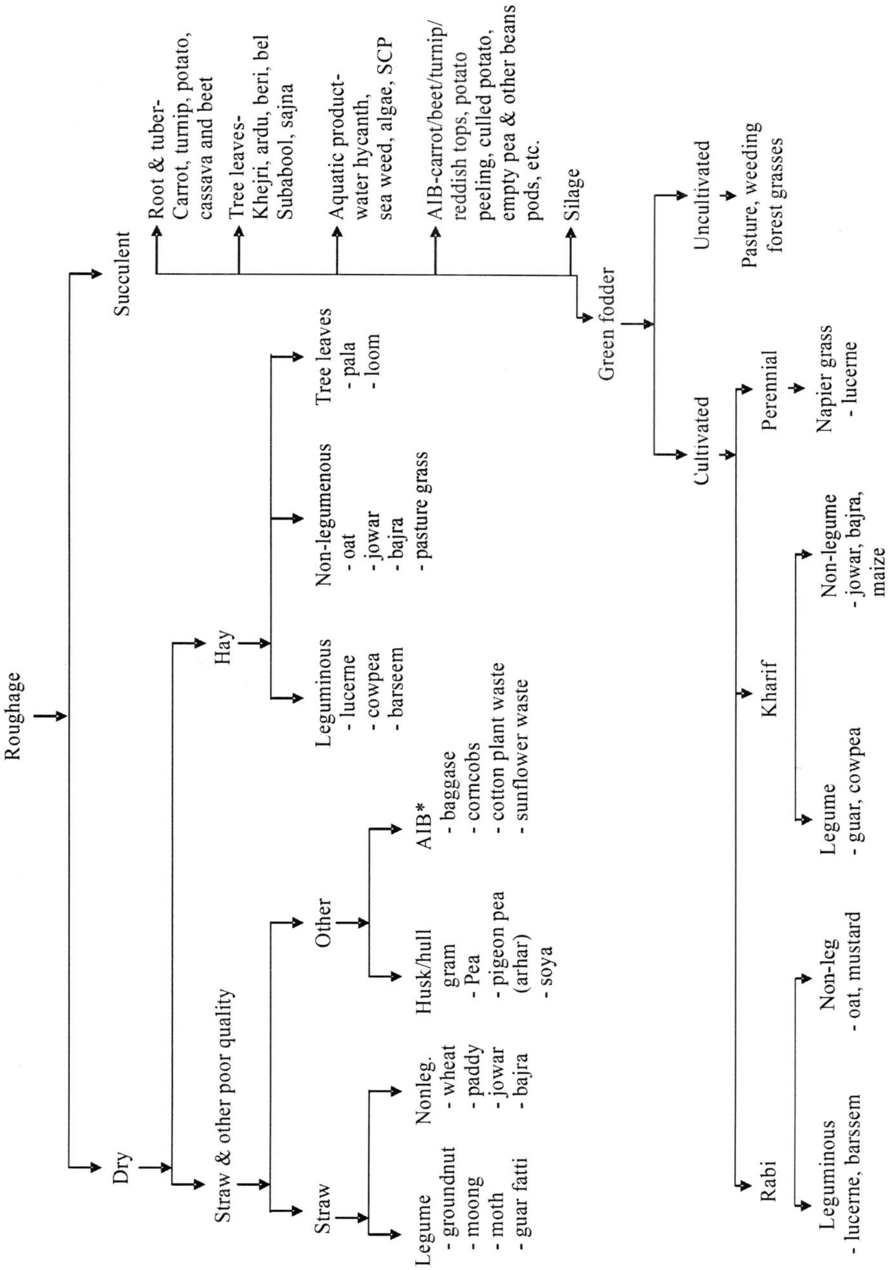

* Agriculture based industry byproducts

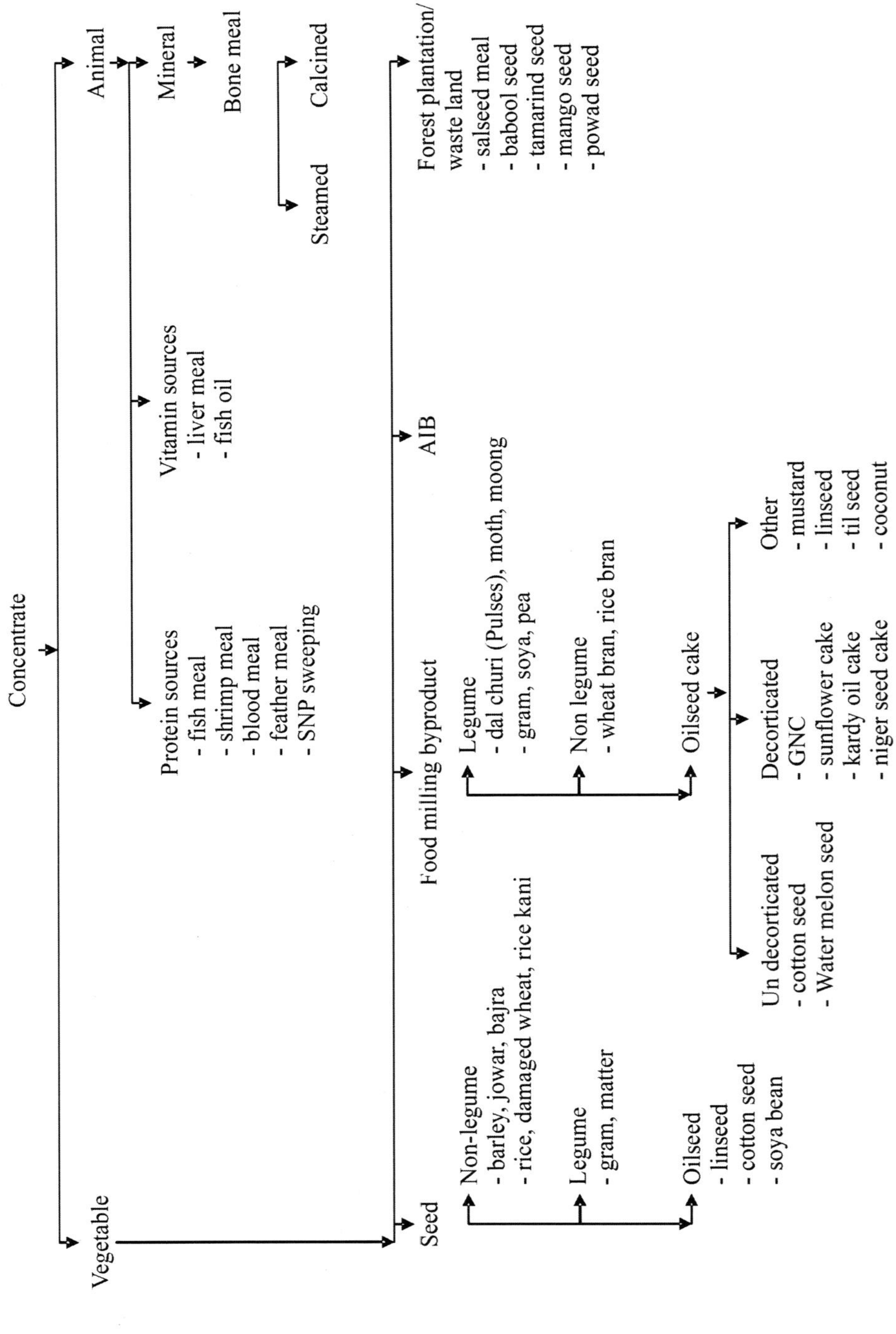
Concentrate
Animal
Vegetable
Protein sources
- fish meal
- shrimp meal
- blood meal
- feather meal
- SNP sweeping
Vitamin sources
- liver meal
- fish oil
Mineral
Bone meal
Steamed
Calcined
Seed
Non-legume
- barley, jowar, bajra
- rice, damaged wheat, rice kani
Legume
- gram, matter
Oilseed
- linseed
- cotton seed
- soya bean
Food milling byproduct
Legume
- dal churi (Pulses), moth, moong
- gram, soya, pea
Non legume
- wheat bran, rice bran
Oilseed cake
Un decorticated
- cotton seed
- Water melon seed
Decorticated
- GNC
- sunflower cake
- kardy oil cake
- niger seed cake
Other
- mustard
- linseed
- til seed
- coconut
AIB
Forest plantation/
waste land
- salseed meal
- babool seed
- tamarind seed
- mango seed
- powad seed

AIB (Agriculture based Industry byproducts)

- Gum ind.
  - guar korma
- Sugar ind.
  - molasses
  - beet pulp
- Liquor ind.
  - brewers grain
  - yeast powder
  - yeast sludge
- Starch ind.
  - maize gluten
  - maize bran
  - maize germ
  - corn spentliquor
- Fruit & veg. Preservation ind.
  - peeling
  - culled
  - waste
- Solvent extraction & refinery
  - DORB
  - deoiled cake
  - acid oil fatty acid
- Farm waste
  - poultry dropping
  - litter

Feed supplement

- NPN
  - Urea
  - DAP
  - Amines
  - Biuret
- Mineral
  - common salt
  - lime stone
  - calcite
  - chalk
  - oyster shell
  - DCP
  - complex minerals
    - Chelated minerals*
    - Non-chelated minerals
- Vitamins
  - proprietor preparation
  - AD preparation
  - AD_3K preparation
  - AD_3KE&B complex
- Bypass nutrient
  - bypass protein
  - bypass fat
  - bypass starch

* Chelation of minerals refers to the process of binding a mineral to an organic moiety called ligands e.g. amino acids, carbohydrates, etc. Chelated mineral is a complex consisting of a mineral element and an organic compound carrier, such as protein or polysaccharide.

Feed additive/nutraceuticals

The word 'nutraceutical' was first coined by Stephen DeFelice. A nutraceuical is a food or food ingredient having some health benefit including disease treatment and prevention.

- Microbial-Probiotics, prebiotics, antibiotics, ionophore
- Enzymes-Phytase, amylase, cellulose
- Hormone-Growth hormone, sex hormone, steroids
- Amino acid preparations
- Buffers
- Arsenicals
- Coccidiostat
- Antioxidant
- Antifungal
- Binder- Cement, bentonite, gum
- Colour, flavouring and sweetener agents
- Glactogauge
- Appetizer
- Cleansing/ ecbolic group

Chapter 3

Thumb Rules in Animal Feeding & Other General Information

- Dry Matter Intake (DMI) in Dairy animals = 2.5-3.5 % of body weight or formula of DMI = 2.2x Body weight (kg)+ 20 X Milk in litre/day/100
- The average DM (Dry matter) requirement of desi cow is 2 (dry) to 2.5 (lactating) Kg/100 Kg body weight/day while it is 2.5 (dry) to 3.0 Kg. (lactating) in cross breed cows and buffaloes and for high yielding it may go up to 3.5%
- The roughage requirement : About 2/3rd of DM through dry fodder and remaining 1/3rd from green fodder
- The concentrate requirement of animal for maintenance production and pregnancy is as follows :
  - a) Maintenance requirement of indigenous cow and crossbreed cow / buffalo is 1 and 1.5 Kg respectively.
  - b) Lactating animal should be given 1 Kg additional concentrate for every 2.5 Kg (Buffalo) to 3 Kg (Cow) milk produced.
  - c) Pregnant cows/ buffaloes should receive 1.5 -2.0 Kg per day extra concentrate allowance during advance pregnancy to meet extra need of nutrients for growth of foetus
  - d) Breeding bulls in service should get 1 Kg per day extra concentrate.
  - e) Mineral mixture and common salt each @ 25-50 gm should be given to fulfill mineral requirements of animal.
- As a thumb rule, 1 kg of concentrate mixture is fed for each 2.0 litre of buffalo milk and 2.5 litre of cow milk. This difference is

because buffalo milk contains higher amounts of fat as compared to cow milk

- Other thumb rule is to feed 400 gm concentrate/Kg of milk of 4% fat. For above 4% fat, 0.075Kg additional concentrate should be given for each 1% higher fat.
- Large animal will eat more than a small one. Animal producing a lot of milk will eat more than one producing little milk.
- Immediately after calving, cows are able to eat less feed than usual.
- Cattle will typically eat no more than about 0.1% of their body weight of salt/day.
- Quantity of colostrum to be fed to newly born calf is $1/10^{th}$ of its body weight.
- Thumb rule of green fodder feeding to daily animals = 10 % of body weight.
- 6-8 kg of leguminous fodder is nutritionally equal to 1 Kg of concentrate.
- 12.5 kg non-leguminous fodder is nutritionally equal to 1 Kg of concentrate.
- Average water consumption per bovine is 10% of their body weight. Slight variation in consumption may be due to environmental, physiological and reproductive needs.
- In adult cows, the volume of the three pre-stomachs is about 14 times larger than the abomasum. A well developed rumen has a volume of 100-150 litres. The four stomachs together fill about $3/4^{th}$ of the abdominal cavity.
- Around 45-50 Kg green berseem/lucerne/cow pea/maize/jowar/bajra is sufficient for maintenance of 450-500kg cow.
- Add $1/10^{th}$ straw in leguminous fodder like berseem/ lucerne/ cow pea before feeding.
- Thumb rule of straw/stubble feeding = 1.75% of body weight.
- A concentration of about 2-5 mg NH_3-N/100 ml of rumen liquor is sufficient for the rumen bacterial growth.

- 5 mg NH_3-N/100 ml of rumen liquor can be occurred with ration of 13% CP.
- More than 80 mg NH_3-N/100 ml of rumen liquor can lead to urea toxicity.
- 80% of microbial protein is true protein and remaining 20% consists of nucleic acid.
- The saliva produced by cattle contain 125 meq/litre of bicarbonate.
- Protein makes 17-20% of animal body and 3.6% of the milk.
- For one Kg of milk production, 3-4 kg water is required.
- About 35 gm urea/day is considered sufficient for a 400 kg cow.
- Total Volatile Fatty Acid (VFA) concentration in rumen varies between 2-15 g/litre.
- On one acre, 8-10 large ruminant animals can be kept to fulfill their nutritional needs.
- Painting in summer can lead to respiratory alkalosis.
- The amount of calcium in adult animal body is 1.2 to 1.5 % of body weight.
- High calcium in the diet can lead to Zn deficiency.
- 450-500 gm CP is required per day for the maintenance requirement of adult milch animal.
- 70gm CP/Kg milk is required as production requirement.
- The ratio of Rumen degradable protein : Un-degradable protein should be 60:40 in low to medium yielder, for high yielder it should be 50:50 and for exceptionally high yielder it should be 40:60.
- Area surrounding the industrial complex or brick kiln is supposed to be rich in Fluorine.
- Leguminous fodder/hay are rich source of calcium but poor in phosphorus.
- Straw in general are poor source of Calcium.
- Maintenance ration required to have 0.254kg DCP and 3.03 KG TDN.

- Molasses contain about 50% sugar and 3.2% CP.
- Molasses is about 1/3rd of the quantity of sugar and about 2-4% of sugarcane.
- In silage, molasses can be added @ 3.5-4% of weight of sugar limited green fodder.
- Urea can be added in silage @ 0.5% of fresh forage.
- Cereal grains, wheat bran, rice bran, polishing, cakes are good source of phosphorus.
- Linseed meal is excellent feed for putting bloom on animals.
- Feed high in fibre i.e. fodder or cakes has higher heat increment (HI) than feed high in starch or fat.
- 1Kg of TDN= 4.4Mcal DE
- Bacterial and protozoal protein in rumen have been determined using α-^{1}-diaminopimelic acid, an amino acid found only in the bacteria and amino ethyl phosphonic acid (AEP) which is present only in protozoa.
- Rumen protozoa contribute 43% cellulose, 58% protease and 38% of amylase of rumen.
- Microbial protein formation range between 90-230 gm per Kg organic matter digested in the rumen.
- On the average 20 gm of bacterial protein is synthesized per 100 gm of organic matter fermented in rumen.
- Approximately 60% of the amino acid absorbed through the small intestine is from bacterial protein and remaining 40% is from ruminally undegraded dietray protein.
- The threshold size of particles in cattle to filter through reticulo-omasal orifice lies in the range of 3-5 mm.
- The percentage of protein in bacteria varies from 38 to 55% (Average = 47.7%).
- About 3% of animal body consists of minerals.
- Rumen size varies from 3 to 15 litres in sheep and 35 to 100 litres in cattle and buffaloes.

- Contrast to monogastric stomach abomasum secrete lysozyme which catalyse the hydrolysis of specific glycosidic bond in muco polysaccharides present in bacterial cell wall.
- *Selenomonas ruminantium* scavenge the oxygen enter via feed in rumen.
- Rumen bacteria are superoxide dismutase and catalase negative, so oxygen is toxic to rumen microbes due to production of peroxide or free radicals.
- Copra meal (coconut meal) has the properties of absorbing upto half of its weight of molasses.
- Til cake is richest among all oilcakes in calcium content being 2.3% but due to high phytic acid, it appears to bind Ca.
- Maize and sorghum grains have higher level of naturally protected starch than barley grains.
- Wheat has the highest content of starch for the grain (77%) followed by corn and sorghum (72%) and then by barley (57%) and oats (58%).
- Oldest method of rumen protection of protein is "Heat treatment".
- Cotton seed should not be fed at more than 3 kg per cow per day.
- Feed pass through fastly in GIT tract of horse as compared to ruminants.
- As a rule of thumb if butter fat production is to maintained, the fibre content of the total Dry matter of diet should consist of not less than 16% Crude fibre, 21% ADF and 28% NDF or roughage component of the diet should not be less than 35 to 40% of the total DM.
- To assess if fibre levels in the diet are adequate, 50% of the herd should be chewing their cud when resting, if less than 30%, then fibre content is too low, if greater than 70%, the fibre content is too high.
- The rumen requires fibre particles of 2-5 cm long that promote cud chewing and rumination to produce saliva and to maintain milk fat percentage.

- Splitting the concentrates into more than two feeds per day is usually beneficial only when the concentrate proportion of the diet exceed 60% or an amount equivalent to approximately 2% of body weight.
- Dry cow should not normally be fed more concentrate than about 0.5 % of their body weight per day.
- For dry cows more than 21 days before calving DMI will be about 2% of body weight.
- Dry cow should not be fed diet which are high in calcium or phosphorus. So, legume like lucerne, berseem should be avoided.
- After calving increase the concentrate at the rate of a kg/day from the day of calving until the desired maximum rate has been reached.
- It is normal for high yielding adult cow to lose 30 to 60 Kg body mass during the first 80 days of lactation representing a drop of 1 to 1.5 point in body condition score.
- For HF cows-one body condition score is about 44 kg.
- Generally, the amount of weight gain required to increase the cow's condition by one condition score is about 8% of the cow's live weight.
- One Kg of live mass can be converted to about 5-8 kg of milk.
- Body condition score at calving = 3 to 3.5
- Target body condition score at service = 2+
- Target body condition score at drying = 2.5 to 3
- The efficiency of conversion of dietary energy to milk energy is 0.62 but when this energy is stored in body fat and later used for milk production, the efficiency factor is 0.5%. This indirect route is still less efficient if body reserve are laid down during the dry period. The dry period is not the time to condition cows. Body recovery should take place from mid to late lactation while cow is still in milk. Cow in milk are about 25% more efficient at feed conversion than are dry cows. So, it is more cost effective to regain lost condition during lactation.
- Few days before calving, feeding of about 2 kg of wheat bran in lieu of concentrate will prevent the constipation and facilitate calving.

- Guideline for supplemental fat feeding is up to a maximum of 2% of the total diet DM.
- 50% of milk fat synthesized in the mammary gland is derived from fat sources in diet.
- The total fat in lactating dairy cow diets should be limited to 6% of the diet DM.
- During dry period cow receive a forage based ration which cause rumen papillae to shorten to less than 0.5 cm, when cow receive ration higher in fermentable carbohydrate, the papillae elongate to 1.2 cm increasing surface area of the rumen. The time for total elongation of papillae is 4-6 weeks.
- Excess NH_3 has to be excreted from blood stream at an energy cost of 22.8 kilojoules per gram of nutrition.
- The rumen has limited capacity to convert ammonia to microbial protein. The maximum limit of conversion is considered to be 30-32 g N per kg digestible organic matter consumed by the animals.
- Most of the B - Vitamins are synthesized by rumen and intestinal bacteria.
- Vitamin C is synthesized by the cow in the liver and kidneys.
- The feed usually remains in the rumen reticulum complex for upto 60 hours, in the omasum for 8 hours and in the abomasum, it remains for about 3 hours.
- About 8% of total digestible dietary energy is lost as methane.
- Common buffers include sodium bicarbonate and magnesium oxide. These buffers help in stabilizing rumen pH and thereby prevent incidence of acidosis. Generally, they are in ratio of 2:1 to 3:1 (sodium bicarbonate: magnesium oxide).
- Provide buffers at 1-1.5% of ration DM or 100-200gm/animal/day.
- The microbial population in the rumen consists of bacteria, protozoa and fungi. The majority of the concentration is as bacteria which can number 10^{10} to 10^{11} cells/gram of rumen contents. The protozoa in the rumen number about 10^5 to 10^{16} cells/gram of rumen contents.

- Legumes are generally higher in lignin and lower in NDF.
- Milk fever is more common in older cows than in first calvers since older cows are less able to mobilize calcium from the skeleton.
- Number of chewing cycle/cud is 55-65.
- About 30 minute of cud chewing time per day for each kilogram of dry matter ingested is required.
- Calcium and phosphorus together formed the 75% of the total body mineras (Calcium 46% and Phosphorus 29%)
- In close up dry cow, DCAD level should be -10 to -15 meq/100g diet DM. Urine pH should be between 6.0-6.5 for last 2-3 weeks before calving.
- In lactating cow, DCAD should be 25-35 meq/100gm DM.
- DCAD (milliequivalent/100gm of dietary DM) = (% Sodium x 43.5 + % Potassium x 25.6) - (% Chloride x 28.2 + % Sulphur x 62.5).
- Approximately 1.8 - 2.0 kg of feed is required by a broiler to produce 1kg of broiler meat.
- Likewise a laying pullet needs 2.5 to 3.0 kg feed to produce 1 kg of eggs.
- Wool is rich in cystine and contains about 4% of sulphur.
- Calcium carbonate ($CaCO_3$) is heated to form quicklime (CaO) which is then added to water. This forms another material known as slaked lime ($Ca(OH)_2$).
- Sulphur is present in 3 amino acids (Cystine, Cysteine and Metionine), 2 vitamins (Biotin and thiamine) and one hormone (insulin).
- Lactose is made only by mammals. It is found only in milk.
- 6 inches silage layer needs to be removed from the opened surface every day to prevent heating and mould growth.
- A target packing density of 15 lb of DM per ft^3 or 240 kg of DM per m^3 is required to minimize shrinkage in silage.
- Milk fat globules are the largest particles in milk and are also the lightest.

- Caseins make up over 80% of the total protein content of milk and can be further divided into five groups – the alphas 1, alphas 2, beta, gamma and kappa caseins. Caseins do not have an organized structure, thus they cannot be denatured by heating of milk.
- Cracked grain should be used in concentrate mixture as whole seed /grain will pass through the digestive tract intact.
- Blend of different cakes should be used in concentrate mixture rather than single cake.
- Bypass protein and fat must be used in high yielding animals ration to meet the nutrient requirement.
- In summer season add more energy and protein through grains, cakes and bypass feet in the ration to compensate low dry matter intake in milch animals.
- The jaw moments per cud should be around 50.
- About 450-500 gm crude protein per day is required for maintenance requirement of adult milch animals.
- Treatment of selenium poisoning or degnella disease : with pentasulphate mixture comprising of :

  Magnesium sulphate = 100gm

  Ferrous sulpahte = 16.6 gm

  Zinc sulphate = 7.5 gm

  Copper sulphate = 2.4 gm

  Cobalt sulphate = 1.5 gm

  Adminsister this mixture @ 15-40 gm/day.
- Rice straw contains 2.14 ppm Selenium compared to 0.21 ppm in wheat straw.
- Wheat straw contains negligible amount of total oxalate (0.17%) while paddy straw has 1.54%.
- Grain fed at 0.5% body weight is the acceptable level
- About 4-6% fat in total feed is optimum for maximum production.
- Rumen temperature is genreally higher than 1 degree than rest of the body.

- Rumination generally starts after 0.5 to 1.5 hour after feed intake.
- Too much of protein in feed will lead to loose motion and reproductive problems.
- If more undigested maize comes in dung, then check grain size, quantity of grain, intake of degradable protein and soluble protein in the ration.
- Forage dry matter consumption is around 1.25-1.50% cows body weight.
- Tree leaves are good source of calcium.
- Milk is deficient in magnesium, iron and copper.
- High level of calcium in the diet can cause zinc deficiency.
- Higher nitrate content in the fodder can lead to vitamin A deficiency.
- Supplementation of Niacin lessen the risk of ketosis.
- Feed 6 gm Niacin/day during the last 21 days before calving and 3 months after calving.
- Gaines devised an equation for calculaing energy value from fat content. He proposed the following formula for expressing milks of different fat content in terms of 4% fat milk:

  4% milk = 0.4M+ 15F

  M = weight of milk and F = weight of fat.
- Sheep has both pregastric and hindgut fermentation.

Note: Information is intentionally written in haphazard manner to sustain the interest of readers.

❑❑❑

Chapter 4

Animal Nutrition and 70 Figures

1. Carbohydrate is the largest component in the ration and contribute 60-70% of the net energy used for milk production.
2. Carbohydrate -the single largest component (60-70%) of a buffalo diet.
3. The Volatile fatty acid in ruminants supply the 60-70% the energy needed by the animals.
4. Out of the total microbial nucleic acid entering the small intestine, 60-70% is RNA.
5. 70-75% of the growth of ruminant foetus occur during the last trimester of gestation.
6. 70-80% iodine reserve in body is stored in thyroid gland.
7. 70% of the total magnesium in the body is in skeleton.
8. In ruminants between 70-80% of daily iodine intake is absorbed directly from the rumen and 10% from abomasums.
9. Dressing percentage in poultry is around 70-75% and in pig is 68-72%.
10. Approximate 70% crude protein entering the small intestine is of microbial origin.
11. Microbial protein tends to have biological value of 60-70%.
12. The average human body contains 70 % water.
13. Cattle water content is 75 to 80 % at birth, 68 to 72 % at five month and 50 to 60 % in the mature animal.

14. Feed costs representing upto 70% of the overall cost of farm production.
15. The proportion of Acetic acid in total volatile fatty acid produced is around 65-70%.
16. Thumb rule of cattle feeding is to feed 70% DM from concentrate and 30% DM from roughage.
17. 70 gm crude protein is required per Kg milk production.
18. The percentage of water in leen adult dog is approximatily 70%.

❑❑❑

A. NUTRIENTS

by Dr Jaswinder Singh

Chapter 5

Carbohydrate

Q 1 Major constituents of plants body is __________

a) **Carbohydrate** b) Protein

c) Lignin d) None of these

Q 2 Which of the following is the sugar of blood __________

a) **Glucose** b) Ribose

c) Xylose d) Arabinose

Q 3 Principle function of the carbohydrate in the body is ________

a) **Furnish energy** b) Structural

c) Nervous integrity d) None of these

Q 4 Which of the following is a carbohydrate __________

a) Thromboxane b) **Heparin**

c) Waxes d) Terpenes

Q 5 Which of the following sugar is present in every living cell _____

a) Galactose b) Xylose

c) **Ribose** d) Fructose

Q 6 Which of the following is not a pentoses sugar?

a) Ribose b) Xylose

c) Arabinose d) **Mannose**

Q 7 End product on hydrolysis of glucose is __________

a) Glucose & Galactose b) Glucose

c) **Galactose*** d) Glucose & Fructose

* Galactose is a monosaccharide

Q 8 Which of the following is not a hexose sugar?

a) Glucose
b) Mannose
c) Fructose
d) **Arabinose***

* Arabinose is a pentose sugar

Q 9 Which of the following is not a disaccharides?

a) Sucrose
b) Lactose
c) **Mannose**
d) Maltose

Q 10 End product on hydrolysis of maltose is ________

a) Glucose + Galactose
b) **Glucose + Glucose**
c) Glucose + Fructose
d) Glucose + Galactose + Fructose

Q 11 The sweet taste of sugarcane molasses is due to ________

a) **Sucrose**
b) Maltose
c) Fructose
d) Mannose

Q 12 Which of the following is a reserve carbohydrate in plants ________?

a) Dextrin
b) Cellulose
c) **Starch**
d) Glycogen

Q 13 The reserve carbohydrate in animal body is ________

a) Dextrin
b) Cellulose
c) Starch
d) **Glycogen**

Q 14 End product on hydrolysis of glycogen is ________

a) Starch
b) **Glucose**
c) Glucose + Fructose
d) Fructose

Q 15 End product on hydrolysis of starch is ________

a) **Glucose**
b) Fructose
c) Mannose
d) Galactose

Q 16 End product on hydrolysis of dextrin is ________

a) Fructose
b) **Glucose**
c) Maltose
d) None of these

Q 17 Sugar found in Nucleic acid of all living cells ________

a) Xylose b) Glucose
c) **Ribose** d) Galactose

Q 18 The sugar of the body is ________

a) **Glucose** b) Fructose
c) Galactose d) Mannose

Q 19 The circulating carbohydrate in animal body is ________

a) Fructose b) **Glucose**
c) Galactose d) None of the above

Q 20 The most abundant sugar found in nature is ________

a) **Glucose** b) Galactose
c) Fructose d) Mannose

Q 21 Which of the following is known as "Grape sugar"?

a) Galactose b) Sucrose
c) **Glucose** d) Maltose

Q 22 Dextrose is also known as ________

a) Galactose b) **Glucose**
c) Sucrose d) Lactose

Q 23 The only naturally occurring Ketohexose ________

a) Glucose b) Galactose
c) **Fructose** d) Mannose

Q 24 The predominant sugar in germinating grain is ________

a) Glucose b) Cellobiose
c) **Maltose** d) Fructose

Q 25 Levulose is an other name of which sugar?

a) Glucose b) Dextrose
c) **Fructose** d) Galactose

Q 26 The most abundant carbohydrate found in nature ________

a) **Polysaccharides** b) Disaccharides
c) Monosaccharides d) None of these

Q 27 Starch is a mixture of two polymer amylase and amylopectin, which statement is true pertaining to above?

a) Generally, Amylose constitutes greater percentage in starch

b) **Generally, Amylopectin constitute greaters percentage in starch**

c) Both Amylose and amylopectin contribute equally in starch

d) None of the above

Q 28 α 1-6 glucosidic linkage is present in ________

a) Amylose

b) **Amylopectin**

c) Both amylase and amylopectin

d) None of these

Q 29 Which of the following is known as Animal starch?

a) Starch b) **Glycogen**

c) Cellulose d) Glucose

Q 30 Cotton fibre consists of ________

a) **Cellulose** b) Starch

c) Hemicellulose & Lignin d) Glycogen

Q 31 Grass hemicellulose is a polymer of which sugar ________

a) Glucose b) Fructose

c) **Xylose** d) Galactose

Q 32 Hemicellulose is digested relatively more in which of the following?

a) Pig b) Dog

c) **Man** d) Horse

Q 33 Intermediate product of the hydrolysis of starch is ________

a) **Dextrin** b) Glucose

c) Galactose d) Xylose

Q 34 Pectin is present in which of the following?

a) Orange peel off b) Sugarbeet pulp

c) Jam d) **All the above**

Q 35 Smallest carbohydrates are trioses, which of the following is a triose?

a) Glucose
b) Ribulose
c) Ribose
d) **Glyceraldehyde**

Q 36 Starch consists of __________

a) **Unbranched amylase and branched amylopectin**
b) Branched amylase and branched amlopectin
c) Branched amylase and unbrached amylopectin
d) Unbranched amylase and unbranched amylopectin

Q 37 Cellulose is made up of repeating units of __________

a) **β1-4 Linkage between D-glucose unit**
b) β 1-2 Linkage between D-glucose unit
c) α 1-4 Linkage between D-glucose unit
d) a 1-2 linkage between D glucose unit

Q 38 Amylopectin has __________

a) **α 1-4 and α 1-6 Linkage**
b) β 1-4 linkage
c) b 1-2, α 1-6 Linkage
d) α 1-2 linkage

Q 39 Chitin consists of __________

a) **N-acetyly glucosamine**
b) N-acetyl muramic acid
c) D-glucose unit
d) L-arabinose

Q 40 Carbohydrates are __________

a) Polyhydroxy aldehyde and phenols
b) **Polyhydroxy aldehyde and ketones**
c) Polyhydroxy ketones and phenols
d) Polyhydroxy phenols and alcohols

Q 41 The most abundant bio molecule on the earth is __________

a) Protein
b) Lipid
c) **Carbohydrate**
d) Nucleic acid

Q 42 The polysaccharide used in assessing the glomerular filteration rate is __________

a) Glycogen
b) Agar
c) **Inulin**
d) Hyaluronic acid

Q 43 Which of the following is/are correct combination of monosaccharides to form disaccharides?

i) Glucose + Glucose = Maltose

ii) Glucose + Fructose = Lactose

iii) Glucose + Fructose = Sucrose

iv) Glucose + Galactose = lactose

a) i,ii and iii only b) ii only

c) **i, iii and iv only** d) All the above

Q 44 Which test is used for reducing sugar?

a) Biuret test b) Ninhydrin test

c) **Benedicts test** d) None of these

Q 45 What is the name of bond formed between glucose and galactose sugar to produce the lactose __________?

a) α 1-2 glycosidic bond b) **β 1-4 glycosidic bond**

c) Alpha 1-4 glycosidic bond d) β 1-2 glycosidic bond

Q 46 Which of the following sugar is absorbed by active transport?

a) Fructose b) Mannose

c) **Glucose** d) Xylose

Q 47 Which of the following sugar has the fastest absorption rate?

a) **Galactose** b) Glucose

c) Fructose d) All have equal

Q 48 Boat and chair conformation are found in __________

a) **Pyranose sugar**

b) Furanose sugar

c) Only in a D Glucopyranose

d) In any sugar without axial – OH group

Q 49 Which of the following is a polymer of fructose?

a) **Inulin** b) Dextrin

c) Cellulose d) Glycogen

Q 50 The carbohydrate of blood group substance is __________

a) **Fucose** b) Xylose

c) Lyxose d) Fructose

Q 51 A disaccharides produced on hydrolysis of starch is called __________

a) Sucrose b) Lactose
c) **Maltose** d) Trehalose

Q 52 Galactose and glucose are __________

a) **Epimers** b) Isomers
c) Anomers d) None of these

Q 53 The sugar which form major component of nucleic acid is __________

a) **Ribose** b) Galactose
c) Mannose d) Maltose

Q 54 Which of the following is not a disaccharide?

a) **Amylose** b) Cellobiose
c) Lactose d) None of these

Q 55 Structural polysaccharides includes __________

a) **Cellulose, hemicellulose, chitin**
b) Cellulose, starch and chitin
c) Cellulose, starch and glycogen
d) Cellulose, glycogen and chitin

Q 56 Nutritional polysaccharides are __________

a) **Starch and glycogen** b) Starch and chitin
c) Starch and cellulose d) Starch and Glucose

Q 57 Which of the following is not a reducing sugar

a) Fructose b) Glucose
c) Ribose d) **Sucrose**

Q 58 Which pair are both structural carbohydrate molecules?

a) Starch and glycogen b) Starch and cellulose
c) Glycogen and cellulose d) **Cellulose and chitin**

Q 59 Which carbohydrate is found in the cell walls of plants?

a) Starch b) Chitin
c) **Cellulose** d) Glycogen

Q 60 Which carbohydrate is used in the liver for energy storage?

a) Starch b) Chitin
c) Cellulose d) **Glycogen**

Q 61 Which carbohydrate is found in the exoskeleton of insects and crabs?

a) Starch b) **Chitin**
c) Cellulose d) Glycogen

Q 62 The edible bacteria are also known as __________

a) **Probiotics** b) Prebiotics
c) Xenobiotic d) Synbiotics

Q 63 The process in which glycogen/monosaccharides are broken down to pyruvic acid and lactic acid is known as __________

a) **Glycolysis** b) Glycogenesis
c) Glycogenolysis d) Gluconeogenesis

Q 64 In Anaerobic condition, the glycolysis of one mole of glucose yields __________

a) **2 Moles of ATP** b) 4 Moles of ATP
c) 8 Moles of ATP d) 12 Moles of ATP

Q 65 In Glycolysis,one mole of glucose yields __________

a) **2 Moles of lactic acid** b) 4 Moles of lactic acid
c) 6 Moles of lactic acid d) 8 Moles of lactic acid

Q 66 The synthesis of glycogen from the simple sugar is known as __________

a) **Glycogenesis** b) Glycogenolysis
c) Gluconeogensis d) Glycolysis

Q 67 The degradation of glycogen to glucose is known as __________

a) Glycogenesis b) **Glycogenolysis**
c) Gluconeogensis d) Glycolysis

Q 68 The synthesis of glucose from non-carbohydrate source is known as __________

a) Glycogenesis b) Glycogenolysis
c) **Gluconeogensis** d) Glycolysis

Q 69 The oxidation of one mole of glycerol yields __________

a) **22 moles of ATP** b) 21 Moles of ATP

c) 20 Moles of ATP d) 24 moles of ATP

Q 70 The conversion of ammonia into urea through urea cycle uses __________

a) **3 Moles of ATP** b) 2 Moles of ATP

c) 1 Moles of ATP d) 4 Moles of ATP

Q 71 The more active site of deamination is __________

a) Liver b) Kidney

c) **Both a & b** d) Brain

Q 72 Under aerobic condition, glycolysis yields ____________ moles of ATP

a) 2 b) 4

c) 6 d) **8**

Q 73 The conversion of NAD into NADH leads to production of ____________ moles of ATP.

a) 2 b) **3**

c) 4 d) 5

Q 74 The conversion of FAD into $FADH_2$ leads to production of ____________ moles of ATP

a) **2** b) 3

c) 4 d) 5

Q 75 Conversion of GDP into GTP leads to production of _______ mole(s) of ATP

a) **1** b) 2

c) 3 d) 4

Q 76 The process of citric acid cycle takes place in __________

a) **Mitochondria** b) Cytosol

c) Golgi bodies d) Endoplasmic reticulum

Q 77 Glycolysis is also known as __________

a) **Embden mayerhof pathway**

b) Hexose monophosphate shunt

c) Pentose phosphate pathway

d) Alternate pathway

Q 78 Which of the following is not a synonymus?

a) **Embden mayerhof pathway**

b) Hexose monophosphate shunt

c) Pentose phosphate pathway

d) Alternate pathway

Q 79 The chief site for gluconeogenesis is __________

a) **Liver** b) Kidney

c) Brain d) Both a & b

Q 80 In TCA cycle, total ATP produced per molecule of pyruvic acid __________

a) **15** b) 30

c) 20 d) 5

Q 81 The chief sites for glycogensis are __________

a) **Liver & Muscle** b) Muscle & Kidney

c) Kidney & Brain d) None of the above

Q 82 The tentative amount of methane formed per 100 gram of digested carbohydrate in ruminant is __________

a) 1.5g b) **4.5g**

c) 15 g d) 25 g

Q 83 Amongst the VFA's produced in the rumen, which acid is formed in higher amount in general __________

a) **Acetic acid** b) Butyric acid

c) Propionic acid d) Valeric acid

Q 84 When cow is kept exclusively on fodder/roughages, which VFA production exceed the others?

a) **Acetic acid** b) Butyric acid

c) Propionic acid d) Lactic acid

Q 85 Which of the following volatile fatty acid is produced in higher amount, when cow fed predominately on concentrate diet?

a) Acetic acid b) Butyric acid

c) **Propionic acid** d) Valeric acid

Q 86 Raffinose is a __________

a) Disaccharides
b) **Trisaccharides**
c) Tetrasaccharides
d) Monsaccharides

Q 87 Stachyose is a __________

a) Disaccharides
b) Trisaccharides
c) **Tetrasaccharides**
d) Monsaccharides

Q 88 Lactulose - a synthetic sugar used in the treatment of constipation in human is a __________

a) **Disaccharides – consist of fructose and galactose**
b) Disaccharides - consist of fructose and sucrose
c) Trisaccharides - consist of glucose, galactose and fructose
d) Trisaccharides - consist of glucose, sucrose and fructose

Q 89 Sucralose (Splenda)- an artificial sweetener is a __________

a) Monosaccharides
b) **Disaccharides**
c) Trisaccharides
d) Tetrasaccharides

Q 90 Non-starch polysaccharides (NSP) used in preparation of jam and jellies is __________

a) Glucans
b) Fructans
c) **Pectin**
d) Inulin

Q 91 Carbohydrate of animal origin is __________

a) **Lactose**
b) Fructans
c) Inulins
d) Pectin

Q 92 How many vitamins function in the citric acid cycle?

a) 1
b) 2
c) 3
d) **4***

* Thiamine, pantothenic acid, niacin and riboflavin

Q 93 Which of the following is a misnomer?

a) Bypass protein
b) Milk fever
c) Ketone bodies*
d) **All the above**

* β-hydroxy butyrate is not a ketone

Q 94 Ball like masses of undigested plant fibre that obstruct the digestive tract is known as ________

a) **Phyotobezoars** b) Trichobezoars*

c) Both of these d) None of these

* It is a mass of hair that obstruct the tract

Q 95 The word " Glycans" is mostly used as synonymous for which of the following?

a) Monosaccharides b) Disaccharides

c) Oligosaccharides d) **Polysaccharides**

Q 96 Which of the following sugar is a ketose sugar?

a) Glucose b) Galactose

c) **Fructose** d) Mannose

Q 97 Which of the following sugar is a ketose sugar?

a) Arabinose b) Xylose

c) Ribose d) **Ribulose**

Q 98 Which of the following is a grape sugar?

a) **Glucose** b) Fructose

c) Mannose d) Laevulose

Q 99 The exceptionally sweet taste of honey is due to _______ sugar.

a) Glucose b) Sucrose

c) **Fructose** d) Galactose

Q 100 Which of the following is also called milk sugar?

a) Sucrose b) Glucose

c) **Lactose** d) Fructose

Q 101 Lactose is formed from ________

a) 1 Molecule of glucose+ 1 Molecule of fructose

b) **1 Molecule of glucose + 1 Molecule of galactose**

c) 1 Molecule of glucose + 1 Molecule of manoose

d) 2 Molecule of glucose

Q 102 Which of the following is not a reducing sugar?

a) **Sucrose** b) Lactose

c) Maltose d) Cellibiose

Q 103 Which of the following sugar is formed during the germination of barley?

a) Sucrose b) **Maltose**
c) Laevulose d) Cellobiose

Q 104 Raffinose on hydrolysis yields __________

a) **One molecule of each glucose, galactose and fructose**
b) One molecule of each glucose, galactose and mannose
c) 2 molecule of glucose and 1 molecule of galactose
d) 2 molecule of galactose and 1 molecule of glucose

Q 105 Stachyose on hydrolysis yields __________

a) **2 molecule of galactose + 1 glucose + 1 fructose**
b) 2 molecule of glucose + 1 galactose + 1 fructose
c) 2 molecule of glucose + 2 molecule of galactose
d) 2 molecule of glucose + 2 molecule of fructose

Q 106 On keeping the honey in refrigerator, a white crystalline precipitate are formed which is due to presence of __________

a) **Fructose** b) Sucrose
c) Mannose d) Stachyose

Q 107 Blood sugar of vertebrate is __________

a) Fructose b) Sucrose
c) **Glucose** d) Lactose

Q 108 Nutrients absorbed into blood of intestinal villi goes to _______

a) Aorta b) Precaval vein
c) **Hepatic portal vein** d) Hepatic artery

Q 109 Which organism is responsible for metabolism in the "first pass effect"?

a) Brain b) Heart
c) Kidney d) **Liver**

Q 110 The precursor of ketone bodies is __________

a) Acetyle CoA b) Acetoacetic acid
c) Beta-hydroxy butyric acid d) **Cholesterol**

Q 111 Aldosterone causes __________

a) Decreased K+ in urine
b) Increased Na+ in urine
c) Increased urine output
d) **Decreased urine output**

Q 112 Glucose is __________

a) Filtered, reabsorbed and secreted
b) **Filtered, reabsorbed but not secreted**
c) Filtered, secreted but not reabsorbed
d) Filtered, neither secreted nor reabsorbed

Q 113 In starving animal catabolism of body reserve occurs in the following order __________

a) **Glycogen-fat- protein**
b) Fat- glycogen- protein
c) Fat- protein- glycogen
d) Protein-glycogen- fat

Q 114 A young growing animal will store energy positively in the form of __________

a) **Protein**
b) Fat
c) Glycogen
d) All the above

Q 115 The quantity of heat produced on complete oxidation of unit weight of a food is known as __________

a) Metabolic energy
b) **Gross energy**
c) Net energy
d) All the above

Q 116 Which of the following acid has higher gross energy?

a) Acetic acid
b) Propionic acid
c) **Butyric acid**
d) Lactic acid

Q 117 Which of the following has the higher energy value than the other?

a) Propionic acid
b) Acetic acid
c) Butyric acid
d) **Methane**

Q 118 Which of the following nutrient has the higher gross energy than the others?

a) Carbohydrates
b) Protein
c) **Fat**
d) Mineral

Q 119 Digestible energy is ________

a) **GE-FE** b) ME- NE

c) GE-FE-UE d) GE-FE+NE

Q 120 What percentage of gross energy of food is lost as methane in ruminants?

a) 3-4% b) 5-6%

c) **7-9%** d) 11-13%

Q 121 What percentage of digestible energy of food is lost as methane in cow?

a) 3-4% b) 5-6%

c) 7-9% d) **11-13%**

Q 122 Metabolizable energy value of maize is higher in ________

a) Cow b) Buffalo

c) Sheep d) **Pig**

Q 123 Which of the following fraction is generally considered as a "tax" on the energy of food?

a) **Heat increment** b) Methane energy

c) Faecal energy d) Urinary energy

Q 124 Tick the wrong statement ________

a) **Energy has mass and it occupies the mass**

b) Energy exist in two forms- kinetic and potential

c) Study of energy is covered under bioenergetic

d) Total energy of feed is known as gross energy

Q 125 One calorie is equal to ________

a) 2.326 joules b) **4.1868 joules**

c) 1055.06 joules d) 5.932 joules

Q 126 One BTU (British thermal unit) is equal to ________

a) 1055.06 Joules b) 251.996 calories

c) **Both a & b** d) None of the above

Q 127 Which of the following is not the part of bomb calorimeter?

a) Bucket
b) Insulating jacket
c) Bomb
d) **Water bath**

Q 128 The number of heat unit liberated by a unit mass of a sample when burned with oxygen in an enclosure of constant volume is known as __________

a) Calorific value
b) Heat of combustion
c) Gross energy
d) **All the above**

Q 129 Oxidative phosphorylation occurs in __________

a) **Mitochondria**
b) Endoplasmic reticulum
c) Cytoplasm
d) Golgi bodies

Q 130 Embden - Meyerhof Pathway takes place in __________

a) **Cytosol**
b) Golgi bodies
c) Both of these
d) Non of these

Q 131 The net production of ATP per moles of glucose is anaerobes glycolytic pathway is __________

a) 4
b) **2**
c) 6
d) 8

Q 132 When glucose is used as energy source under anaerobic condition, which of the following substances accumulate in the tissue?

a) Urea
b) Glycogen
c) **Lactate**
d) Pyruvate

Q 133 Embden Meyerhof Pathway is also known as __________

a) Pentose phosphate pathway
b) TCA cycle
c) **Glycolytic pathway**
d) All the above

Q 134 Pentose phosphate pathway is also known as __________

a) Phosphogluconate pathway
b) Hexose phosphate shunt
c) **Both of these**
d) None of these

Q 135 Hexose phosphate shunt occur in the cytosol of the cells of __________

a) Liver
b) Adipose tissue
c) Mammary gland
d) **All the above**

Q 136 How many molecules of Pyruvic acid are produced, when one molecule of glucose is oxidized?

a) **2**
b) 4
c) 3
d) 5

Q 137 Amount of energy received from one ATP is __________

a) 8.9 Kcal
b) **7.3 Kcal**
c) 73 Kcal
d) 89 Kcal

Q138 Glycolysis pathway can proceed in __________

a) Anaerobic condition only
b) Aerobic condition only
c) **Both aerobic & anaerobic condition**
d) None of these

Q 139 How many moles of ATP are generated during the conversion of NAD into NADH?

a) 4
b) **3**
c) 2
d) 5

Q 140 How many moles of ATP are generated during the conversion of GTP into GDP?

a) 4
b) 3
c) **1**
d) 2

Q 141 How many moles of ATP are generated during the conversion of FAD into $FADH_2$?

a) 4
b) 3
c) **2**
d) 5

Q142 Which of the following is more efficient in term of providing energy to cell?

a) Anaerobic glycolysis
b) **Aerobic glycolysis**
c) Both are equal
d) Depends upon situation

Q143 Net yield of ATP in aerobic glycolysis is ________

a) 2 b) 6

c) **8** d) 10

Q 144 The total ATP production from the oxidation of one mole of glucose aerobically is ________

a) 16 b) 20

c) 30 d) **38**

Q 145 Tricarboxylic acid cycle is also known as ________

a) Krebs cycle b) Citric acid cycle

c) TCA cycle d) **All the above**

Q 146 The entire TCA cycle takes place in the ________

a) Cytosol b) **Mitochondria**

c) Golgi apparatus d) Endoplasmic reticulum

Q 147 Which of the following compound required to initiate the TCA cycle and is regenerated at the end of TCA cycle?

a) Citric acid b) Malic acid

c) **Oxaloacetic acid** d) Acetyl CoA

Q 148 Indirect method of measuring methane production in ruminant animal is ________

a) **8% of gross energy** b) 81% of gross energy

c) 18% of gross energy d) 28 % of gross energy

Q 149 Which of the following equation can be used to estimate the ME value of ruminant feed?

a) **DE x 0.81** b) GE x 0.81

c) NE x 0.81 d) GE x 0.81/DE

Q 150 Net gain of ATP Moles per moles of propionic acid, when later is used as source of energy via glucose ________

a) 30 b) 27

c) **13.5** d) 14.5

Q 151 Net gain of ATP moles per moles of propionic acid, when later is directly used as source of energy ________

a) 30 b) 27

c) 13.5 d) **14.5**

Q 152 Which of the following VFA is present in significant amount in the peripheral blood of cow?

a) Propionic acid b) **Acetic acid**

c) Butyric acid d) Valeric acid

Q 153 Net yield of ATP per mole of Acetate, when later is used as source of energy ________

a) **8** b) 10

c) 12 d) 14

Q 154 Most of the urea fermented in the liver of ruminant is ________

a) **Excreted via urine**

b) Recycled via saliva

c) Re-enter into rumen via rumen wall

d) Excreted via gall bladder

Q 155 Gross energy content of 4% fat corrected milk is ________

a) 24.9 MJ/Kg DM b) 104.18 Claorie/Kg DM

c) **Both of the above** d) None of the above

Q 156 Which of the following factor effect the ME value of food?

a) Type of digestion b) Frequency of feed

c) Species of animal d) **All the above**

Q 157 Carbohydrate content of an egg is around ________

a) **less than 1%** b) 3-5%

c) 5-10% d) 10-15%

Q 158 Presence of glycolysis ad its key enzymes in the chicken embryo was first reported by ________

a) **Meyerhof & Perdigon** b) Embden & Meyerhof

c) Eijkman d) Funk & Mccollum

Q 159 Average Gross energy content of 1 gram of carbohydrate is __________

a) 9.5 Kcal
b) 5.3 Kcal
c) **4.2 Kcal**
d) 15.3 Kcal

Q 160 Average gross energy content of 1 gram fat is __________

a) 4.2 Kcal
b) **9.5 Kcal**
c) 5.3 Kcal
d) 14.4 Kcal

Q 161 Average gross energy content of 1 gram of protein is _______

a) 4.2 Kcal
b) 9.5 Kcal
c) **5.3 Kcal**
d) 18.5 Kcal

Q 162 Gross energy content of fat is approximately________ time greater than that of starch.

a) 1.15
b) **2.25**
c) 2.56
d) 2.85

Q 163 NE (maintenance) of the adult hen can be calculated by the following equation __________

a) **NEm = 83 x BW(Kg)$^{0.75}$**
b) NEm = 16 x BW(Kg)$^{0.75}$
c) NEm = 183 x BW(Kg)$^{0.75}$
d) NEm = 193 x BW(Kg)$^{0.75}$

Q 164 ME value is generally __________ % higher than NE value.

a) **18%***
b) 28%
c) 38%
d) 48%

* ME (m) = NE(m)/0.82

Q 165 The per day ME requirement for maintenance of a newly hatched chicks weighing 40 g is around __________

a) 40-45 Kcal
b) **8-10 Kcal**
c) 70-80 Kcal
d) 90-100 Kcal

Q 166 Under normal condition activity allowance for the adult hen is __________

a) 37% of BMR
b) **50% of BMR**
c) 70% of BMR
d) 90% BMR

Q 167 Activity allowance in the caged layer is __________

a) **37% of BMR**
b) 50% of BMR
c) 67% of BMR
d) 87% of BMR

Q 168 β-oxidation of fatty acid is promoted by which of the following?

a) ATP
b) **NAD+**
c) $FADH_2$
d) Acetyl CoA

Q 169 In mammals, the main site for urea cycle is ________

a) **Liver**
b) Kidney
c) Spleen
d) Small Intestine

Q 170 RQ in hibernating animal is about ________

a) 1.0
b) **0.7**
c) 0.89
d) 1.5

Q 171 As a cow process the gross energy consumed, the energy is partition among various outputs. Which of the following energy output is the greatest?

a) Maintenance energy
b) Faecal energy
c) Milk energy
d) **Heat energy**

Q 172 The amount of food energy required to keep the animal at a constant body weight and composition is called ________

a) **Maintenance energy**
b) Net energy
c) Gross energy
d) Heat Increment

Q 173 The method adopted to arrive at energy requirement for maintenance as well as growth is ________

a) Fasting metabolism
b) Feeding trial method
c) Comparative slaughter
d) **All the above**

Q 174 One megacalorie is equivalent to ________

a) 100 Kilocalorie
b) **1000 Kilocalorie**
c) 1000 Calorie
d) 10 Kilocalorie

Q 175 Tick the wrong statement regarding energy ________

a) **Carbohydrate feed have more gross energy than high fat feeds**
b) Digestible energy (DE) is less accurate and less precise than measuring GE
c) ME (metabolisable energy) is less accurate and less precise than DE
d) Measuring of NEL is the least accurate and precise measure of energy.

❏❏❏

Chapter 6

Protein

Q 1 Which of the following is an amino acid because it contains amino group (NH) instead of NH_2 group?

a) Valine
b) Serine
c) **Proiline**
d) Cysteine

Q 2 The simplest amino acid is __________

a) **Glycine**
b) Proline
c) Arginine
d) Histidine

Q 3 Which of the following is sulphur containing amino acid?

a) Glutamine
b) Asparagine
c) **Cysteine**
d) Proline

Q 4 Out of the 20 commonly found amino acid, how many contain sulphur in them?

a) 5
b) 4
c) **2**
d) 1

Q 5 Tick the sulphur containing amino acid __________

a) Glutamine
b) **Methionine**
c) Tyrosine
d) Proline

Q 6 Which of the following is not the basic amino acid?

a) Lysine
b) Histidine
c) Arginine
d) **Alanine**

Q 7 Which of the following contain disulphide bridge?

a) Cysteine
b) Phenyl alanine
c) **Cystine**
d) Thyroxine

Q 8 Tick the wrong statement __________

a) Amino acid are amphoteric

b) In aqueous solution, amino acid exist as zwitter ion

c) **All amino acids involved in protein structure have D-configuration***

d) Except glycine all amino acids are optically active

* They have L configuration

Q 9 Which of the following is not a cyclic amino acid?

a) Phenyl alanine b) Tyrosine

c) Tryptophan d) **Arginine**

Q 10 Which of the following amino acid has dicarboxylic group in it?

a) Isoleucine b) Threonine

c) Serine d) **Glutamic acid**

Q 11 Which of the following animal was used to study the essentiality of the amino acids?

a) Cat b) **Rat**

c) Dog d) Horse

Q 12 How many essential amino acids are required in the diet of growing chicken?

a) 10 b) **11**

c) 15 d) 18

Q 13 The amino acids which can not be synthesized by the animal body and are must be included in the diet for proper growth are termed as __________

a) **Indispensible amino acid** b) Dispensible amino acid

c) Both a & b d) Semi-essential amino acid

Q 14 Number of essential amino acid required in Pig is __________

a) **10** b) 15

c) 20 d) 25

Q 15 Nature of enzyme protein is __________

a) Fibrous b) **Globular**

c) Conjugated d) Simple

Q 16 Which of the following is not an example of fibrous protein?

a) Collagens
b) Elastin
c) **Prolamins**
d) Keratins

Q 17 Depending upon density, lipoprotein can be classified into how many categories?

a) 2
b) 3
c) **5**
d) 9

Q 18 Which of the following amino acid is not present in collagens?

a) Cystine
b) Tryptophan
c) **Both a & b**
d) Proline

Q 19 The primary structure of protein represents __________

a) **Linear sequence of amino acid joined by peptide bond**
b) 3- Dimensional structure of protein
c) Helical structure of protein
d) All the above

Q 20 All the following statements are true for protein denaturation except that it __________

a) Is a shape change
b) **Is always reversible**
c) May be caused by pH change
d) Could result from temperature change

Q 21 The purine base present in nucleic acid is __________

a) Cytosine
b) Thymine
c) Uracil
d) **Adenine**

Q22 Which of the following amide is also classed as amino acid?

a) Asperagine
b) Glutamine
c) **Both a & b**
d) None of the above

Q 23 Which of the following is an amide?

a) Putrescine
b) **Urea**
c) Tyramine
d) Cadaverine

Q 24 The amine "cadaverine" is formed from which amino acid?

a) Arginine
b) Histidine
c) **Lysine**
d) Tryptophan

Q 25 The term "protein" was coined by ________

a) L. Spallanzani b) **G.J. Mulder**

c) F. Magendie d) A. Lavoisier

Q 26 In birds, principle end product of nitrogen metabolism is ______

a) Urea b) **Uric acid**

c) Allantoin d) None of the above

Q 27 In mammals, the main end product of nitrogen metabolism is ________

a) **Urea** b) Uric acid

c) Allantoin d) None of the above

Q 28 Urea cycle consists of how many reaction?

a) 2 b) 3

c) 4 d) **5**

Q 29 Urea cycle comprises of ________

a) **Two mitochondrial and three cytosolic reaction**

b) Three mitochondrial and two cytosolic reaction

c) One mitochondrial and four cytosolic reaction

d) Four mitochondrial and one cytosolic reaction

Q 30 Urea cycle is also known as ________

a) Ornithine cycle b) Kreb- Henseleit cycle

c) **Both a & b** d) None of the above

Q 31 How many nitrogen are eliminated in every urea cycle?

a) 1 b) **2**

c) 3 d) 4

Q 32 Which of the following statements about urea cycle is correct?

a) Arginosuccinate is lysed to urea and ornithine in urea cycle

b) Carbamoyl phosphate supplies both of the nitrogen atom in urea cycle

c) The formation of urea in urea cycle yield energy

d) **Arginine is hydrolysed to urea and ornithine in the urea cycle**

Q 33 Based upon the fate of carbon skeleton of amino acid,which of the following is ketogenic in nature?

a) Alanine
b) Arginine
c) **Leucine**
d) Glycine

Q 34 Tick the wrong statement __________

a) Both rumen bacteria and protozoa actively deaminate amino acid
b) **Like bacteria, ruminal protozoa can also synthesize amino acid from ammonia**
c) Defaunation decreseas ruminal ammonia concentration
d) Protolytic activity of protozoa is higher than that of bacteria

Q 35 Which of the following is critical amino acid for poultry?

a) **Lysine**
b) Phenylalanine
c) Leucine
d) Histidine

Q 36 The first limiting amino acid in poultry diet is __________

a) **Methionine**
b) Lysine
c) Tryptophan
d) Arginine

Q 37 The second limiting amino acid in poultry diet is __________

a) Methionine
b) **Lysine**
c) Arginine
d) Phenylalanine

Q 38 First limiting amino acid in most of the practical swine diet is __________

a) **Lysine**
b) Methionine
c) Threonine
d) Tryptophan

Q 39 The second limiting amino acid in most practical diet in swine is __________

a) Lysine
b) Methionine
c) **Threonine**
d) Valine

Q 40 Which of the following is a cat specific amino acid?

a) **Taurine**
b) Lysine
c) Methionine
d) Arginine

Q 41 In cat, majority of ornithine is synthesized from which amino acid?

a) **Arginine***
b) Lysine
c) Methionine
d) Taurine

* Deficiency of arginine can lead to accumulation of ammonia in the blood

Q 42 The first limiting amino acid in corn-soyabean based poultry diet is __________

a) Methionine
b) **Lysine**
c) Tryptophan
d) Threonine

Q 43 Deficiency symptoms of taurine in cat includes __________

a) Reproductive problem
b) Retinal Degeneration
c) Cardiomyopathy
d) **All the above**

Q 44 Number of essential amino acid in dog is __________

a) **10**
b) 12
c) 8
d) 14

Q 45 Number of essential amino acid in cat is __________

a) 10
b) **11**
c) 12
d) 14

Q 46 Which of the following is not a fibrous protein?

a) Collagen
b) Elastin
c) **Globulins**
d) Keratin

Q 47 Which of the following is not a globular protein?

a) Albumin
b) Globulins
c) Histones
d) **Collagen**

Q 48 Which of the following is not an example of conjugated protein?

a) Mucoprotein
b) Protamines
c) **Albumin**
d) Glycoprotein

Q 49 The first limiting amino acid for wool production is ________

a) Methionine
b) **Cysteine**
c) Arginine
d) Histidine

Q 50 The first limiting amino acid in microbial protein for growing cattle is __________

a) **Methionine** b) Cysteine
c) Arginine d) Lysine

Q 51 The first limiting amino acid in microbial protein in sheep is __________

a) **Methionine** b) Cysteine
c) Lysine d) Argine

Q 52 Which of the following amino acid is used as reference amino acid for calculating ideal amino acid ratio?

a) Methionine b) **Lysine**
c) Arginine d) Tryptophan

Q 53 Mimosine is a (an) __________

a) Polysaccharide b) Polypeptide
c) **Amino acid** d) None of the above

Q 54 The bacterium responsible for metabolization of DHP (3 hydroxy-4 (IH)pyridine) – product of mimisine in the rumen is __________

a) ***Synergisted Jonesii*** b) *Ruminococcus albus*
c) *Fibrobacter succinogens* d) *Lactobacillus Spp.*

Q 55 3- Methyindole-a product formed in the rumen from the metabolism of __________

a) Mimosine b) **Tryptophan**
c) Pyruvic acid d) Acetic acid

Q 56 "Fog fever" occur due to accumulation of which of the following in the rumen?

a) **3-methyindole (skatole)*** b) Mimosine
c) Lactic acid d) None of the above

* Skatole is formed from the tryptophan

Q 57 Which of the following amino acid is commercially available in the rumen protected form?

a) Arginine b) Biotin
c) Choline d) **Methionine**

Q 58 Which of the following amino acid does not exist in D & L (Isomer) forms?

a) Methionine
b) Lysine
c) **Glycine**
d) Alanine

Q 59 Storage protein in grains are __________

a) Albumins
b) Glutelins
c) **Prolamines**
d) Globulins

Q 60 Collagen does not have __________

a) Cysteine
b) Cystine
c) Tryptophan
d) **All the above**

Q 61 Gelatin comes from __________

a) **Collagens**
b) Elastin
c) Keratins
d) Prolamines

Q 62 Which of the following protein is soluble in water?

a) **Albumin**
b) Collagens
c) Keratins
d) Prolamines

Q 63 Which of the following has higher requirement for arginine?

a) Cow
b) Dog
c) Sheep
d) **Poultry**

Q 64 Which of the following amino acid has sulhydryl group in it?

a) Methionine
b) **Cysteine**
c) Cystine
d) Arginine

Q 65 Which of the following amino acid has disulphide bond in it?

a) Methionine
b) Cysteine
c) **Cystine**
d) Mimosine

Q 66 Which of the following sulphur containing compound are excreted in cat urine for territorial marking?

a) Taurine
b) Felinine
c) Isovalthine
d) Skatole
e) **Both b & c**

Q 67 The unpleasant odour (Boar taint) of pig meat is due to _______

a) **Skatole** b) Isovalthine

c) Picolinic acid d) Taurine

Q 68 Amino acid containing an indole group _________

a) Arginine b) Methionine

c) **Tryptophan** d) Cysteine

Q 69 Which amino acid is most affected by the maillard reaction?

a) **Lysine** b) Methionine

c) Tryptophan d) Arginine

Q 70 Which of the following did not suffer from gout?

a) Dalmation dog b) Poultry birds

c) **Pig** d) Human

Q 71 In a tripeptide, how many amino acids and peptide bonds are there?

a) 3 & 3 b) **3 & 2**

c) 2 & 3 d) 3 & 1

Q 72 In 57 g standard egg, the amount of protein is around _______

a) **6.7g** b) 15 g

c) 19 g d) 20 g

Q 73 High amount of which of the following amino acid has deleterious effect on the birds arginine status _________

a) Lysine b) Histidine

c) Leucine d) **All the above**

Q 74 The minimum recommended level of methionine in broiler starter diet is _________

a) **0.50%** b) 0.35%

c) 1.0% d) 1.5%

Q 75 The minimum recommendation level of lysine by BIS (1992) in broiler starter diet is _________

a) 0.5% b) 0.35%

c) **1.2%** d) 1.7%

Q 76 The minimum recommended level of methionine in broiler finisher diet is ________

a) 0.25% b) **0.35%**

c) 0.50% d) 0.75%

Q 77 The minimum recommended level of lysine in broiler finisher diet is ________

a) 1.2% b) **1.0%**

c) 0.5% d) 0.35%

Q 78 The minimum recommended level of methionine in layer is ________

a) 0.10 % b) 0.20%

c) **0.30%** d) 1.0%

Q 79 The minimum recommended level of lysine in layer is ________

a) 0.25% b) **0.65 %**

c) 1.75% d) 1.50%

Q 80 Poultry need one more essential amino acid ________ than cattle.

a) Lysine b) Methionine

c) **Glycine** d) Cysteine

Q 81 Bovine bunker is synonymous to ________

a) **Urea toxicity** b) salt toxicity

c) Oxalate toxicity d) Selenium toxicity

Q 82 The digestibility of bypass protein of most of the concentrate is in the range of ________

a) 30-40% b) 50-60%

c) **80-90 %** d) 100%

Q 83 Which of the following feedstuff has highest percentage of UDP (bypass protein)?

a) **Solvent extracted cottonseed cake**

b) Linseed cake

c) Mustard cake

d) Ambadi cake

Q 84 Feedstuff whose ruminal protein degradability value range from 0-30% has ________

a) **High bypass protein value**
b) Medium bypass protein value
c) Low bypass protein value
d) No bypass protein value

Q 85 Feedstuff whose ruminal protein degradability value range from 31 to 60% has ________

a) High bypass protein content
b) **Medium bypass protein content**
c) Low bypass protein content
d) Very high bypass protein content

Q 86 Feedstuff whose ruminal protein degradability value ranging from 61 to 100% ________

a) High bypass protein content
b) Medium bypass protein content
c) **Low bypass protein content**
d) Very high bypass protein content

Q 87 Tick the right answer about the amino acids ________

a) Amphoteric in nature
b) At isoelectric point exhibit zwitterion structure
c) Mostly occur in L - configuration
d) **All are right**

Q 88 Which of the following is basic amino acid?

a) Aspartic acid b) Glutamic acid
c) Glycine d) **Lysine**

Q 89 Which of the following is not a basic amino acid?

a) Lysine b) Arginine
c) **Alanine** d) Hydroxylysine

Q 90 Which of the following is acidic amino acid?

a) Lysine b) Arginine
c) **Aspartic acid** d) Serine

Q 91 Which of the following is an example of aromatic amino acid?

a) Phenylalanine b) Tyrosine
c) **Both a & b** d) None of these

Q 92 Which of the following is not an example of sulphur containing amino acid?

a) Methionine b) Cystine
c) Cysteine d) **Serine**

Q 93 Which of the following amino acid is bitter in taste?

a) Glycine b) Alanine
c) Serine d) **Arginine**

Q 94 Which of the following amino acid is sweet in nature?

a) Glycine b) Alanine
c) Serine d) **All the above**

Q 95 Enzyme is a type of ________

a) **Catalyst** b) Substance
c) Product d) Metabolite

Q 96 Broadly enzymes are divided into how many groups?

a) **6** b) 5
c) 4 d) 3

Q 97 Natures of enzymes are ________

a) **Protein** b) Carbohydrate
c) Cellulose d) Lipid

Q 98 The enzyme which catalyse the transfer of hydrogen, oxygen or electron from one molecule to another is known as ______

a) **Oxidoreductase** b) Transferase
c) Hydrolases d) Lyases

Q 99 Enzymes which catalyse nonhydrolytic decomposition are known as ________

a) Hydrolases b) Ligases
c) **Lyases** d) Oxidoreductase

Q 100 All the following are protein in nature except __________

a) Deaminase
b) Esterase
c) Kinases
d) **Ribozymes**

Q 101 Certain enzymes require some substance to activate them. These enzymes are known as __________

a) **Apoenzyme**
b) Coenzyme
c) Holoenzyme
d) Ribozymes

Q 102 The substance required to activate the apoenzyme is known as __________

a) Coenzymes
b) Cofactors
c) **Both of the above**
d) None of the above

Q 103 The organic cofactors are known as __________

a) **Coenzymes**
b) Apoenzymes
c) Holoenzymes
d) None of the above

Q 104 The inactivate precursor of enzymes are known as __________

a) Apoenzymes
b) **Zymogen**
c) Coenzymes
d) Holoenzymes

Q 105 Enzymes accelerate the reaction by __________

a) **Lowering activation energy of the reaction**
b) By increasing reactant
c) By removal of product
d) None of the above

Q 106 Rate of enzyme action is influenced by __________

a) Substrate concentration
b) Enzyme concentration
c) Temperature
d) Acidity
e) **All the above**

Q 107 The main structural component of animal body is __________

a) Protein
b) Mineral
c) Fat
d) **Both a and b**

Q 108 The main structural component of plant body is __________

a) Protein
b) Fat
c) **Carbohydrate**
d) Mineral

Q 109 Which of the following protein is heat coagulable in nature?

a) Histone b) **Albumin**

c) Keratins d) All the above

Q 110 Which of the following protein contain pigment as a prosthetic group?

a) Phosphoprotein b) Glycoprotein

c) Lipoprotein d) **Chromoprotein**

Q 111 Urea nitrogen is frequently determined in all of the following except __________

a) Urine sample b) **Faecal sample**

c) Milk sample d) Serum sample

Q 112 Which of the following scientists classified amino acid into essential or non-essential amino acids?

a) **Rose** b) Osborne and Mendel

c) Hopkins d) Magendie

Q 113 Number of essential amino acid requirement for adult pig is __________

a) 10 b) 13

c) **9** d) 12

Q 114 Most toxic amino acid is __________

a) **Methionine** b) Tryptophan

c) Lysine d) Threonine

Q 115 Least toxic amino acid is __________

a) Methionine b) Lysine

c) Valine d) **Threonine**

❑❑❑

Chapter 7

Fat

Q 1 The most abundant fatty acid in plant kingdom is ________

a) **Linolenic acid** b) Palmitic acid

c) Oleic acid d) None of these

Q 2 The most common saturated fatty acid is ________

a) Linolenic acid b) Linoleic acid

c) Oleic acid d) **Palmitic acid**

Q 3 The most common monounsaturated fatty acid is ________

a) Linolenic acid b) Linoleic acid

c) **Oleic acid** d) Palmitic acid

Q 4 Fat is insoluble in ________

a) Benzene b) Ether

c) Chloroform d) **Water**

Q 5 Which of the following is a non-glycerol based lipid?

a) Glucolipid b) Lecithins

c) Cephalins d) **Waxes**

Q 6 Which of the following is an example of lipid?

a) Pectin b) Chitin

c) Gum d) **Steroids**

Q 7 The product of saponification of fat is ________

a) Sodium salt of fatty acid b) Potssium salt of fatty acid

c) Calcium salt of fatty acid d) **Both a & b**

Q 8 Lipids are readily soluble in __________

a) Water b) Alcohol

c) **Benzene** d) None of these

Q 9 Which of the following is/are unsaturated acid?

a) Linoleic acid b) Oleic acid

c) Palmitoleic acid d) **All of these**

Q 10 The synthesis of glucose from fat is known as __________

a) Glycolysis b) Saponification

c) **Gluconeogensis** d) All the above

Q 11 Hydrolysis of fat by alkali into fatty acid and glycerol is called __________

a) **Saponification** b) Rancidity

c) Colloidal d) Suspension

Q 12 Which of the following is a phospholipid?

a) **Lecithin** b) Cholesterol

c) Sterols d) Steroids

Q 13 The number of double bond in arachidonic acid is __________

a) 1 b) 2

c) 3 d) **4**

Q 14 Which of the following is an example of essential fatty acid?

a) Linoleic acid b) Arachidonic acid

c) Linolenic acid d) **All of these**

Q 15 Example of monounsaturated fatty acid is __________

a) **Oleic acid** b) Arachidonic acid

c) Palmitic acid d) Linolenic acid

Q 16 The presence of free fatty acid in a fat (which can cause rancidity) can be determined by __________

a) **Acid value** b) Iodine Number

c) Both of these d) None of these

Q 17 Which of the following is a measure of unsaturation of fatty acid in the fat?

a) Acid value b) **Iodine Number**

c) Saponification d) All of these

Q 18 Omega system of fatty acid nomenclature was given by ______

a) **R.T.Holman** b) R.E. Hungate

c) C.G. Orpin d) T.Bauchop

Q 19 Which of the following is an example of non-saponifiable lipid?

a) Waxes b) Phosphoglycerides

c) Sphingolipid d) **Steroids**

Q 20 Which of the following is an example of saponifiable lipid?

a) Terpenes b) Steroids

c) **Sphingolipids** d) Prostaglandin

Q 21 Cholesterol belongs to which of the following group?

a) **Steroids** b) Neutral fats

c) Waxes d) Phospholipid

Q 22 Ceramide is a type of __________

a) Carbohydrate b) Protein

c) **Lipid** d) None of these

Q 23 Tick the right statement __________

a) Cholesterol is the part of both vegetable and animal food

b) It is dietary essential

c) **Egg yolk has high cholesterol level**

d) All are right

Q 24 Which of the following thing is the major form of energy storage in the animal body?

a) Glycogen b) Protein

c) **Fat** d) Glucose

Q 25 Majority of naturally occurring unsaturated fatty acid have ________________ configuration.

a) **Cis** b) Trans

c) Both in equal ratio d) None of these

Q 26 Which of the following fatty acid abbreviation is belong to omega-6 family?

a) N-9-18:1 b) **N-6,9-18:2**

c) N-3,6,9-18:3 d) None of these

Q 27 Which of the following represents essential fatty acid in true sense?

a) Linoleic acid b) Linolenic acid

c) Arachidonic acid d) **Both a & b**

Q 28 Which of the following represents the essential fatty acid for animal in general?

a) Linoleic acid b) Linolenic acid

c) Arachidonic acid d) **All the above**

Q 29 According to thumb rule, to fulfill the requirement of EFA in mammals, how much percentage of energy is in the form of linoleic acid?

a) 10% b) 5%

c) **3%** d) 0.5%

Q 30 Which of the following mammals has limited Δ6 desaturase activity which is required for conversion of linoleic and linolenic acid to arachidonic acid?

a) Cow b) Buffalo

c) Goat d) **Cat**

Q 31 Tick the wrong statement __________

a) In rumen, hydrogenation of unsaturated fatty acid can result in trans fatty acid

b) **Trans fatty acid possess essential fatty acid activity**

c) Trans fatty acid can possess the risk of cardiovascular disease, cancer and diabetes.

d) Trans fatty acid has higher melting point than their cis analogues.

Q 32 Which of the following is not the breakdown product of galactolipid in rumen?

a) **Glucose** b) Galactose

c) Fatty acid d) Glycerol

Q 33 Which of the following is not an example of glycolipid?

a) Sphingosine b) Cerebrosides

c) Gangliosides d) **Cephalins**

Q 34 Which of the following fatty acid is unsaturated in nature?

a) Myristic acid
b) Palmitic acid
c) Stearic acid
d) **Oleic acid**

Q 35 Which of the following is monounsaturated fatty acid?

a) Linoleic acid
b) Linolenic acid
c) **Oleic acid**
d) Myristic acid

Q 36 Chemically fat and oils are __________

a) Acids
b) Alcohols
c) **Esters**
d) Alkones

Q 37 Which of the following is classified as "Steroid"?

a) Phospholipid
b) Glycolipid
c) Wax
d) **Cholesterol**

Q 38 Which of the following is an example of Steroid?

a) Cholesterol
b) Bile acid
c) Cortisol
d) **All the above**

Q 39 Which of the following is not an example of terpenes?

a) Vitamin A
b) Vitamin E
c) Vitamin K
d) **Ergosterol**

Q 40 Tick the wrong statement __________

a) Saturated fatty acid increases the serum cholesterol
b) **Polyunsaturated fatty acid increases the serum cholesterol**
c) Omega-6 fatty acid decreases the serum cholesterol
d) High level of low density lipoprotein (LDLP) increases the chances of coronary disease.

Q 41 A person on a fat free carbohydrate rich diet continuous to grow obese, which of the following lipoprotein is likely to be elevated in his blood?

a) Chylomicron
b) **VLDL**
c) LDL
d) HDL

Q 42 HDL's are synthesized in __________

a) Blood b) Liver

c) Intestine d) **Both b & c**

Q 43 Fatty acid synthesis takes place in __________

a) Mitochondira b) Cell membrane

c) **Cytosol** d) Endoplasmic reticulum

Q 44 Cholesterol is a precursor of __________

a) Steroid hormone b) Vitamin A

c) Bile salt d) **Both a & c**

Q 45 VLDL are synthesized in __________

a) Blood b) **Liver**

c) Intestine d) Pancreases

Q 46 How many lipoproteins are there on the basis of density?

a) 2 b) 3

c) 6 d) **5**

Q 47 Which of the following is not included in PUFA?

a) **Monoenoic acid** b) Dienoic acid

c) Trienoic acid d) Polyenoic acid

Q 48 Tick the wrong statement __________

a) Naturally occurring fats and oils are mixture of mixed triacylglycerols

b) Most of naturally occurring fatty acids have an even number of carbon atoms

c) **Most naturally occurring fatty acid have trans configuration***

d) Trans fat is considered as bad for health

* They have cis configuration.

Q 49 The cerebrosidess is an example of __________

a) **Glycilipid** b) Phospholipid

c) Terpenes d) Steroids

Q 50 The gangaliosides is an example of _________

a) **Glycolipid** b) Phospholipid

c) Waxes d) Terpenes

Q 51 Glycolipid is mainly found in which animal part?

a) **Brain** b) Kidneys

c) Heart d) None of the above

Q 52 Lecithin is a _________

a) Glycolipid b) **Phospholipid**

c) Terpenes d) Steroid

Q 53 You are doing proximate analysis of a plant based feed having high content of waxes. Which of the following proximate fraction is then overestimated?

a) Crude protein b) Nitrogen free extract

c) **Ether extract** d) Crude fibre

Q 54 Transport of cholesterol from tissue to liver occur with the help of _________

a) Chylomicron b) VLDL

c) LDL d) **HDL**

Q 55 The major fatty acid in coconut oil is _________

a) **Lauric acid** b) Oleic acid

c) Linoleic acid d) Linolenic acid

Q 56 A standard weight egg (57g) contain how much lipid?

a) 10.2g b) **5.7 g**

c) 15.7 g d) 1.4 g

Q 57 The percentage of shell, albumin and yolk in standard egg is _________

a) **11,57 & 32 %** b) 57,11 & 32

c) 32,11 & 57 % d) 11,32 & 57

Q 58 Which of the following fatty acid is not a omega-3 fatty acid?

a) Eicosapentaenoic acid b) Docosaentaenoic acid

c) Docosahexaenoic acid d) **Arachidonic acid***

* Arachidonic acid is omega-6 fatty acid

Q 59 Which of the following is omega-6 fatty acid ________

a) **Linoleic acid** b) Gamma- linolenic acid

c) Docosapentaenoic acid d) Eicosapentaenoic acid

Q 60 Which of the following is used as an antioxidants preservative to prevent the auto-oxidation of lipid in foods and feeds?

a) Butylated hydroxyanisole b) Butylated hydroxytoluene

c) Ethoxquin d) **All the above**

Q 61 Which of the following antioxidant reduces the initiation of lipid peroxidation?

a) Superoxide dismutase b) **Catalase**

c) Vitamin E d) All the above

Q 62 Which of the following oil is high in monounsaturated fatty acid?

a) **Canola oil** b) Safflower oil

c) Sunflower oil d) Coconut oil

Q 63 Which of the following oil is rich in omega-3 fatty acid?

a) Canola oil b) **Linseed oil**

c) Rapeseed oil d) Soybean oil

Q 64 Which of the following lipoprotein is considered as bad cholesterol?

a) Chylomicrons b) VLDL

c) **LDL** d) HDL

Q 65 Which of the following lipoprotein is considered as good cholesterol?

a) Chylomicron b) VLDL

c) LDL d) **HDL**

Q 66 Conjugated fatty acids are those in which double bonds are ________

a) Separated by a methylene group

b) **Not separated by a methylene group**

c) Separated by two methylene group

d) Separated by – SH group

Q 67 Cholesterol is a _________

a) **Steroids**
b) Eicosanoids
c) Terpenes
d) Phospholipid

Q 68 Tick the wrong statement _________

a) **Trans fatty acids are good for human health**
b) Trans fatty acids have extended half life and flavour stability
c) Conjugated linoleic acid is an anticarcinogenic
d) Naturally occurring trans fatty acids arise from bacterial synthesis.

Q 69 Bile acids are produced in _________

a) Gall bladder
b) **Liver**
c) Intestine
d) Pancrease

Q 70 Which of the following is not an example of terpenes?

a) Vitamin A
b) Carotenoid pigments
c) Giberellic acid
d) **Cortisol**

Q 71 High density lipoprotein (HDL) has _________

a) High protein and high lipid content
b) **High protein and low lipid content**
c) Low protein and high lipid content
d) Low protein and low lipid content

Q 72 Chylimicron consists of _________

a) 98-99% Protein and 1-2 % lipid
b) **98-99 % lipid and 1-2 % protein**
c) 50% protein and 50 % lipid
d) 80% lipid and 20% protein

Q 73 Which of the following lipids does not contain glycerol as its constituent unit?

a) Lecithin
b) Cephalins
c) Cerebrosides
d) **Waxes**

Q 74 Iodine number of saturated fatty acid is __________

a) 100 b) **0**

c) 90 d) 274

Q 75 Which of the following fatty acid is omega-3 type?

a) Oleic acid b) Arachidonic acid

c) **α-linolenic acid** d) Linoleic acid

Q 76 Elaidic acid ia a trans isomer of __________

a) **Oleic acid** b) Linoleic acid

c) Linolenic acid d) Arachidonic acid

Q 77 During the splitting off of the two carbon acetyl CoA from the fatty acid acyl CoA, how many ATP's are produced?

a) 2 b) 3

c) **4** d) 8

Q 78 Fatty acid synthesis occur in __________

a) Mitochondria b) **Cytosol**

c) Golgi bodies d) Endoplasmic reticulum

Q 79 The proportion of unsaturated fatty acid in a lipid is estimated by __________

a) **Iodine value** b) Acid value

c) Peroxide value d) Anisidine value

Q 80 Measuring the milligram of KOH required to neutralize 1g of fat is known as __________

a) Iodine value b) **Acid value**

c) Peroxide value d) Anisidine value

Q 81 Which of the following value is a measurement of the proportion of free fatty acids in a given sample?

a) Iodine value b) **Acid value**

c) Peroxide value d) Anisidine value

Q 82 Which of the following value is an indicator of the product of primary oxidation of lipid?

a) Iodine value b) Acid value

c) **Peroxide value** d) Anisidine value

Q 83 Thiobarbituric acid (TBA) test for lipid is used to measure the extent of __________

a) Unsaturation b) Free fatty acid present

c) **Peroxidation** d) Impurities

Q 84 Which of the following test is used to estimate the oxidation of lipid?

a) Peroxide value b) Thiobarbituric acid

c) Anisidine values d) **All the above**

Q 85 The brown colour of brown fat is due to presence of large quantity of __________

a) Oil b) Vitamin A

c) **Mitochondria** d) Pigments

Q 86 Majority of body cholesterol is produced by __________

a) **Liver** b) Diet

c) Pancreas d) Spleen

Q 87 Which country developed the idea of functional food for the first time?

a) India b) USA

c) Australia d) **Japan**

Q 88 Number of millilitres of decinormal alkali required to neutralize the steam volatile fatty acid from 5 gram of fat is known as __________

a) Polenske number

b) **Reichert Meissl Number**

c) Iodine Number

d) Saponification Number

Q 89 Number of millilitres of 0.1N KOH required to neutralize the insoluble fatty acid obtained from 5 gram of fat is known as __________

a) **Polenske number** b) Reichert Meissl number

c) Iodine number d) Saponification number

Q 90 Hydrolysis of fat into glycerol and fatty acid is also known as

a) Hydrogenation b) Halogentaion

c) **Saponification** d) Acetylation

Q 91 Millilitres of KOH required to neutralize the free fatty acid present in 1 gram of fat is called as ________

a) Acetyl number
b) **Acid number**
c) Iodine number
d) Polesnke number

Q 92 Which of the following has the lowest heat increment?

a) Fibre
b) Protein
c) **Fat**
d) All have equal

Q 93 Carbon percentage in fat is ________

a) 77%
b) 57%
c) **47%**
d) 37%

❑❑❑

Chapter 8

Minerals

Q 1 Which of the following mineral is present in the enzymes succinate dehydrogenase?

a) Cu b) **Fe**

c) Zn d) Mn

Q 2 The mineral present in cytochrome a, b, & c is __________

a) Cu b) **Fe**

c) Zn d) Mn

Q 3 Which of the following mineral is present in the enzymes Glutathione peroxidases?

a) **Se** b) Cu

c) Zn d) Mo

Q 4 Superoxide dismutase enzyme contain which of the following mineral?

a) **Cu** b) Se

c) Zn d) Mn

Q 5 The excess of anion in the animal body give rise to _________

a) **Metabolic acidosis** b) Metabolic alkalosis

c) Both of these d) None of these

Q 6 The excess of cation in the animal body give rise to _________

a) Metabolic acidosis b) **Metabolic alkalosis**

c) Both of these d) None of these

Q 7 Panting under heat stress lead to __________

a) **Respiratory alkalosis** b) Respiratory acidosis

c) Both of these d) None of these

Q 8 Feeding of ammonium chloride (nishader) before 4-5 weeks of calving is often recommended to avoid the __________

a) **Milk fever** b) Retention of placenta

c) Abortion d) Metritis

Q 9 High molasses diet before calving prone the animal for ______

a) **Milk fever** b) Retention of placenta

c) Abortion d) Metritis

Q 10 In mammalian blood plasma, Calcium is around __________

a) **80-120 mg/litre** b) 40-60 mg/litre

c) 200-300 mg/litre d) 150-200 mg/litre

Q 11 Pica or depraved appetite is generally associated with the deficiency of following mineral __________

a) Ca b) **P**

c) Na d) K

Q 12 Efficiency of conversion of ß carotene to vitamin A is in the order __________

a) Rat>Ruminants> Pig> Poultry

b) Rat>Poultry>Pig>Ruminants

c) **Rat>Poultry>Ruminants>Pig**

d) Pig>Poultry>Ruminants>Rat

Q 13 Cage layer fatigue occur due to deficiency of __________

a) **Ca** b) Cl

c) Mg d) Na

Q 14 Cannibalism in poultry bird can be due to __________

a) Calcium deficiency b) **Salt deficiency**

c) Salt excess d) Iodine deficiency

Q 15 Perosis (slipped tendon) disease in poultry is due to deficiency of __________

a) Manganese b) Choline

c) Biotin d) **All the above**

Q 16 Nutritional muscular dystrophy in poultry bird is due to deficiency __________

a) Selenium

b) Vitamin E

c) Sulphur containing amino acid

d) **All the above**

Q 17 Selenium deficiency in poultry bird causes __________

a) Exudative diathesis

b) Nutritional muscular dystrophy

c) Pancreatic dystrophy

d) **All the above**

Q 18 The enzyme ATPase is activated by the mineral __________

a) **Mg^{+2}** b) Ca^{+2}

c) Na^{+} d) K^{+}

Q 19 The enzyme ATPase is inhibited by the mineral __________

a) Mg^{+2} b) **Ca^{+2}**

c) Na^{+} d) K^{+}

Q 20 Which of the following is a source of calcium sulphate?

a) Chalk b) Limestone

c) Marble d) **Gypsum**

Q 21 Which of the following hormone lower the blood calcium level?

a) Thyroid hormone b) Parathyroid hormone

c) **Thyrocalcitonin** d) Aldosterone

Q 22 The calcium in laying hens ranged between v

a) 9-12 mg/100 ml b) **30-40 mg/100ml**

c) 5-10 mg/100 ml d) 2-5 mg/100ml

Q 23 The optimum Ca :P ratio in farm animals for effective absorption of Ca & P lies in the range of ________

a) **1:1 to 2:1** b) 3:1 to 6:1

c) 6:1 to 8:1 d) 8:1 to 10:1

Q 24 The amount of phosphorus present in blood of farm animal is ________

a) **4-12 mg/100 ml** b) 12-24 mg/100 ml

c) 2-5 mg/dl d) 1-2 mg/dl

Q 25 Which is the chief cation of intracellular fluid?

a) Na b) **K**

c) Cl d) Mg

Q 26 Iron is transported in blood as ________

a) Apoferritin b) Ferritin

c) **Transferrin** d) Hemosiderin

Q 27 Excess of Ca feeding to cattle can lead to deficiency of ______

a) **Zn** b) Na

c) Cl d) Cu

Q 28 Sulphur is present in how many amino acid?

a) **3** b) 4

c) 5 d) 6

Q 29 Which of the following amino acid contain sulphur?

a) Cystine b) Cysteine

c) Methionine d) **All the above**

Q 30 How many vitamins contain sulphur as their structural part?

a) **2** b) 3

c) 4 d) 5

Q 31 Which of the following vitamins contain sulphur?

a) **Biotin and thiamine** b) Thiamine and choline

c) Choline and niacin d) Biotin and riboflavin

Q 32 Which of the following does not contain sulphur?

a) Coenzyme A b) **Riboflavin**
c) Chondroitin sulphate d) Cystine

Q 33 The commonest enzyme activator mineral is __________

a) Ca b) **Mg**
c) Cu d) Mn

Q 34 Hypomagnesmia is also known as __________

a) Magnesium tetany b) Lactation tetany
c) Grass staggers d) **All the above**

Q 35 Which of the following does not contain iron in it?

a) Ferritin b) Transferrin
c) Haemosiderin d) **Ceruloplsmin**

Q 36 "Thumps" in piglets occur due to deficiency of __________

a) Ca b) F
c) P d) **Fe**

Q 37 Mucosal block theory is associated with __________

a) Ca b) F
c) Mn d) **Fe**

Q 38 Which mineral is required for normal colour of wool?

a) **Cu** b) Mn
c) S d) Mo

Q 39 Stringy wool condition is caused by deficiency of __________

a) **Cu** b) Mn
c) Co d) Mo

Q 40 Copper deficiency in ruminants can lead to __________

a) Enzootic atexia b) Sway back
c) Falling disease d) **All the above**

Q 41 Which of the following organism is affected mostly in copper poisoning?

a) **Liver** b) Kidney
c) Spleen d) Heart

Q 42 The physiological active form of thyroid hormone is __________

a) T1 b) T2

c) **T3** d) T4

Q 43 Selenium deficiency in ruminant leads to __________

a) Ill thrift b) Blind staggers

c) Alkali disease d) **All the above**

Q 44 "Pinning Condition" occur due to deficiency of __________

a) **Cobalt** b) Zinc

c) Copper d) Sulphur

Q 45 Salt lick disease occur due to deficiency of __________

a) Salt b) **Copper**

c) Sodium d) Choline

Q 46 Big neck disease occur due to deficiency of __________

a) Salt b) **Iodine**

c) Copper d) Cobalt

Q 47 Dagnala disease occur due to __________

a) **Excess of selenium** b) Deficiency of selenium

c) Excess of fluorine d) Deficiency of flourine

Q 48 "Teartness" condition occur due to excess of __________

a) **Molybdenum** b) Magnesium

c) Manganese d) Sodium

Q 49 Feeding of paddy straw exclusively can lead to deficiency of __________

a) **Ca** b) Na

c) Cl d) K

Q 50 Perakeratosis oocur due to deficiency of __________

a) Ca b) **Zn**

c) P d) S

Q 51 "Lechsucht" disease occur due to deficiency of __________

a) **Cu** b) Ca

c) Na d) K

Q 52 Copper is transported in which of the following form in the body?

a) Erythrocuprin
b) **Ceruloplasmin**
c) Cerebrocuprin
d) None of these

Q 53 Iodine deficiency can cause __________

a) Goiter
b) Cretinism
c) Myxedima
d) **All the above**

Q 54 The ratio of Ca :P in the bone is generally __________

a) 1:1
b) 1:2
c) **2:1**
d) 2:3

Q 55 Among the following part of body, which has highest amount of Calcium?

a) **Cartilage**
b) Muscle
c) Heart
d) Spleen

Q 56 The percentage of calcium in pure calcium carbonate is ______

a) 15
b) 30
c) 35
d) **40**

Q 56 How many vitamin contain cobalt in their structure?

a) 2
b) **1**
c) 3
d) 5

Q 57 If a dairy cow is fed on ration low in protein, calcium and phosphorus, then she will secrete milk __________

a) Low in protein
b) Low in energy
c) Low in Ca & P
d) **Normal composition**

Q 58 Which of the following is not a good source of calcium?

a) Legume feeds
b) Milk
c) Colostrums
d) **Straw**

Q 59 The most abundant mineral in animal body is __________

a) **Ca**
b) P
c) Mg
d) K

Q 60 The second most abundant mineral in animal body is ______

a) Ca b) **P**

c) Mg d) K

Q 61 Tick the odd one out ________

a) Chalk b) limestone

c) Marble d) **Gypsum**

* Gypsum is $CaSO_4$ other are $CaCO_3$

Q 62 The calcium content in the body of adult animal is _______

a) 1.2-1.5 % calculated in term of fresh tissue

b) 3.5-4.0 % calculated on dry tissue

c) 26-30 % calculated on the ash

d) **All the above**

Q 63 A 600 kg cow's body contain how much calcium?

a) **6-7 kg** b) 1-2 kg

c) 10-15 kg d) 20-25 kg

Q 64 Which of the following is not the source of calcium?

a) Fluorite b) Fluoroapatite

c) Dolomite d) **Felspar**

Q 65 The bulk of calcium in the animal body is found in ________

a) Blood b) Muscle

c) **Bone** d) Lymph

Q 66 Extra Calcium requirement in the laying hens is fulfilled by the following ________

a) **Medullar bone** b) Skin

c) Blood d) Diet

Q 67 Ca :P ratio in the bone is nearly ________

a) **2:1** b) 5:1

c) 1:1 d) 3:1

Q 68 Who discovered that earthy matter of bone was calcium phosphate?

a) Boussingalt
b) **Scheele and Gahn**
c) Sir Humphrey Davey
d) Mccay

Q 69 Which of the following has negative effect on calcium absorption in gut?

a) Lactose
b) Parathyroid
c) Vitamin D
d) **Calcitonin**

Q 70 The most prevalent mineral deficiency in grazing livestock across the world is of __________

a) Calcium
b) **Phosphorus**
c) Selenium
d) Sulphur

Q 71 Peg Leg Condition in grazing cattle is due to __________

a) **Calcium deficiency**
b) Phosphorus deficiency
c) Selenium deficiency
d) All the above

Q 72 The most abundant metal in the earth crust is __________

a) **Aluminium**
b) Iron
c) Magnesium
d) None of these

Q 73 The second most abundant metal in the earth crust is ________

a) Aluminium
b) **Iron**
c) Magnesium
d) None of these

Q 74 The third most abundant mineral in body is __________

a) Ca
b) P
c) **K**
d) Zn

Q 75 The highest concentration of zinc is found in __________

a) **Skin**
b) Brain
c) Lungs
d) None of these

Q 76 Which of the following increases the zinc absorption?

a) Copper
b) Phytate
c) Clay
d) **Casein**

Q 77 Which of the following is the function of zinc?

a) Stabilizing the quaternary structure of enzymes

b) Stabilizing the structure of DNA and RNA

c) Zinger finger formulation

d) Initiate apoptosis

e) **All the above**

Q 78 Which of the following state in relation to zinc is/are correct?

a) Zinc decline as plant mature

b) Bran is good source of zinc

c) Animal products, meat, seafood are rich source of zinc

d) **All the above are correct**

Q 79 Which of the following is the ore of zinc?

a) Sphalerite or blende b) Smithsonite

c) Calamine d) Franklinite

e) **All the above**

Q 80 Which of the following substances is also known as "Philosopher wool"

a) **ZnO** b) $ZnCO_3$

c) $ZnSO_4$ d) None of the above

Q 81 Which of the following is known as stainable iron of the tissue?

a) **Hemosiderin** b) Ferritin

c) Tranferrin d) None of these

Q 82 The highest iron concentration amongs the following organ/tissue occur in __________

a) **Liver** b) Kidney

c) Skeletal muscle d) Brain

Q 83 Which of the following is iron carrier in blood?

a) **Transferrin** b) Haemoglobin

c) Hemosiderin d) None of these

Q 84 Storage form of iron in body is ________

a) Ferritin b) Hemosiderin

c) **Both of the above** d) None of the above

Q 85 Which of the following iron containing compound is secreted by mammary gland and has reported to have antibiotic effect?

a) **Lactoferrin** b) Uteroferrin

c) Holotransferrin d) None of these

Q 86 Milk of which animal is low in iron ________

a) **Cow** b) Rat

c) Rabbit d) Kangroo

Q 87 Approximately how much iron a chicken egg contain?

a) **1 mg** b) 3 mg

c) 6 mg d) 9 mg

Q 88 The most common method to assess the iron status of the body is ________

a) **Measurement of haemoglobin**

b) Evaluation of bone marrow

c) Dietary analysis

d) Urinary analysis

Q 89 Which of the following statement in relation ot iron is not correct?

a) Gossypol,Phytic acid and Tannin decrease iron absorption

b) **Vitamic C inhibit iron absorption**

c) Histidine, Lysine, cysteine and iron absorption

d) High P, Zn, Cu interfere in iron absorption

Q 90 The laboured and spasmodic breathing (thumps) occur in piglet due to deficiency of ________

a) **Iron** b) Zinc

c) Copper d) Sodium

Q 91 Which of the following is correctly matched?

A	Milk	i)	Lactoferrin
B	Uterus	ii)	Uteroferrin
C	Egg Albumen	iii)	Ovo transferrin
D	Egg yolk	iv)	Phosphovitin

a) **A-i, B-ii, C-iii, D-iv** b) A-i, B-ii, C-iv, D-iii
c) A-iv, B-iii, C-ii, D-i d) A-I,B-iii, C-iv, D-ii

Q 92 Which of the following mineral is known as master mineral?
a) Ca b) **P**
c) Mg d) I

Q 93 Phosphorus is discovered by ________
a) **Hennig Brand** b) Tillman and Brethour
c) Wadsworth and Cohen d) None of these

Q 94 What percentage of phosphorus in body is found in bone and teeth?
a) 40% b) 60%
c) **80%** d) 20%

Q 95 % "Super juice" is used in some countries as a source of __________
a) **Phosphorus** b) Calcium
c) Vitamins d) Manganese

Q 96 How much phosphorus is secreted in cows saliva/day?
a) **30-60 gm** b) 10-20 gm
c) 90-150 gm d) No phosphorus in saliva

Q 97 How many minerals are involved directly in blood production?
a) **2** b) 4
c) 5 d) 6

Q 98 How many minerals are directly involved in vitamin formation?
a) **2** b) 4
c) 5 d) 6

Q 99 In Ruminants major route of phosphorus excretion is ________

a) **Faeces**
b) Urine
c) Sweat
d) Equally through urine and faeces route

Q 100 Deficiency of P in animals can lead to __________

a) Pica
b) Sarcophagia
c) Rupturing of achillus tendons
d) Haemoglobinurea
e) **All the above**

Q 101 Percentage of P in DCP is __________

a) 22-25%
b) **18-19%**
c) 10-15%
d) 30-35%

Q 102 Which of the following mineral is assumed to be culprit for eutrophication due to its indiscriminate use in animal agriculture?

a) **P**
b) F
c) N
d) S

Q 103 "Parturient paresis" is a metabolic disease occur due to deficiency of __________

a) **Ca**
b) P
c) Na
d) Se

Q 104 "Big head disease" in horse occur due to __________

a) Phosphorus deficiency
b) **Phosphorus excess**
c) Calcium excess
d) None of these

Q 105 Excessive feeding of P along with low calcium feeding in horse can lead to __________

a) Big head disease
b) Brain disease
c) Nutritional secondary hyperparathyroidism
d) **All the above**

Q 106 "Manchester wasting disease, enteque saco, and humpy back diseases are related with which mineral?

a) **Ca** b) K
c) Na d) Mg

Q 107 Brans are good source of __________

a) **P** b) Ca
c) Both of these d) None of these

Q 108 The most expensive item in cows ration is __________

a) **Energy** b) Fat
c) Vitamin d) Carbohydarte

Q 109 The most expensive nutrient in cows ration is __________

a) **Protein** b) Carbohydrate
c) Fat d) Vitamin

Q 110 The costliest mineral in mineral mixture is __________

a) Ca b) **P**
c) Fe d) S

Q 111 The most expensive mineral fed to cattle is __________

a) Ca b) Fe
c) **P** d) F

Q 112 "Pica" in dairy animals can occur due to deficiency of ______

a) Na b) P
c) Cl d) **All the above**

Q 113 Which of the following animal is salt (NaCl) sensitive and having less maximum tolerance level?

a) Cattle b) Swine
c) Sheep d) **Poultry**

Q 114 "Potash" is __________

a) **Potassium carbonate** b) Potassium chloride
c) Potassium sulphate d) All of these

Q 115 Which statement is wrong in context to potassium?
- a) Act as break in regulating heart beat
- b) **Ruminant have lesser K requirement than non-ruminant**
- c) Potassium deficiency decrease the feed intake
- d) Potassium maintain osmatic pressure

Q 116 Milk fever in cattle can occur if prepartum diet is __________
- a) **High in K**
- b) Low in Sodium
- c) High in Cl
- d) High in S

Q 117 Epsomite is ore of __________
- a) **Mg**
- b) Na
- c) Cl
- d) Mn

Q 118 The major absorption site for Magnesium in ruminant is _____
- a) **Reticulorumen**
- b) Small intestine
- c) Large intestine
- d) Abomasum

Q 119 Which of the following has antagonistic effect on magnesium absorption?
- a)` High Ca
- b) High P
- c) High K
- d) **All the above**

Q 120 Excessive use of NPK fertilizer in soil can decrease which mineral in the fodder
- a) **Mg**
- b) P
- c) Both a & b
- d) N

Q 121 "Stepping Syndrome" in Pig is caused by deficiency of ______
- a) Ca
- b) S
- c) Fe
- d) **Mg**

Q 122 Hypomagnesmia is dairy animal can lead to __________
- a) Grass staggers
- b) Lactation tetany
- c) Winter tetany
- d) **All the above**

Q 123 Grass tetany in ruminant animals occur due to deficiency of __________
- a) **Mg**
- b) Mn
- c) Ca
- d) P

Q 124 Which of the following statement is wrong in context to Mg?

a) **Rice bran is a poor source of Mg**

b) Mature animals are more susceptible for stagger than young ones

c) Egg shall contain more magnesium than its content

d) Mg is required for DNA & RNA synthesis

Q 125 Which trace mineral is present in highest amount in body?

a) **Fe** b) Zn

c) Mn d) I

Q 126 The major cation in sweat of ruminant is __________

a) **K** b) Na

c) Mg d) Ca

Q 127 How many atoms of sulphur are present per molecule of methionine?

a) **1** b) 2

c) 3 d) 4

Q 128 How many atoms of sulphur are present in Biotin?

a) **1** b) 2

c) 3 d) 4

Q 129 How many sulphur atoms are present in thiamine?

a) **1** b) 2

c) 3 d) 4

Q 130 In " cystine" how many atoms of sulphur are present?

a) 1 b) **2**

c) 3 d) 4

Q 131 Which of the following contain sulphur?

a) Insulin b) Oxytocin

c) **Both of these** d) None of these

Q 132 Cu-Mo-S interrelationship was first reported by __________

a) **Dick and Bull** b) Schwarz and Foltz

c) Underwood & Suttle d) McCollum

Q 133 S-Se interrelationship was first reported by ________

a) Dick and Bull
b) **Schwarz and Foltz**
c) Underwood & Suttle
d) McCollum

Q 134 Which of the following statement is wrong in context to sulphur?

a) Non ruminant can utilize sulphur from organic source only
b) Ruminant can utilize Sulphur from both inorganic and organic sources
c) **S is not present in heparin and lipoic acid**
d) N:S ratio in wool is 5:1

Q 135 High Dietary sulphur intake by ruminants can cause ________

a) Copper deficiency
b) Polioencephalomalacia
c) **Both a & b**
d) None of these

Q 136 Which mineral is in abundant in saline water?

a) **Sodium**
b) Potassium
c) Magnesium
d) Chlorine

Q 137 How many atom of Cobalt is present in Vitamin B_{12}?

a) **1**
b) 2
c) 3
d) 4

Q 138 Cobalt is a component of how many vitamins?

a) **1**
b) 2
c) 3
d) 4

Q 139 Cobalt is a component of which vitamin?

a) Vitamin B_1
b) Vitamin B_2
c) Vitamin B_6
d) **Vitamin B_{12}**

Q 140 Which animal is more susceptible for cobalt deficiency?

a) Cow
b) Pig
c) **Sheep**
d) None of these

Q 141 Which of the following is not a good source of vitamin B_{12}?

a) **Leafy things**
b) Meat
c) Fermentation residue
d) Egg

Q 142 'Xanthine oxidase' enzyme contain which mineral?

a) Mn b) Mg
c) Zn d) **Mo**

Q 143 Cobalt content in Vitamin B_{12} is ________

a) **4.5%** b) 1.0%
c) 7.5% d) 9.5%

Q 144 What percentage of absorbed Cobalt in ruminant is converted to Vitamin B_{12}?

a) 1% b) 2%
c) **3%** d) 7%

Q 145 Salt sick condition in ruminants can occur due to deficiency of?

a) Cu b) Co
c) Fe d) **All the above**

Q 146 The per cent cobalt in cobalt sulphate is ________

a) **21.3%** b) 46%
c) 70% d) 25.4%

Q 147 Which of the following element is present in highest amount in body?

a) **Oxygen** b) Carbon
c) Hydrogen d) Nitrogen

Q 148 Percentage of Ca and P in total body mineral is ________

a) **75%** b) 50%
c) 25% d) 95%

Q 149 Which of the following is a correct statement?

a) 99% of the calcium occur in bone
b) 85% of the total P occur in bone
c) 70 % of the total magnesium occur in bone
d) **All the above**

Q 150 Who discovered that iron was present in blood?

a) **Menghini** b) Brand
c) Duncan & Huffman d) McCollum

Q 151 Iodine was discovered by ________

a) Menghini
b) **B. Courtois**
c) McCollum
d) Brand

Q 152 Cobalt deficiency can cause ________

a) Bush sickness
b) Salt sick
c) Coast disease
d) Pinning disease
d) **All the above**

Q 153 Intrinsic factor required for the absorption of Vitamin B_{12} is secreted by ________

a) Small intestine
b) Large intestine
c) **Stomach**
d) None of the above

Q 154 White liver disease and phalaris staggers disease occur due to deficiency of which mineral?

a) **Co**
b) Cu
c) Cl
d) Cd

Q 155 Which of the following mineral is recycled to rumen via saliva as of N system?

a) S
b) P
c) Zn
d) Both a & b

Q 156 Who suggested the concept of N:S ratio?

a) **Loosli**
b) Funk
c) Steenbock
d) Moore

Q 157 Which mineral is present in high amount in lush green pasture which when fed to animal lead to hypomagnesmia?

a) **K**
b) Zn
c) Na
d) Cl

Q 158 How many vitamin contains Sulphur in their structure?

a) 1
b) **2**
c) 3
d) 4

Q 159 Which mineral is called as the "maternal mineral"?

a) P b) Se

c) **Mn** d) Cu

Q 160 Iodization of salt to prevent goiter was first suggested by _____

a) **Boussingault** b) Courtois

c) Proust D) Kendall

Q 161 Active form of Thyroxine hormone is __________

a) **Triiodothyronine** b) Tetraiodothyronine

c) Diiodotyrosine d) Monoidotyrosine

Q 162 The conversion of thyroxine to triiodothyroxine is catalysed by deiodinase enzyme. Which element is present in this enzyme?

a) **Se** b) Zn

c) Mn d) Fe

Q 163 Which of the following element is involved in thyroxine synthesis?

a) **Se** b) Ca

c) F d) Mn

Q 164 Iodine is stored in thyroid gland as __________

a) **Thyroglobulin** b) Thyroxine

c) Triiodothyroxine d) Mono idotyrosine

Q 165 The major route of iodine excretion is through __________

a) **Urine** b) Faeces

c) Sweat d) Equally in faeces & urine

Q 166 Which of the following substance is goitrogenic in nature?

a) Glucosinolate b) Hydrocyanic acid

c) Thiouracil d) **All the above**

Q 167 Which animal is more prone for iodine toxicity?

a) **Horse** b) Cattle

c) Poultry d) Pig

Q 168 Deficiency of which mineral leads to perosis in chick ________

a) **Mn** b) Mg
c) Zn d) F

Q 169 "Nutritional Chondrodystrophy" in chick occur due to deficiency of __________

a) **Mn** b) Mg
c) Zn d) F

Q 170 Wearing of tires on the road can contaminate the nearby soil with __________

a) **Zn** b) Mn
c) Mg d) Mo

Q 171 The active form of selenium in selenoenzymes is __________

a) **Selenocysteine** b) Seleno methionine
c) Selenite d) Selenate

Q 172 Who discovered the Selenium?

a) **J.J. Berzelius** b) Marco polo
c) Loosli d) Dick and Bull

Q 173 Which of the following is "selenate" state of selenium?

a) Se^{-2} b) Se^{0}
c) Se^{+4} d) **Se^{+6}**

Q 174 Mulberry heart disease or Nutritional microangiopathy in pig occur due to deficiency of __________

a) **Se** b) Mn
c) Mo d) Co

Q 175 "Selenide" state of selenium is represented by __________

a) **Se^{-2}** b) Se^{0}
c) Se^{+4} d) Se^{+6}

Q 176 "Hepatosis dietetica" in swine occur due to deficiency of _____

a) **Se** b) Co
c) Cu d) Zn

Q177 Selenium deficiency in poultry birds can lead to __________
a) Exudative diathesis
b) Nutritional muscular dystrophy
c) Nutritional pancreatic dystrophy
d) **All the above**

Q 178 "White Muscle disease" in cattle occur due to deficiency of __________
a) **Se** b) Cu
c) Co d) Zn

Q 179 "Flying scapula or shoulder lameness" condition in cattle occur due to deficiency of __________
a) **Se** b) Cu
c) P d) F

Q 180 Yellow discolouration of adipose tissue (yellow fat) condition in swine occur due to deficiency of __________
a) **Se** b) S
c) Zn d) Mn

Q 181 Alkali disease or blind staggers is related to toxicity of __________
a) **Selenium** b) Flourine
c) Lead d) Cadmium

Q 182 Match the correct answer __________
a) Peat scour i) Undivided India
b) Teart ii) New Zealand
c) Degnala disease iii) England
a) **a-ii,b-iii,c-i** b) a-i, b-ii-c-iii
c) a-iii, b-i, c-ii

Q183 Fluorine was discovered by __________
a) **Scheele** b) Ampere
c) Courtois d) Dean

Q 184 Urine is not the major route for the excretion of which element?
a) K b) Mg
c) **Fe** d) F

Q 185 Which of the following animals exhibits the greatest tolerance to fluorosis?

a) **Poultry** b) Swine
c) Horse d) Cattle

Q 186 Which of the following statement is wrong in context to fluorine?

a) **Ruminants are less susceptible to Fluorine toxicosis than non ruminants**
b) F-toxicosis can lead to mottling of teeth
c) F is beneficial element rather than essential
d) Excessive F interfere with Ca metabolism

Q 187 "Degnala disease" in bovine occur due to ________

a) Selenium deficiency b) **Selenium excess**
c) Se & Vitamin E deficiency d) Zn excess

Q 188 Quch-Quch disease in human occur due to toxicity of ______

a) Lead b) **Cadmium**
c) Arsenic d) Mercury

Q 189 Which of the following toxic mineral is used as growth promoters in poultry?

a) **Arsenic** b) Lead
c) Cadmium d) Mercury

Q 190 "Drunken Hog syndrome" in swine occur due to toxicosis of ________

a) **Arsenic** b) Lead
c) Cadmium d) Mercury

Q 191 Which of the following animals is most susceptible for lead poisoning?

a) **Cattle** b) Horse
c) Pig d) Dog

Q 192 "Saturinism" is the toxicity of ________

a) **Pb** b) Hg
c) Cd d) As

Q 193 "Plumbism" is the toxicity of ________

a) **Pb**
b) Hg
c) Cd
d) As

Q 194 Which of the following toxic mineral is least transferred across the placenta?

a) Arsenic
b) Lead
c) **Cadmium**
d) Mercury

Q 195 Which animal among the following is least susceptible for lead poisoning?

a) Cattle
b) Poultry
c) Horse
d) **Pig**

Q 196 "Hydragyria" is the toxicity of ________

a) Arsenic
b) Lead
c) Cadmium
d) **Mercury**

Q 197 "Degcure" mixture used for the treatment of degnella disease is a ________

a) **Penta sulphate mineral mixture**
b) Tetra sulphate mineral mixture
c) Hexa sulphate mineral mixture
d) Tri sulphate mineral mixture

Q 198 Cigarette smoke is a source of which toxic element ________

a) **Cadmium**
b) Arsenic
c) Lead
d) Mercury

Q 199 In the process of DCP making,Rock phosphate is treated with which acid to form phosphoric acid?

a) **Sulphuric acid**
b) Nitric acid
c) Hydrochloric acid
d) Acetic acid

Q 200 Which acid is generally used for demineralization of bone for making DCP?

a) Sulphuric acid
b) Nitric acid
c) **Hydrochloric acid**
d) Acetic acid

Q 201 Which of the following statement is wrong in context to Dicalcium Phosphate (DCP)?

a) It is also known as Calcium Monohydrogen phosphate

b) **It has two calcium molecules**

c) It contains about 22% calcium

d) It can be prepared from bone or inorganic material

Q 202 "Mucosal block theory" of iron absorption was advocated by __________

a) **Hahn and coworkers**

b) McCance and Widdowson

c) Sydenham & Willis

d) Fischer & Zeile

Q 203 Higher amount of iron is present in which of the following compound?

a) Haemoglobulin b) **Hemosiderin**

c) Ferritin d) Apoferritin

Q 204 Which of the following is insoluble form of storage iron?

a) **Hemosiderin** b) Ferritin

c) Both of the above d) None of the above

Q 205 "Bunny Hopping", Pacing Gait and Pigeon Toed conditions in ruminants occur due to the deficiency of __________

a) Ca b) **Cu**

c) Na d) Mn

Q 206 Percentage of phosphorus in tri calcium phosphate* $(Ca_3(PO_4)_2$ is __________

a) 10 % b) **20%**

c) 30 % d) 40%

* 3x40+2x31+2x4x16=120+62+128+310, 62/310 x100=20%

Q 207 Ratio of Ca:P in the tri calcium phosphate is __________

a) 3:2.02 b) **2:1.03**

c) 2:3.02 d) 1:2.03

Q 208 The molecular formula for the amino acid lysine is $C_6H_{14}N_2O_2$. What is the percentage of amino acid?

a) 16.18% b) 17.18%
c) 18.18% d) **19.18%**

Q 209 The most abundant mineral in wool is __________

a) **Sulphur** b) Phosphorus
c) Sodium d) Potassium

Q 210 About how much percentage of Sulphur is present in wool __________

a) 1% b) 2%
c) 3% d) **4%**

Q 211 The atomic weight of Sulphur(S) is __________

a) **32** b) 24
c) 23 d) 56

Q 212 The atomic weight of Calcium (Ca) is __________

a) 32 b) **40**
c) 23 d) 56

Q 213 The atomic weight of Magnesium (Mg) is __________

a) **24** b) 32
c) 40 d) 56

Q 214 The atomic weight of Phosphorus (P) is __________

a) 24 b) **31**
c) 40 d) 32

Q 215 Percentage of salt usually included in a ruminant ration is _____

a) **1** b) 2
c) 3 d) 4

Q 216 Percentage of salt usually included in a poultry ration is ______

a) **0.5-0.6** b) 2.5-3.5
c) 3.5-4.5 d) 4.5-5.5

Q 217 Percentage of salt usually included in a swine ration is ______

a) **0.5** b) 1
c) 2 d) 3

Q 218 High feeding of which of the following mineral is sometimes used to induced moulting in layer?

a) Ca b) Na

c) **Zn** d) P

Q 219 Which of the following mineral feeding starategies can be helpful to induce moulting in layer?

a) Low Ca diet b) Low Na Diet

c) High Zn diet d) **All the above**

Q 220 For hydrogenation of vegetable and fish oil in the manufacturing of margarine, which of the following is used as catalyst?

a) **Nickel** b) Iron

c) Copper d) Sulphur

Q 221 An average 57gm egg contain how much ash?

a) 15.7 gm b) 2.1 gm

c) **6.1 gm** d) 17.4 gm

Q 222 "Scabby hip syndrome" in chicken occur due to deficiency of __________

a) Na b) **Mo**

c) Cu d) Zn

Q 223 Ideal DCAD (milliequivalent/100 gm ration DM) in the last three weeks of pregnancy should be __________

a) **-10 to -15** b) -10 to 0

c) 0 to 10 d) 10 to 15

Q 224 Beside high calcium intake during prepartum, what should be other possible reason for hypocalcemia?

a) Low Na in diet b) High Na in diet

c) **High K in diet** d) Low K in diet

Q 225 Normal Blood calcium in a dairy cow (mg/100ml) is ________

a) 6-8 b) **9-11**

c) 3.5 d) 0-2

Q 226 For how long, should anionic salt be fed for before calving?

a) **Minimum of 10 days**
b) Maximum of 2 weeks
c) At least 21 days
d) Not more than 5 days

Q 227 Which macro-minerals are used for DCAD calculation?

a) Na,Ca,P and S
b) **Na,K,Cl and S**
c) Ca,K,Cl and P
d) Ca,K,Cl and P

Q 228 Which of the following salt can be used to lower the DCAD of a diet?

a) NaCl
b) KCl
c) **NH_4Cl**
d) All the above

Q 229 Wilson disease in human being is due to faulty metabolism of which mineral?

a) **Cu**
b) Ca
c) Zn
d) Se

Q 230 Dental caries can occur due to deficiency of ________

a) **F**
b) Ca
c) Mg
d) Cl

Q 231 To prevent dental caries, which mineral is added to tooth paste?

a) Ca
b) **F**
c) Cl
d) Na

Q232 The birth of hairless or dead piglets occur due to deficiency of ___________

a) **I**
b) F
c) S
d) Mn

Q 233 Goiter can occur due to ________

a) Deficiency if Iodine
b) Excess of iodine
c) **Both deficiency and excess of iodine**
d) Salt deficiency

Q 234 Which of the following animal is prone to iodine toxicity?

a) Cattle
b) Swine
c) Poultry
d) **Horse**

Q 235 A condition of " Parrot mouth" is horse can occur due to excess of ___________

a) **I** b) F

c) Ca d) Cu

Q 236 Which of the following species can tolerate the higher F level (About 200 ppm)?

a) Cattle b) Horse

c) Sheep d) **Chicken**

Q 237 The maximum tolerable level (MTL) for calcium in dairy animal as per latest NRC ___________

a) **1.5%** b) 3.0%

c) 4.0% d) 5.5 %

Q 238 The maximum tolerable level for P in dairy animal is ________

a) 1.0% b) **0.7%**

c) 1.5 % d) 2.0 %

Q 239 Maximum tolerable level for salt in dairy animal is ___________

a) 2% b) **3%**

c) 5% d) 8%

Q 240 Maximum tolerable level for zinc in dairy animal is ___________

a) 5 ppm b) 50 ppm

c) **500 ppm** d) 5000 ppm

Q 241 Maximum tolerable level for selenium in dairy animal is _____

a) 50 ppm b) **5 ppm**

c) 500 ppm d) 70 ppm

Q 242 Which of the following mineral functions in the maintaining of osmotic pressure, acid base balance and body fluid balance?

a) **Na** b) Se

c) S d) Zn

Q 243 Mineral necessary for hemoglobin formation is ___________

a) Zn b) **Cu**

c) Se d) I

Q 244 Ideal DCAD (milliequivalent/100gm of ration DM) in the last three weeks of lactation should be ________

a) **-10 to -15**
b) -10 to 0
c) 0 to 10
d) 10 to 15

Q 245 Which macrominerals are used for DCAD calculations?

a) Na, Ca, P & S
b) **Na, K, Cl & S**
c) Ca, K,Cl & P
d) Ca, K, Cl & S

Q 246 There is evidence that cow fed anionic salt pre-partum ______

a) Have less subclinical hypoglycemia
b) Have lower incidence of retained placenta
c) Produce more milk
d) **All the above**

Q 247 What is expected urinary pH when DCAD is about 50 meq/ 100 g DM?

a) Less than 5.0
b) Between 5.0 and 6.0
c) Between 6.0 and 7.5
d) **Between 7.5 and 8.5**

Q 248 For how long should anionic salt be fed before calving?

a) **Minimum of 10 days**
b) Maximum of 2 weeks
c) At least 21 days
d) Not More than 5 days

Q 249 Which of the following condition in animal is related with subclinical hypocalcemia and milk fever?

a) Low Na in diet
b) High Na in diet
c) **High K in diet**
d) Low K in diet

Q 250 Which of the following salts can be used to lower the DCAD of the diet?

a) NaCl
b) KCl
c) NH_4Cl
d) $(NH_4)_2SO_4$
e) **All the above**

Q 251 Which is the optimum range of urine pH that indicates good effectiveness of anionic salt in reducing risk of milk fever?

a) Urinary pH less than 5.0
b) **Urinary pH 6.0 to 6.5**
c) Urinary pH 6.5 to 8.0
d) Urinary pH 8 to 10

Q 252 Milk fever occur in dairy cow, when blood calcium is ________

a) 8-9 mg/100 ml
b) 9-11 mg/100 ml
c) **5-7 mg/100 ml**
d) 0.5 to 1.0 mg/100 ml

Q 253 High potassium intake will decrease a cows ability to mobilize what?

a) Bone phosphorus
b) Lymphocytes
c) **Bone calcium**
d) Immunoglobulins

Q 254 99% calcium is present in the __________ and 1% of the total body calcium is present in the __________ & __________

a) Bone, teeth and liver
b) **Bone, blood and tissue**
c) Blood, bone & tissue
d) Blood, teeth and tissue

Q 255 As per standard classification, how many macro minerals are there?

a) 5
b) **7**
c) 8
d) 10

Q 256 Out of total iodine found in the body, majority of it is found in __________

a) Brain
b) Liver
c) Kidney
d) **Thyroid**

Q 257 Micro elements which can cause toxicity are

a) **Mo, Se and F**
b) Mg, Se and F
c) S, Se and Mo
d) Fe, Mo and Se

Interesting Knowledge

- Manganese is considered as "Maternal Mineral" because Mn deficiency in female cause a reduced maternal caring for her young.
- Excessive Cu & Fe = Decrease Mn
- Excessive Mn = Deplete Fe and Cu
- Tea is a good source of Mn and also contain appreciable amount of K
- Coffee is better source of K than tea and has appreciable amount of Mg and Mn.

❑❑❑

Chapter 9

Vitamins

Q 1 Which of the following is known as "Sunshine vitamin"?

a) Vitamin A b) **Vitamin D**

c) Vitamin E d) Vitamin K

Q 2 Which of the following is known as "antirachitic vitamin"?

a) Vitamin A b) **Vitamin D**

c) Vitamin E d) Vitamin K

Q 3 Crazy chick disease (encephalomalacia) occur due to deficiency of __________

a) **Vitamin E** b) Vitamin B2

c) Vitamin C d) Vitamin A

Q 4 Polyneuritis in birds occur due to deficiency of __________

a) **Thiamine** b) Riboflavin

c) Niacin d) Choline

Q 5 Curled toe paralysis in birds occur due to deficiency of _______

a) Thiamine b) **Riboflavin**

c) Niacin d) Choline

Q 6 Black tongue in poultry birds occur due to deficiency of ______

a) Thiamine b) Riboflavin

c) **Niacin** d) Choline

Q 7 Club down condition in chicks occur due to deficiency of ____

a) Thiamine b) **Riboflavin**

c) Niacin d) Choline

Q 8 Vitamin H is synonymous for __________

a) **Biotin**
b) Pantothenic acid
c) Choline
d) Thiamine

Q 9 Which of the following vitamin is synthesized in poultry?

a) **Vit C**
b) Folic acid
c) Choline
d) Thiamine

Q 10 Vitamin B_1 is also known as __________

a) Thiamine
b) Thiamine
c) Aneurine
d) **All the above**

Q 11 The oldest vitamin is __________

a) **Thiamine**
b) Cobalamin
c) Vitamin B_6
d) Vitamin E

Q 12 Continuous feeding of boiled polished rice to chick can lead to deficiency of __________

a) **Vitamin B_1**
b) Vitamin B_6
c) Vitamin B_{12}
d) Vitamin B_2

Q 13 The term Vitamin (e) was coined by __________

a) **Funk**
b) Eijkman
c) Loosli
d) Grijns

Q 14 Which of the following vitamin has sulphurous odour?

a) **Thiamin**
b) Riboflavin
c) Cyanocobalamin
d) Niaicn

Q 15 The sulphur containing vitamin is __________

a) **Vitamin B_1**
b) Vitamin B_6
c) Vitamin B_{12}
d) Vitamin B_2

Q 16 Excessive feeding of amprolium salt (Coccidiostat) in poultry can lead to deficiency of __________

a) **Vitamin B_1**
b) Vitamin A
c) Vitamin B_{12}
d) Vitamin D

Q 17 Excessive feeding of raw fish to carnivorous animal can lead to deficiency of __________

a) **Vitamin B_1**
b) Vitamin B_6
c) Vitamin B_{12}
d) Vitamin B_2

Q 18 Majority of thiamine of the body is present in which form?

a) **Thiamine pyrophosphate**
b) Thiamine triphosphate
c) Thiamine monophosphate
d) Free thiamine

Q 19 The richest known natural source of thiamine is __________

a) Corn germ meal
b) **Brewer's grain**
c) Rice bran
d) Egg

Q 20 Thiamine deficiency in poultry leads to __________

a) **Polyneuritis**
b) Curled toe paralysis
c) Perosis
d) All the above

Q 21 Thiamine deficiency in ruminants leads to __________

a) **Polioencephalomalacia**
b) Rickets
c) Osteoporosis
d) Pellegra

Q 22 "Chastek paralysis" in foxes occur due to deficiency of _______

a) **Vitamin B_1**
b) Vitamin B_2
c) Choline
d) Vitamin B_6

Q 23 " Star gazing posture" in chicks occur due to deficiency of ___

a) **Thiamine**
b) Niacin
c) Choline
d) Riboflavin

Q 24 Which of the following animal was responsible for the discovery of thiamine?

a) **Chicken**
b) Pig
c) Rabbit
d) Cattle

Q 25 "Secadera" a wasting disease of ruminants occur due to deficiency of __________

a) **Vitamin B_1**
b) Vitamin B_6
c) Vitamin B_{12}
d) Vitamin B_2

Q 26 Which vitamin was earlier known as Vitamin F?

a) **B_1**
b) B_2
c) Niacin
d) B_{12}

Q 27 The term "Flavin" was coined by ________

a) Funk
b) **Kuhn**
c) Karrers
d) Warburg

Q 28 Riboflavin in feed occur as ________

a) FAD
b) FMN
c) Free riboflavin
d) **All the above**

Q 29 Deficiency of riboflavin in poultry birds causes ________

a) **Curled toe paralysis**
b) Polyneuritis
c) Perosis
d) All the above

Q 30 Vitamin G is synonymous for ________

a) Thiamine
b) **Riboflavin**
c) Niacin
d) Pantothenic acid

Q 31 Riboflavin is known as Vitamin ________

a) B_1
b) **B_2**
c) B_6
d) B_{12}

Q 32 The precursor of niacin is ________

a) **Tryptophan**
b) Arginine
c) Methionine
d) Lysine

Q 33 Which of the following animal lack the ability to convert tryptophan to niacin?

a) Cattle
b) Rat
c) **Cat**
d) Poultry

Q 34 Niacin deficiency in poultry birds leads to ________

a) **Black tongue**
b) Black leg
c) Curled toe paralysis
d) None of the above

Q 35 Which of the following animal has highest requirement of niacin?

a) Pig b) Chick
c) **Duck** d) Calf

Q 36 "Pellagra" in human being occur due to deficiency of _______

a) **Niacin** b) Pyridoxin
c) Folic acid d) Choline

Q 37 Niaicn is also known as __________

a) Vitamin B_3 b) Nicotinic acid
c) Vitamin PP d) **All the above**

Q 38 3M's (Meal, meat, molasses) and 4 D's (dermatitis, diarrohea, dementia and death) concept is related with vitamin _______

a) **Niacin** b) Thiamin
c) Riboflavin d) Pyridoxin

Q 39 Which statement about niacin is wrong?

a) Its deficiency causes black tongue in poultry.
b) Tea and coffee are good source of niacin
c) Tryptophan is precursor of niacin
d) **It promote lipid mobilization**

Q 40 Vitamin B_6 occur in how many forms __________

a) 3 b) 4
c) **5** d) 2

Q 41 The name "pyridoxine" for vitamin B_6 was proposed (coined) by __________

a) **Szent-Gyorgy** b) Eijkman
c) Funk d) Goldberger & Lillie

Q 42 Vitamin B_6 is also known as __________

a) **Pyridoxine** b) Niacin
c) Biotin d) Pantothenic acid

Q 43 Which of the following is also known as "Code Carboxylase"?
a) Pyridoxal b) Pyridoxamine
c) **Pyridoxal phosphate** d) Pyridoxamine phosphate

Q 44 Commercial preparation of vitamin B_6 contain which of the following?
a) **Pyridoxine hydrochloride** b) Pyridoxal phosphate
c) Pyridoxamine phosphate d) Pyridoxal

Q 45 Which vitamin is required for amino acid transport/ metabolism?
a) **B_6** b) B_5
c) B_7 d) B_9

Q 46 Which vitamin is involved in conversion of tryptophan to niacin?
a) **Pyridoxine** b) Pantothenic acid
c) Biotin d) Folic acid

Q 47 Pantothenic acid is synonymous with ________
a) Vitamin B_5 b) Filtrate factor
c) Chick antidermatitis factor d) Eluate factor
e) **All the above**

Q 48 Which if the following is vitamin B_5?
a) **Pantothenic acid** b) Pyridoxine
c) Biotin d) Niacin

Q 49 Which vitamin is also known as "Anti-grey hair factors"?
a) **Pantothenic acid** b) Pyridoxine
c) Biotin d) Niacin

Q 50 Pantothenic acid is a component of ________
a) Coenzyme A b) Acyl carrier protein
c) **Both of the above** d) +None of the above

Q 51 The richest source of Vitamin B_6 and pantothenic acid ________
a) **Royal jelly of bees** b) Clover hay
c) Blood meal d) Polished rice

Q 52 Goose stepping in pigs occur due to deficiency of __________

a) **Pantothenic acid** b) Niacin
c) Biotin d) Pyridoxine

Q 53 A pig having scurfy skin, brownish secretion around eye and sit in a posture of a sitting dog indicate the deficiency of __________

a) Niacin b) **Pantothenic acid**
c) Biotin d) Folic acid

Q 54 Burning feet syndrome in human being occur due to deficiency of __________

a) Vitamin E b) Vitamin B_1
c) Vitamin B_2 d) **Vitamin B_5**

Q 55 The word "Biotin" was coined by __________

a) **Kogl & Tonnis** b) Minot & Murphy
c) Funk d) Eijkman

Q 56 Biotin is also known as __________

a) Vitamin B_2 b) Vitamin B_5
c) **Vitamin B_7** d) Vitamin B_9

Q 57 Which of the following is known as vitamin H?

a) **Biotin** b) Pantothenic acid
c) Folic acid d) Niacin

Q 58 Biotin is synonymous with __________

a) Vitamin H b) Coenzyme R
c) Vitamin B_W d) **All the above**

Q 59 Sulphur containing vitamin is __________

a) Thiamine b) Biotin
c) **Both of the above** d) Niacin

Q 60 Vitamin required for transfer of carbon dioxide from one substance to another is __________

a) Thiamine b) **Biotin**
c) Folic acid d) Riboflavin

Q 61 Continuous feeding of raw egg can lead to deficiency of _____

a) **Biotin** b) Riboflavin

c) Pantothenic acid d) Ascorbic acid

Q 62 Egg white injury occur due to deficiency of _________

a) **Biotin** b) Riboflavin

c) Niacin d) All the above

Q 63 Biotin antagonist present in raw egg is _________

a) **Avidin** b) Oxybiotin

c) Desthiobiotin d) All the above

Q 64 Which of the following statement regarding biotin is wrong?

a) Grain are poor source of biotin

b) Its deficiency causes perosis in poultry

c) It is required for hoof health

d) **It is the cheapest vitamin**

Q 65 The most expensive vitamin in B-complex series is _________

a) **Biotin** b) Riboflavin

c) Niacin d) Pyridoxine

Q 66 Scaly dermatitis occur due to deficiency of _________

a) **Biotin** b) Thiamine

c) Folic acid d) Niacin

Q 67 Fatty Liver and Kidney Syndrome in chick occur due to deficiency of _________

a) Thiamine b) **Biotin**

c) Folacin d) Riboflavin

Q 68 Pteroylglutamic acid is the chemical name of which vitamin?

a) Nicotinic acid b) **Folic acid**

c) Biotin d) Pantothenic acid

Q 69 Vitamin B_9 is synonymous with _________

a) **Folic acid** b) Niaicn

c) Biotin d) Choline

Q 70 Folic acid is known as _________

a) Vitamin M
b) Vitamin Bc
c) Factor U
d) **All the above**

Q 71 *Lactobacillus casei factor* is now known as _________

a) Nicotinic acid
b) Cyanocobalamin
c) **Folic acid**
d) Choline

Q 72 Which vitamin has PABA in its structure?

a) **Folic acid**
b) Cyanocobalamin
c) Niacin
d) Riboflavin

Q 73 Which of the following vitamin has more biological active form than any other vitamin?

a) Thiamine
b) Riboflavin
c) **Folic acid**
d) Ascorbic acid

Q 74 Which vitamin consist of combination of glutamic acid and pteroic acid?

a) **Folic acid**
b) Riboflavin
c) Cyanocobalamin
d) Niaicn

Q 75 Deficiency of which vitamin can lead to functional folacin deficiency even when folacin intake and absorption are normal?

a) Thiamine
b) Riboflavin
c) Niaicn
d) **Cyanocobalamin**

Q 76 Which of the following vitamin is required for purine and pyrimidine synthesis?

a) Niacin
b) **Folic acid**
c) Biotin
d) None of these

Q 77 Which of the following animal is more susceptible for folic acid deficiency?

a) Cow
b) Swine
c) Horse
d) **Poultry birds**

Q 78 Deficiency of which vitamin leads to megaloblastic anemia?

a) Folic acid b) Vitamin B_{12}

c) **Both of the above** d) None of the above

Q 79 For human being,the most common vitamin deficiency in the world is of ________

a) Vitamin C b) Vitamin B_1

c) **Vitamin B_9** d) Vitamin D

Q 80 Urinary excretion of FIGLU (formimino glutamic acid) can be measured to assess the status of which vitamin ________

a) **Folic acid** b) Pantothenic acid

c) Nicotinic acid d) Ascorbic acid

Q 81 Coenzyme A contain which vitamin?

a) Folic acid b) Thiamine

c) **Pantothenic acid** d) Riboflavin

Q 82 Last vitamin discovered was ________

a) Folic acid b) Vitamin E

c) Vitamin C d) **Vitamin B_{12}**

Q 83 Which vitamin is only synthesized by microorganism?

a) Vitamin B_1 b) Folic acid

c) Choline d) **Vitamin B_{12}**

Q 84 Which of the following vitamin usually not found in the plant feedstuff?

a) B_1 b) B_5

c) B_6 d) **B_{12}**

Q 85 Cobalt is an integral part of which vitamin?

a) B_1 b) Choline

c) B_6 d) **B_{12}**

Q 86 Vitamin B_{12} is also known as ________

a) Cyanocobalamin b) Animal protein factor

c) Chick growth factor d) **All the above**

Q 87 Among all the vitamin, which has the most complex structure?

a) Vitamin A
b) Vitamin C
c) **Vitamin B_{12}**
d) Vitamin D

Q 88 Which vitamin has cyanide (-CN) in it?

a) **Vitamin B_{12}**
b) Vitamin A
c) Vitamin B_5
d) Vitamin D

Q 89 An intrinsic factor is required for the absorption of which vitamin?

a) B_5
b) B_6
c) B_7
d) **B_{12}**

Q 90 Intrinsic factor required for the absorption of vitamin B_{12} is secreted by __________

a) **Gastric mucosa**
b) Pancreatic cell
c) Intestinal mucosa
d) Gall bladder

Q 91 The percentage of cobalt in vitamin B_{12} structure is ________

a) **4.5%**
b) 6.5%
c) 8.5%
d) 1.0%

Q 92 How much percentage of ingested cobalt is converted into Vitamin B_{12} in the rumen?

a) 15
b) **3**
c) 9
d) 10

Q 93 Deficiency of which vitamin lead to pernicious anemia ______

a) **B_{12}**
b) Folic acid
c) Ascorbic acid
d) All the above

Q 94 Which vitamin has a "corrin nucleus" in its structure?

a) B_2
b) B_5
c) B_6
d) **B_{12}**

Q 95 Which vitamin involved in the synthesis of DNA?

a) Folic acid
b) B_{12}
c) **Both of the above**
d) None of the above

Q 96 "Squat test" in human being is used to assess the deficiency of which vitamin?

a) **B_1** b) B_2

c) B_5 d) B_6

Q 97 Methyl malonyl CoA isomerase (mutase) – an enzyme required for conversion of propionate to succinate need which vitamin for its functioning?

a) B_1 b) B_2

c) B_5 d) **B_{12}**

Q 98 Oxidation of biotin converts it into __________

a) **Sulfone** b) Oxybiotin

c) Desthiobiotin d) None of the above

Q 99 Which of the following vitamin is red in colour?

a) Folic acid b) **B_{12}**

c) Pyridoxine d) Choline

Q 100 Which of the following vitamin can be synthesized in the liver?

a) **Choline** b) Riboflavin

c) Thiamine d) All the above

Q 101 Which vitamin is an integral part of lecithin?

a) **Choline** b) Biotin

c) Niaicn d) None of the above

Q 102 Which vitamin is known as " lipotrophic factor"?

a) Biotin b) Thiamine

c) Vitamin E d) **Choline**

Q 103 Which vitamin prevents fatty liver formation?

a) **Choline** b) Vitamin A

c) Niaicn d) Cyanocobalamin

Q 104 "Spraddled leg condition" in swine can occur due to deficiency of __________

a) Biotin b) Thiamine

c) **Choline** d) Niaicn

Q 105 "Scurvy" occur due to deficiency of __________

a) Choline
b) **Ascorbic acid**
c) Niaicn
d) Biotin

Q 106 Vitamin C occur in how many forms?

a) One
b) **Two**
c) Three
d) Four

Q 107 The least stable vitamin is __________

a) **C**
b) B_{12}
c) A
d) D

Q 108 Which vitamin involves in the synthesis of collagen?

a) Vitamin B_{12}
b) **Vitamin C**
c) Vitamin D
d) Vitamin E

Q 109 Which vitamin enhance the absorption of iron?

a) Vitamin A
b) Vitamin B_1
c) **Vitamin C**
d) Vitamin K

Q 110 Which animal can synthesize ascorbic acid?

a) Ruminants
b) Swine
c) Poultry
d) **All the above**

Q 111 Deficiency of vitamin C can lead to __________

a) Bleeding gum syndrome
b) Naval bleeding syndrome
c) High retained placenta incidence
d) **All the above**

Q 112 Which of the following vitamin is not found in plant feedstuffs?

a) Vitamin A
b) Vitamin D
c) **Vitamin B_{12}**
d) Vitamin C

Q 113 The most important vitamin from practical stand point is __________

a) **Vitamin A**
b) Vitamin D
c) Vitamin C
d) Vitamin K

Q 114 Which of the following has the highest Vitamin A activity?

a) α - Carotene
b) **β - Carotene**
c) g - Carotene
d) Cryptoxanthin

Q 115 Theoretically, hydrolysis of one molecule of β - Carotene yield how many molecule of Vitamin A (retinol)?

a) One
b) **Two**
c) Three
d) Four

Q 116 Which of the following animal is unable to convert carotene to vitamin A?

a) **Cat**
b) Pig
c) Goat
d) Buffalo

Q 117 The major storage organ for vitamin A is __________

a) **Liver**
b) Kidney
c) Lungs
d) Blood

Q 118 Major storage form of vitamin A is __________

a) Carotene
b) **Retinyl ester**
c) Retinoic acid
d) Retinol

Q 119 Which form of vitamin A is not involved in Vision Cycle?

a) Retinol
b) **Retinoic acid**
c) Retinol
d) All involved

Q 120 Xerophthalmia occur due to deficiency of __________

a) Vitamin C
b) Vitamin D
c) **Vitamin A**
d) Vitamin K

Q 121 Which of the following form is unable to fulfill the function of vitamin A in reproduction?

a) Retinol
b) **Retinoic acid**
c) Retinol
d) Both b & c

Q 122 Which animal is more efficient in conversion of carotene to vitamin A?

a) Cattle
b) Horse
c) Pig
d) **Poultry birds**

Q 123 Which vitamin is known as " Anti-infective vitamin"?

a) **Vitamin A** b) Vitamin D
c) Vitamin C d) Vitamin E

Q 124 "Pink eye condition" in ruminant occur due to deficiency of __________

a) Vitamin B_1 b) Vitamin E
c) **Vitamin A** d) Folic acid

Q 125 Bitot's Spot in conjunctiva occur due to deficiency of __________

a) **Vitamin A** b) Vitamin E
c) Vitamin K d) Vitamin B_9

Q 126 Nyctalopia condition can occur due to deficiency of __________

a) Vitamin B_1 b) **Vitamin A**
c) Vitamin E d) Vitamin C

Q 127 Which statement in relation to vitamin A is wrong?

a) **Vitamin A is present in plant or green food**
b) It is required for vision.
c) Maintain integrity of epithelial cell
d) Required for reproduction

* It is carotene -precursor of vitamin A which is present in plants/green food.

Q 128 "Carotene was precursor to vitamin A" was first reported by __________

a) Morton b) **Moore**
c) Wackenroder d) Steenbock

Q 129 Sunshine Vitamin is __________

a) A b) C
c) **D** d) E

Q 130 Which of the following is known as vitamin D_3?

a) Ergosterol b) Ergocalciferol
c) 7-dehydrocholesterol d) **Cholecalciferol**

Q 131 Vitamin D_2 is synonymous with __________

a) Ergosterol b) **Ergocalciferol**

c) 7-dehydrocholesterol d) Cholecalciferol

Q 132 Cholecalciferol is produced __________

a) Exclusively from plants

b) **Exclusively from animal products**

c) Can be from plants & animals products

e) None of these

Q 133 The major circulating form of vitamin D is __________

a) Cholecalciferol

b) Ergocalciferol

c) **25-hydroxy Vitamin D_3**

d) 1,25 dihydroxy Vitamin D_3

Q 134 Conversion of vitamin D_3 to 25 hydroxy D_3 predominately occur __________

a) **Microsomes** b) Mitochondria

c) Ribosome d) None of these

Q 135 Conversion of Vitamin D_3 to 25 hydroxy D_3 predominately occur in which organ?

a) Lung b) **Liver**

c) Kidney d) Spleen

Q 136 Conversion of 25 OHD_3 to 1,25 $(OH)_2D_3$ occurs in __________

a) Liver b) **Kidney**

c) Spleen d) Lung

Q 137 Which of the following form of vitamin D has hormonal role?

a) Cholecalciferol b) 25, OH D_3

c) **1,25 $(OH)_2D_3$** d) None of these

Q 138 The principal storage of Vitamin D occurs in __________

a) Lungs b) Kidney

c) Liver d) **Blood***

* Blood has higher concentration than other tissue

Q 139 Which statement pertaining to vitamin D is incorrect?

a) Sunlight through glass window is ineffective in producing vitamin D

b) **Sunlight is more potent in temperate than tropic in producing vitamin D**

c) Antirachitic power of sunlight is more potent during summer than winter.

d) Sunlight is more potent at high altitude

Q 140 Which of the following disease is known as first air pollution disease?

a) **Ricket** b) Silo Filler disease

c) Farmer lung disease d) None of these

Q 141 Which vitamin is also called as antirachitic vitamin/factor?

a) A b) **D**

c) E d) C

Q 142 In poultry, term "International chick unit" is use for which vitamin?

a) A b) **D**

c) B_1 d) B_2

Q 143 "Rachitic Rosary" condition occur die to deficiency of ______

a) Vitamin A b) Vitamin C

c) **Vitamin D** d) Vitamin E

Q 144 The rich source of vitamin D is ________

a) Green fodder b) Egg

c) Milk d) **Fish oil**

Q 145 Beading of ribs in chick occur due to deficiency of vitamin ________

a) A b) C

c) **D** d) K

Q 146 "Penguin Like Squat" -a characteristic posture in poultry birds occur due to deficiency of ________

a) **Vitamin D** b) Vitamin A

c) Vitamin E d) Vitamin C

Q 147 In which animal vitamin D_3 has more potency than D_2?

a) Cattle b) Sheep

c) Pig d) **Poultry**

Q 148 "Entequesaco"- calcinosis of soft tissue occur due to ________

a) Deficiency of vitamin D b) **Toxicity of vitamin D**

c) Deficiency of vitamin A b) Both a and c

Q 149 "Humy-back" condition occur due to __________

a) Toxicity of vitamin A b) **Toxicity of Vitamin D**

c) Toxiicty of Vitamin E d) None of these

Q 150 Vitamin E was discovered by __________

a) **Evans & Bishop** b) Scott

c) Ullrey d) None of these

Q 151 The saying "A vitamin looking for a disease" was earlier used for which vitamin?

a) A b) D

c) **E** d) B_1

Q 152 In nature, vitamin E exist in how many forms?

a) 5 b) **8**

c) 10 d) 12

Q 153 Which vitamin function as chain breaking antioxidant

a) A b) C

c) **E** d) All the above

Q 154 Tick the wrong statement regarding vitamin E __________

a) It acts as biological antioxidant

b) **It stimulates platelet aggregation**

c) It is effective in lead toxicity

d) It works in tandem with selenium

Q 155 In silver and arsenic toxicity, which of the following has protective role?

a) Only selenium is effective

b) **Vitamin E along with high dose of selenium is highly effective**

c) Only vitamin E is effective

d) None of these

Q 156 The first line of defence against peroxidation of vital phospholipid in cellular and subcellular membranes is _______

a) Vitamin A
b) Vitamin C
c) **Vitamin E**
d) Vitamin B_{12}

Q 157 Tocopherol exist in how many forms?

a) 1
b) 2
c) 3
d) **4**

Q 158 The most active form of vitamin E is _________

a) **α-Tocopherol**
b) β-Tocopherol
c) g-Tocopherol
d) d-Tocopherol

Q 159 Nutritional muscular dystrophy or white muscle disease in ruminants is caused by deficiency of _________

a) Vitamin E Only
b) Selenium Only
c) **Both vitamin E & Se**
d) None of these

Q 160 Stiff lamb disease occur to _________

a) **Deficiency of vitamin E**
b) Excess of vitamin A
b) Deficiency of vitamin A
d) Excess of vitamin E

Q 161 Toxic liver dystrophy (Hepatosis Dietetica) in swine occur due to _________

a) **Vitamin E deficiency**
b) Vitamin A deficiency
c) Vitamin C deficiency
d) Vitamin B_2 defciency

Q 162. Nutritional Microangiopathy or Mulberry heart disease in swine occur due to _________

a) **Vitamin E- Se deficiency**
b) Vitamin A-Zn deficiency
c) Vitamin B_{12}-Co deficiency
d) None of these

Q 163 Vitamin E deficiency in poultry can lead to _________

a) Exudative diathesis
b) Encephalomalacia
c) Muscular dystrophy
d) **All the above**

Q 164 Crazy chick disease occur due to ________

a) **Deficiency of vitamin E** b) Excess of vitamin E
c) Excess of vitamin A d) Deficiency of vitamin B_{12}

Q 165 Tying up syndrome in horse occur due to ________

a) **Deficiency of vitamin E** b) Deficiency of vitamin A
c) Deficiency of vitamin D d) Deficiency of vitamin C

Q 166 Yellow fat disease(Steatitis) occur due to deficiency of ______

a) **Vitamin E** b) Vitamin D
c) Vitamin C d) Vitamin A

Q 167 Which of the following mineral has sparing effect on vitamin E?

a) **Se** b) Cu
c) S d) Zn

Q 168 The last fat soluble vitamin to be discovered was ________

a) A b) D
c) E d) **K**

Q 169 Antihemorrhagic vitamin is ________

a) A b) B_{12}
c) E d) **K**

Q 170 Vitamin K was also known as ________

a) Coagulation vitamin b) Antihemorrhagic vitamin
c) Prothrombin factor d) **All the above**

Q 171 Which of the following is not a good source of vitamin E?

a) Vegetable oil b) Wheat germ oil
c) Egg d) **Milk**

Q 172 Which vitamin is also known as " Antisterility vitamin"?

a) A b) **E**
c) C d) B_{12}

Q 173 Animal responsible for the discovery of vitamin K is ________

a) Cow b) **Chicken**
c) Pig d) Dog

Q 174 Vitamin K_1 is also known as v

a) **Phylloquinone** b) Menaquinone

c) Menadione d) None of these

Q 175 Vitamin K_2 is also known as __________

a) Phylloquinone b) **Menaquinone**

c) Menadione d) None of these

Q 176 Vitamin K_3 is also known as __________

a) Phylloquinone b) Menaquinone

c) **Menadione** d) None of these

Q 177 Synthetic form of vitamin K is __________

a) K_1 b) K_2

c) $\mathbf{K_3}$ d) All are synthetic

Q 178 Simplest form of vitamin K is __________

a) Phylloquinone b) Menaquinone

c) **Menadione** d) Dicumarol

Q 179 The form of vitamin K extracted from plant is __________

a) **Phylloquinone** b) Menaquinone

c) Menadione d) All the above

Q 180 In blood clotting mechanism,how many factors are vitamin K dependent?

a) 2 b) 3

c) **4** d) 5

Q 181 Which vitamin concentration increases in putrefied meat?

a) Vitamin A b) Vitamin C

c) Vitamin D d) **Vitamin K**

Q 182 Haemorrhagic sweet clover disease is related with ________

a) Vitamin A b) Vitamin C

c) Vitamin D d) **Vitamin K**

Q 183 "Prothrombin time" test is used to measure the deficiency of __________

a) Calcium b) Iron
c) **Vitamin K** d) All the above

Q 184 Haemorrhagic sweet clover disease occur due to __________

a) **Deficiency of Vitamin K** b) Deficiency of Vitamin A
c) Excess of Vitamin K d) Excess of Vitamin A

Q 185 Anti-vitamin K activity exist in __________

a) Warfarin b) Dicumorol
c) Mycotoxin d) **All the above**

Q 186 Water soluble form of vitamin K is __________

a) Phylloquinone (K_1) b) Menaquinone (K_2)
c) **Menadione (K_3)** d) None of these

Q 187 Vitamin K is required for __________

a) Change of prothrombin into thrombin
b) **Synthesis of prothrombin**
c) Change of fibrinogen to fibrin
d) Formation of thromboplastin

Q 188 Continuous bleeding from an injured part of body is due to deficiency of __________

a) Vitamin A b) Vitamin B
c) Vitamin E d) **Vitamin K**

Q 189 Which vitamin is required for carboxylation of clotting factors?

a) A b) D
c) E d) **K**

Q 190 Vitamin K is involved in the post translational modification of __________

a) **Glutamate** b) Aspartate
c) Proline d) Lysine

Q 191 Vitamin K is required for __________

a) Hydroxylation b) Chelation
c) Transamination d) **Carboxylation**

Q 192 "Schilling Test" is performed to detect the deficiency of ______

a) B_1 b) B_2

c) **B_{12}** d) B_6

Q 193 As a hormone vitamin D has three target tissue, which are they?

a) **Kidney, Small intestine, Bone**

b) Heart, Bonemarrow, Blood

c) Kidney, Liver, Brain

d) Small intestine, Liver, Fat cell

Q 194 Deficiency of which vitamin can lead to " Folate trap"?

a) B_1 b) B_2

c) B_6 d) **B_{12}**

Q 195 Intra-dermal dye test is done to detect the deficiency of which vitamin?

a) A b) B_1

c) **C** d) D

Q 196 Transketolase activity is measured for detecting the deficiency of __________

a) **Thiamine** b) Riboflavin

c) Niaicn d) Pyridoxin

Q 197 The active coenzymes form of cobalamin in human being is __________

a) Adenosyl cobalamin b) Methyl cobalamin

c) **Both of these** d) None of these

Q 198 The erythrocyte glutathione reductase activity coefficient is measured for detecting the deficiency of __________

a) Thiamine b) **Riboflavin**

c) Niacin d) Folic acid

Q 199 Which of the following animal is unable to synthesize vitamin C in the body?

a) Cow b) Swine

c) **Guinea pig** d) Poultry

Q 200 L-hexuronic acid was the previous name of __________

a) Vitamin A
b) **Vitamin C**
c) Vitamin E
d) Vitamin K

Q 201 Antiscorbutic factor is __________

a) Vitamin A
b) Vitamin B_{12}
c) **Vitamin C**
d) Vitamin E

Q 202 Synthesis of vitamin C in body mainly occur in __________

a) Small intestine
b) Large Intestine
c) **Liver**
d) Blood

Q 203 Farm Livestock synthesize vitamin C from __________

a) **Glucose**
b) Precursor of vitamin C present in plants
c) Tyrosine
d) Carnitine

Q 204 Vitamin C dietary dependent species lack the following enzymes __________

a) Alkaline phosphatase
b) **L -gulonolactone oxidase**
c) Both of these
d) None of these

Q 205 Wernicke's Syndrome in human being occur due to deficiency of __________

a) **Thiamine**
b) Riboflavin
c) Niacin
d) Folacin

Q 206 Which of the following B-complex vitamin is stored in largest quantity than others?

a) B_2
b) B_6
c) B_7
d) **B_{12}**

Q 207 Which of the following vitamin is excreted in urine?

a) A
b) **C**
c) E
d) K

Q 208 " Bleeding disease" occur due to deficiency of vitamin ______

a) B_1 b) C

c) **K** d) K

Q 209 Enzyme gulonolactone oxidase required in vitamin C synthesis is absent in ______

a) Man b) Monkey

c) Guinea pig d) Indian fruit bat

e) **All the above**

Q 210 "Cheilosis" in human being occur due to deficiency of ______

a) **Riboflavin** b) Choline

c) Ascorbic acid d) Vitamin A

Q 211 The name "Folic acid" was proposed by ______

a) Gyorgy b) **Mitchell et al**

c) William et al d) Funk

Q 212 Folic acid previously known as ______

a) Vitamin M b) Vitamin B_{10}

c) Vitamin B_{11} d) **All the above**

Q 213 "Seborrheic dermatitis" occur due to deficiency of ______

a) Thiamine b) Ascorbic acid

c) **Riboflavin** d) Choline

Q 214 Provitamin are not known for ______

a) Vitamin A b) Vitamin D

c) Vitamin K d) **Vitamin B**

Q 215 One international Unit of vitamin A is equal to ______

a) 0.3 μg retinol b) 0.344 μgretinyl acetate

c) 0.55 mg retinylpalmitate d) **All the above**

Q 216 One retinol equivalent is ______

a) 1 μg retinol

b) 6 μg β – Carotene

c) 3.33 IU vitamin A activity from retinol

d) **All the above**

Q 217 One mg of β - Carotene is equal to how many international unit of vitamin A?

a) 400 b) 555
c) **1667** d) 833

Q 218 The conversion rate of β – Carotene to vitamin A of which animal has been taken as standard value?

a) **Rat** b) Cat
c) Cattle d) Horse

Q 219 One international unit of vitamin D is equal to ________

a) 0.25 μg of vitamin D_3 b) **0.025 μg of vitamin D_3**
c) 0.25 ηg of vitamin D_3 d) 250 ηg vitamin D_3

Q 220 One international chick unit (ICU) is equal to ________

a) **0.025 μg of vitamin D_3** b) 0.25 μg of vitamin D_3
c) 2.5 μg of vitamin D_3 d) 25 μg of vitamin D_3

Q 221 One international unit of vitamin E is equal to ________

a) I mg all - rac - α - tocopherol acetate
b) 0.74 mg RRR- α - tocopherol acetate
c) 0.67 mg RRR α - tocopherol
d) **All the above**

Q 222 Polioencephalomalacia (PEM) in ruminants is also known as __________

a) Cerebrocortical necrosis b) Cerebral necrosis
c) Forage poisoning d) **All the above**

Q 223 Cerebrocortical necrosis in ruminants occur due to deficiency of __________

a) **Thiamine*** b) Riboflavin
c) Biotin d) Ascorbic acid

* Due to bacterial thiaminase production in rumen

Q 224 Bracken fern poisoning in horse causes the deficiency of which vitamin?

a) Pantothenic acid b) Riboflavin
c) **Thiamine** d) Biotin

Q 225 "Nutritional roup" in poultry birds occur due to deficiency of __________

a) **Vitamin A** b) Vitamin E

c) Vitamin C d) Vitamin B

Q 226 "Adermin" was the previous name of __________

a) Pantothenic acid b) **Pyridoxine**

c) Choline d) Biotin

Q 227 " Xerosis" occur due to deficiency of __________

a) **Vitamin A** b) Vitamin E

c) Vitamin D d) Vitamin K

Q 228 Who named the antirachitic factor as vitamin D?

a) Sniadecki b) **McCollum**

c) Mellanby d) Steenbock

Q 229 Spectacle eye appearance due to alopecia in rat occur due to deficiency of __________

a) Thiamine b) Riboflavin

c) **Biotin** d) Choline

Q 230 The name "pantothenic acid" was given by __________

a) **R.J. Williams** b) McCollum

c) Kogl & Tonnis d) Strecker

Q 231 Vitamin B_{12} was also referred as __________

a) Anti pernicious anaemia factor

b) Animal protein factor

c) Chick growth factor

d) Cow manure factor

e) **All the above**

Q 232 "Zoopherin" was the previous name of vitamin __________

a) B_1 b) B_2

c) B_6 d) $\mathbf{B_{12}}$

Q 233 Vitamin C is precursor of __________

a) Acetic acid
b) **Oxalic acid**
c) Phytic acid
d) None of these

Q 234 Vitamin B_T is presently known as __________

a) **Carnitine**
b) Orotic acid
c) Pangamic acid
d) Laetrile

Q 235 Vitamin B_{13} name was assigned to __________

a) Carnitine
b) **Orotic acid**
c) Gerovital
d) Cabagin

Q 236 Vitamin B_{17} synonymous with __________

a) Laetrile
b) Amygdalin
c) **Both of these**
d) None of these

Q 237 Vitamin B_{15} is also known as __________

a) Orotic acid
b) PABA
c) **Pangamic acid**
d) Inositol

Q 238 Vitamin H_3 is synonymous with __________

a) Gerovital
b) Buffered solution of procaine HCl
c) **Both of the above**
d) None of the above

Q 239 Vitamin U is synonymous with __________

a) Cabagin
b) Antiulcer factor
c) **Both of these**
d) None of these

Q 240 Vitamin P name was assigned to __________

a) **Flavonoids**
b) PABA
c) Gerovital
d) Inositol

Q 241 "Corn bred fever" occur due to deficiency of __________

a) **Niacin**
b) Biotin
c) Pantothenic acid
d) Choline

Q 242 Which of the following water soluble vitamin does not contain nitrogen in its structure?

a) Riboflavin
b) Niacin
c) Pyridoxine
d) **Ascorbic acid**

Q 243 The least stable vitamin is __________

a) Vitamin D
b) Cyanocobalamin
c) **Ascorbic acid**
d) Riboflavin

Q 244 Number of vitamin included in B- complex is __________

a) 7
b) **9**
c) 11
d) 13

Q 245 Minimum number of chemical elements found in a typical B-vitamin is __________

a) 3
b) **4**
c) 5
d) 6

Q 246 Which of the following vitamin is synthesized in the rumen?

a) D
b) A
c) $\mathbf{K_2}$
d) E

Q 247 Number of chemical elements found in vitamin D is _________

a) **3**
b) 4
c) 5
d) 6

Q 248 Which vitamin has maximum number of chemical elements in its structure?

a) Pantothenic acid
b) **Cyanocobalamin**
c) Ascorbic acid
d) Biotin

Q 249 Which of the vitamin has " Phosphorus" in its structure?

a) A
b) $\mathbf{B_{12}}$
c) E
d) C

Q 250 Number of chemical elements present in Vitamin B12 is _____

a) 3
b) 4
c) 5
d) **6**

Q 251 The vitamin which can be most easily synthesized in human body is _________

a) A b) B
c) C d) **D**

Q 252 The least stable vitamin is _________

a) **Vitamin C** b) Vitamin D
c) Vitamin B_1 d) Vitamin E

Q 253 How many fat soluble vitamins causes the Hypervitaminosis in farm animals?

a) 1 b) **2**
c) 3 d) 4

Q 254 Hypervitaminosis in farm animals is generally reported for which vitamin?

a) A b) D
c) E d) **Both a & b**

Q 255 Total Number of vitamins that function in animal nutrition __________

a) 9 b) 11
c) **14** d) 17

Q 256 Which of the following vitamin cause Hypervitaminosis in animals?

a) Water soluble vitamin b) **Fat soluble vitamins**
c) Both of the above d) None of the above

Q 257 Which of the following vitamin is not involved in mitochondrial function?

a) B_1 b) B_2
c) **K** d) Niacin

Q 258 Which of the following vitamin is essential for RBC maturation?

a) K b) $\mathbf{B_{12}}$
c) A d) C

Q 259 In ileum which of the following substance is absorbed as such __________

a) Vit K b) Bile salt

c) Protein d) **Monosaccharide**

Q 260 Which vitamin causes mineral deposition?

a) Vitamin A b) Vitamin K

c) **Vitamin D** d) Vitamin C

Q 261 Cows that are at risk of developing ketosis can be fed what vitamin to help prevent ketosis?

a) **Niacin** b) Zinc

c) B-complex d) Vitamin C

Q 262 The last group of dietary essential to be recognized is __________

a) Protein b) Fat

c) Minerals d) **Vitamins**

Q 263 Which of the following period is known as "Golden age" of vitamin research?

a) **1930-1940 AD** b) 1960-1970 AD

c) 1910-1920 AD d) 1880-1890 AD

❑❑❑

Chapter 10

Water

Q 1 Metabolic water produced on oxidation of 1 gram of glucose is __________

a) **0.60 g** b) 1.0g
c) 0.35 g d) 1.1g

Q 2 Metabolic water produced on oxidation of 1gram of starch is __________

a) 0.60g b) **0.56g**
c) 0.42g d) 1.11g

Q 3 Metabolic water produced on oxidation of 1gram of protein is __________

a) 0.60g b) **0.40g**
c) 1.5g d) 1.0g

Q 4 Water produced on the oxidation of carbohydrate, protein and fat is known as __________

a) **Metabolic water** b) Bound water
c) Free water d) Nutrient water

Q 5 Water bound with protein in colloidal system or water present inside cells as hydrated ions is known as __________

a) Free water b) **Bound water**
c) Metabolic water d) Exogenous water

Q 6 Water taken through drinking or from the feed eaten is known as __________

a) Free water b) Bound water
c) **Exogenous water** d) Metabolic water

Q 7 Which of the following hormone control the water balance in the body?

a) Aldosterone
b) **Antidiuretic (Vasopressine) hormone**
c) Thyroid hormone
d) All the above

Q 8 Metabolic water produced on oxidation of 1kg fat is _______

a) **1070 g** b) 550 g
c) 400 g d) 2010 g

Q 9 Dry matter intake: water consumption ratio in adult cattle is __________

a) **1:3-4** b) 1:10-12
c) 1:1 b) 1:1.5

Q 10 Dry matter intake : water consumption ratio in swine is around __________

a) 1:6 b) **1:3**
c) 1:1 d) 1:10

Q 11 Dry matter intake: water consumption ratio in poultry is around __________

a) 1:6 b) 1:7
c) **1:2** d) 1:5

Q 12 DMI: water consumption ratio in calves is around _________

a) 1:3 b) **1:7**
c) 1:2 d) 1:1

Q 13 An average 57 g egg contain how much water?

a) **38g** b) 25 g
c) 50g d) 30 g

Q 14 Which of the following egg part has highest percentage of water?

a) Yolk
b) **Albumin**
c) Shell
d) All have equal water content

Q 15 Moisture content in succulent feed is __________

a) **60-90 %** b) 30-35%

c) 10-15% d) 20-30%

Q 16 Generally, the concentrate feed has moisture content in the range of __________

a) 30-40% b) 1-2%

c) **10-15%** d) 20-30%

Q 17 Water content in blood is __________

a) 70-80% b) **90-92%**

c) 50-60% d) Less than 50%

Q 18 Water content in muscle is __________

a) 40-50% b) 60-65%

c) **72-78%** d) 90-95%

Q 19 Water content in bone is __________

a) 20% b) 30%

c) **45%** d) 35%

Q 20 Water content in enamel is __________

a) 10% b) 20%

c) 15% d) **5%**

Q 21 Hydrogen :oxygen ratio in the water structure is __________

a) 1:1 b) **2:1**

c) 1.5:1 d) 3:1

Q 22 Comparatively greater amount of water is excreted in the faeces when diet is rich in __________

a) **Fibre** b) Fat

c) Protein d) Minerals

Q 23 Upto which level total dissolved solid (TDS) in water can be safely tolerated by animals?

a) **Upto 3000mg/L** b) Upto 5000mg/L

c) Upto 6000mg/L d) Upto 7000mg/L

Q 24 The most abundent salt in saline water is __________

a) Calcium b) Magnesium

c) Fluorine d) **Sodium**

Q 25 Water homeostasis is controlled by __________

a) Antidiuretic hormone b) Aldosterone

c) Sodium Chloride d) **All the above**

Q 26 Which of the following animal use water more efficiently by lowering its excretion in faeces?

a) Cow b) Buffalo

c) Pig d) **Camel**

Q 27 The average figure for the daily water requirement/day of an adult cattle is __________

a) 10-15 litre b) **30-40 litre**

c) 80-100 litre d) 5-10 litre

Q 28 The average figure for the daily water requirement/day of a poultry bird is __________

a) **200-300 ml** b) 500-700 ml

c) 50-100 ml d) 700-900 ml

Q 29 Water content in the body of dairy cow is __________

a) 50-60% b) **70-75%**

c) 90-95% d) 40-50%

Q 30 Water content in milk is __________

a) 50% b) 67%

c) **87%** d) 97%

Q 31 The most abundant nutrient in the body is __________

a) **Water** b) Mineral

c) Carbohydrate d) Protein

Q 32 The most abundant nutrient on the earth is __________

a) **Water** b) Carbohydrate

c) Minerals d) Protein

Q 33 Water constitute about ________ % of the body weight of an adult horse.

a) 30-45 % b) **65-75 %**
c) 40-50 % d) 85-90 %

Q 34 Water content in the foal is about ________

a) **75-80%** b) 20-30%
c) 40-55% d) 25-45%

Q 35 Major constituent of animal body is ________

a) **Water** b) Protein
c) Carbohydrate d) Fat

Q 36 Major constituents of plant body is ________

a) Carbohydrate b) **Water**
c) Fat d) Protein

Q 37 Tick the wrong answer regarding water requirement of animals ________

a) **Adult animals have higher water requirement/unit of body size as compared to young animals**
b) Birds require less water as compared to mammals
c) Salt consumption increases the water intake
d) Higher environmental temperature enhanced the water requirement

Q 38 The age at which concentration of water, protein and mineral matters in the fat free body mass become practically constant is known as ________

a) Puberty b) **Chemical maturity**
c) Geriatric d) Senile

Q 39 The amount of water required for the synthesis of 1 litre milk is ________

a) **5-6 litre** b) 1-2 Litre
c) 10-15 litre d) 20-25 litre

Q 40 The per cent water in milk of most domestic animal is ________

a) 10-20% b) 30-40%
c) 60-70% d) **80-88%**

❑❑❑

B. FEED, FEEDING AND DIGESTION

by Dr Jaswinder Singh

Chapter 11

Feed and Fodder

Q 1 Protein supplements are having following percentage of protein __________

a) Less than 15 % b) Less than 20 %
c) **More than 20%** d) Any of theses

Q 2 Moisture percentage in succulent feed is __________

a) 10-20 % b) 20-40%
c) 40-50% d) **60-90%**

Q 3 The fibre percentage in roughage is __________

a) 5 % b) 10%
c) 15 % d) **> 18%**

Q 4 The fibre percentage in concentrate is __________

a) >18% b) **<18%**
c) Can be above or below 18% d) 0-1%

Q 5 Which of the following is not a leguminous fodder crop?

a) Cow pea b) Cluster bean
c) **Sorghum** d) Lucerne

Q 6 Which of the following is not a non-leguminous fodder crop?

a) Maize b) **Guar**
c) Jowar d) Barley

Q 7 Which of the following is not a rabi fodder crop?

a) Berseem b) Shaftal
c) Oat d) **Teosinte**

Q 8 Which of the following is not a rabi fodder crop?

a) Rye grass b) Lucerne

c) Senji d) **Guar**

Q 9 Kharif fodder crop is ________

a) Sorghum b) Maize

c) Cow pea d) **All the above**

Q 10 Feeds are classified into how many groups of international feed class?

a) 5 b) **8**

c) 12 d) 10

Q 11 Fodder feed is ________

a) **Cow pea** b) Maize

c) Lucerne d) Berseem

Q 12 Excessive feeding of berseem to ruminant can lead to problems of ________

a) **Bloat** b) Nitrate toxicity

c) Oxalate d) Ca- deficiency

Q 13 The fodder with hollow stem is ________

a) **Berseem** b) Lucerne

c) Maize d) Cluster Bean

Q 14 Which of the following is an improved variety of berseem?

a) Ganga b) **Mescavi**

c) Adecuba d) Composite

Q 15 "Kent" is an improved variety of which fodder crop is?

a) **Oat** b) Berseem

c) Lucerne d) Maize

Q 16 Brazilian lucerne is also known as ________

a) White clover b) **Stylo**

c) Both of the above d) None of the above

Q 17 Kharif season belongs to which period?

a) **July-October** b) October- March

c) March- June d) None of these

Q 18 Rabi season belongs to __________

a) July-October b) **October- March**

c) March- June d) None of these

Q 19 Zaid season belongs to __________

a) July-October b) October- March

c) **March- June** d) None of these

Q 20 "Jawahar" is the improved variety of __________

a) Sorghum b) **Maize**

c) Oat d) Lucerne

Q 21 High lysine variety of maize is __________

a) **Shakti*** b) Ganga

c) Adecuba d) Composite

* Others are Ratna, Protina

Q 22 Among all the cereal grain which one is more variable in protein content?

a) **Wheat** b) Maize

c) Bajra d) Rice

Q 23 Safe inclusion level of molasses in ruminant feed is __________

a) **7-8%** b) 11-13%

c) 13-15% d) 15-17%

Q 24 Safe inclusion level of molasses in poultry feed is __________

a) 7-8% b) **4-5%**

c) 10-13% d) 14-15%

Q 25 Triticale is a hybrid of __________

a) **Wheat & Rye** b) Wheat and oat

c) Wheat & sorghum d) Wheat and maize

Q 26 DCP content of maintenance type roughages is ________

a) 0-1% b) 1-1.5%

c) **3-5%** d) None of these

Q 27 DCP content of productive type roughage is ________

a) 0-1% b) 1-2%

c) 2-3% d) **More than 5%**

Q 28 Energy feeds are having ________

a) Less than 20%CP b) Less than 18% CF

c) Less than 35% cell wall d) **All the above**

Q 29 Pasture whether natural or cultivated when cut and fed green to an animal in its stall is known as ________

a) **Soilage** b) Earlage

c) Haylage d) Shredlage

Q 30 Common name of oat is ________

a) **Javi / jaii** b) Jowar

c) Guar d) Bajra

Q 31 Para grass is also known as ________

a) Mautitius grass b) California grass

c) Giant couch d) **All the above**

Q 32 Para grass is a native of ________

a) **Brazil** b) Egypt

c) India d) South Africa

Q 33 Anjan Grass (Cenchrus ciliaris) is a native of ________

a) **India** b) South Africa

c) Maxico d) Egypt

Q 34 Teosinte is synonymous with ________

a) Makchari b) Buffalo grass

c) **Both of these** d) None of these

Q 35 Which of the following fodder crop resembles maize in its morphological character and is also considered as wild ancestor of maize?

a) Guinea grass b) **Teosinte**

c) Bajra d) Dinanath grass

Q 36 Guinea grass is a native of ________

a) America b) Australia

c) **Africa** d) India

Q 37 Napier grass is also known as ________

a) Elephant grass b) Uganda grass

c) **Both of the above** d) None of these

Q 38 In Napier grass or Napier Bajra- the word Napier pertain to __

a) **Name of person** b) Name of laboratory

c) Name of place d) Name of gene

Q 39 Pearl millet is commonly known as ________

a) Milo b) Jowar

c) **Bajra** d) Guinea Corn

Q 40 Bajra is synonymous with ________

a) Pearl millet b) Indian millet

c) Horse millet d) **All the above**

Q 41 DCP content of non-maintenance type roughage is ________

a) **< 3 %** b) 5-7%

c) 7-10% d) > 10%

Q42 Which of the following is not a productive type roughage?

a) Berseem b) Leucerne

c) Cow pea d) **Pearl millet**

Q 43 Common name of sorghum is ________

a) Jowar b) Chari

c) Milo d) **All of these**

Q 44 Maize is a native of _________

a) Brazil
b) Africa
c) **Mexico**
d) Australia

Q 45 Which of the following fodder crop is also known as "crop camel"?

a) **Sorghum**
b) Guar
c) Soybean
d) Napier bajra

Q 46 Common name of cluster bean is _________

a) Jowar
b) Lobia
c) **Guar**
d) Bajra

Q 47 Tick the true statement regarding lucerne _________

a) Native of South-western Asia
b) Also known as alfalfa
c) It is oldest among the cultivated forages crops of the world
d) **All are correct**

Q 48 Queen of fodder crop is _________

a) Maize
b) **Lucerne**
c) Berseem
d) Cow pea

Q 49 Lucerne is also known as _________

a) Alfalfa
b) Snail clover
c) Chilean clover
d) **All the above**

Q 50 Berseem is a native of _________

a) **Egypt**
b) West Indies
c) South Africa
d) Europe

Q 51 Which fodder crop is said to be a "Milk multiplier"?

a) Bajra
b) **Berseem**
c) Soyabean
d) Maize

Q 52 Egyptian clover is _________

a) **Berseem**
b) Lucerne
c) Cow pea
d) Shaftal

Q 53 Cow pea is synonymous with _________

a) Lobia b) Black eye pea

c) **Both a & b** d) None of these

Q 54 Manchurian bean is another name of _________

a) **Soyabean** b) Cluster bean

c) Rice bean d) Moong bean

Q 55 Persian clover is _________

a) Berseem b) **Shaftal**

c) Senji d) Lucerne

Q 56 Indian clover is _________

a) Cow pea b) Teosinte

c) **Senji** d) Shaftal

Q 57 Which of the following is a multicut fodder?

a) Senji b) **Guinea grass**

c) Teosinte d) Maize

Q 58 Crop used for green manuring is _________

a) Sunhemp b) Dhaincha

c) **Both of these** d) None of these

Q 59 Which of the following is not a leguminous crop?

a) Dhaincha b) Sunhemp

c) **Teosinte** d) Lucerne

Q 60 Anjan grass is also known as _________

a) Buffel grass b) African foxtail

c) Dhaman grass d) **All the above**

Q 61 Setaria grass is also known as _________

a) Golden thimothy b) Golden bristle grass

c) **Both of these** d) None of these

Q 62 Which fodder crop is renowned as the outstanding crop for silage?

a) **Maize** b) Oat

c) Guinea grass d) Rye grass

Q 63 Which crop is also known as " Vegetative Meat"?

a) **Cow pea** b) Lucerne

c) Berseem d) Guar

Q 64 Kasni (*Cichroium intybusl*) is a weed in which crop?

a) **Berseem** b) Lucerne

c) Cow pea d) Guar

Q 65 Dodder (*Cuscuta* spp) is a weed in which fodder crop?

a) Berseem b) **Lucerne**

c) Cow pea d) Guar

Q 66 Tick the wrong statement __________

a) All cereals are deficient in Vitamin D and calcium

b) **Bran is a poor source of P**

c) Wheat germ is a good source of thiamine

d) Cereal grains are generally used as source of carbohydrate

Q 67 Maize is deficient in __________

a) Lysine b) Methionine

c) Tryptophan d) **All the above**

Q 68 The richest source of energy among following grain is ________

a) **Maize** b) Wheat

c) Sorghum d) Oat

Q 69 The variety of maize rich in lysine is __________

a) Ganga -2 b) Ganga- 101

c) **Opaque-2** d) Adecuba

Q 70 Wheat bran with a small percentage of wheat flour is known as __________

a) **Pollard**
b) Middlings
c) Groats
d) None of these

Q 71 A byproduct of flour milling industry comprising various proportions of fine bran with high proportion of wheat flour (endosperm and germ) is known as __________

a) Pollard
b) **Middling**
c) Groats
d) None of these

Q 72 Grains from which hulls have been removed are known as ____

a) **Groats**
b) Germs
c) Red dog
d) Gluten

Q 73 Red dog is a byproduct of __________

a) Slaughter house
b) **Wheat milling industry**
c) Sugar industry
d) Beverage industry

Q 74 Blackstrap molasses is a byproduct of which industry?

a) **Cane sugar industry**
b) Beet Sugar industry
c) Fruit Juice industry
d) Paper industry

Q 75 Molasses is generally high in __________

a) Ca
b) Mg
c) Na
d) **K**

Q 76 Unit used for molasses __________

a) Brix
b) Bushel
c) Baume
d) **Both a & c**

Q 77 Brix value of molasses reflects the __________

a) **Level of sugar (Sucrose) in molasses**
b) Volume of molasses
c) Both of these
d) None of these

Q 78 The Brix value of cane molasses is generally __________

a) 75.5° b) **79.5°**

c) 85.5° d) 89.5°

Q 79 The term " Treacle" can also be used for __________

a) **Molasses** b) Table scrap

c) Teosinte d) Rice bran

Q 80 Molasses in ruminant feed act as __________

a) Sweetner b) Appetiser

c) Binder for pelleting d) **All the above**

Q 81 Which of the following is a tuber?

a) Turnip b) Sugarbeet

c) **Potato** d) Carrot

Q 82 The most expensive nutrient in livestock ration is __________

a) Carbohydrate b) **Protein**

c) Minerals d) Fat

Q 83 On the basis of oil seed processing, cakes are classified into how many types?

a) 2 b) **3***

c) 4 d) 5

*Ghani, expeller and solvent extracted

Q 84 Cotton seeds are processed into cake by ghani, expeller and solvent method, then the protein content will be highest in __________

a) Ghani pressed cake

b) Expeller cake

c) **Solvent extracted cake**

d) Equal in all the three type cakes

Q 85 In above question, the highest amount of fat will be in _______

a) **Ghani pressed cake**

b) Expeller cake

c) Solvent extracted cake

d) Equal in all the three type cakes

Q 86 In solvent extracted cake, the oil content is generally ______

a) **< 1%** b) 2-5 %

c) 5-10% d) 10-15%

Q 87 Tick the wrong statement ______

a) **Cakes are good source of carotene and vitamin A**

b) Root and tuber are poor in Ca and P

c) Bran are good source of P

d) Molasses is good source of K

Q 88 The first limiting amino acid in soyabean meal is ______

a) Lysine b) **Methionine**

c) Arginine d) Tryptophan

Q 89 The first limiting amino acid in cottonseed meal is ______

a) **Lysine** b) Methionine

c) Arginine d) Tryptophan

Q 90 Which of the following meal has the property of absorbing the molasses upto half of its own weight?

a) Soyabean meal b) Linseed meal

c) **Coconut meal** d) Cottonseed meal

Q 91 The first limiting amino acid in groundnut meal is ______

a) **Lysine** b) Methionine

c) Arginine d) Tryptophan

Q 92 Cake prone to fungal infestation is ______

a) Cottonseed b) Mustard

c) **Groundnut** d) Linseed

Q 93 "Alsi" is the common name for ______

a) **Linseed** b) Coconut

c) Rapeseed d) Sunflower

Q 94 Feeding of which cake is generally done by the farmers to bring shining on the skin (bloom) of animal before taking them to show or mandi?

a) Cottonseed cake b) **Linseed cake**

c) Mustard cake d) Soyabean cake

Q 95 Popular name of Sesame cake is __________

a) **Til cake** b) Copra cake

c) Alsi cake d) Binola cake

Q 96 Copra meal is synonymous with __________

a) Linseed meal b) **Coconut meal**

c) Sesame meal d) Safflower meal

Q 97 Which cake is richest in calcium among all oilcakes?

a) Coconut b) **Sesame**

c) Linseed d) Mustard

Q 98 Flaxseed is also known as __________

a) Linseed b) Toad flex

c) Lint bell d) **All the above**

Q 99 The highest nutritive value of any plant protein source is of __________

a) **Soybean meal** b) Linseed meal

c) Canola meal d) Sesame meal

Q 100 The fat percentage in full fat soyabean is generally __________

a) 5-7% b) **18-20%**

c) 25-30% d) 45-50%

Q 101 The most widely used energy feed is __________

a) **Maize** b) Wheat

c) Oat d) Barley

Q 102 "Binola cake" is the common name of __________

a) Rapeseed cake b) **Cottonseed cake**

c) Groundnut cake d) Sunflower cake

Q 103 Whole cottonseed are also referred as __________

a) Linted cottonseed
b) Fuzzy seed
c) **Both of the above**
d) None of the above

Q 104 Tick the wrong statement regarding whole cottonseed ______

a) Linters are the short fibers remain on the cottonseed.
b) **Fibres on whole cottonseed are not digestible in ruminant**
c) Whole cottonseed contain around 18% oil.
d) It contains about 20 % CP

Q 105 Tick the wrong statement about cottonseed hulls __________

a) They are outer covering of the cottonseed
b) Can be used as roughage source for ruminant
c) It can easily mix with feed
d) **It is an excellent protein source**

Q 106 To convert the percentage figure to ppm, decimal has to move __________

a) Three points toward left
b) **Four points toward right**
c) Three point toward right
d) Two points toward left

Q 107 Which of the following practice was adopted by dairy farmers of northern India especially of Punjab to get rid their animals from ticks?

a) **Feeding of Taramira seed**
b) Feeding of molasses + ajwain + fennel
c) Feeding of colocynth
d) None of these

Q 108 Crude protein content in groundnut cake is around _________

a) 20-25%
b) 25-30%
c) **40-45%**
d) 10-15%

Q 109 Crude protein content in solvent extracted soyabean meal is __________

a) **44%**
b) 34%
c) 54%
d) 64%

Q 110 Crude protein content of dehulled solvent extracted soyabean meal is ________

a) 44% b) **48%**
c) 67% d) None of these

Q 111 Soy hulls is a good source of ________

a) Protein b) Fat
c) **Fibre** d) All the above

Q 112 The first limiting amino acid in soyabean meal is ________

a) Lysine b) **Methionine**
c) Arginine d) Tryptophan

Q 113 Kunitz and Bowman-Birk factors are present in ________

a) Coconut meal b) Kranz meal
c) **Soyabean meal** d) Linseed meal

Q 114 Inclusion of which meal in the layer ration may cause olive-green discolouration of the yolk ________

a) Soybean b) **Cottonseed**
c) Groundnut meal d) All the above

Q 115 Which of the following cake contain mucilage?

a) Coconut b) Sesame
c) **Linseed** d) Mustard

Q 116 Crude protein content in Til (sesame) cake is ________

a) **40-45%** b) 20-25%
c) 30-35% d) 55-60%

Q 117 Which of the following meal has the highest nutritive value?

a) **White sesame meal** b) Black sesame meal
c) Red sesame meal d) All have the same

Q 118 Crude protein content of sunflower seed meal is around _____

a) 20% b) 30%
c) **40%** d) 60%

Q 119 "Surajmukhi" is the popular name of which oilseed crop ____

a) **Sunflower** b) Safflower

c) Canola d) None of these

Q 120 The largest producer of safflower in the world is ________

a) Australia b) **India**

c) Argintina d) Pakistan

Q 121 The protein content of undecorticated safflower meal is around

a) **20-22%** b) 30-35%

c) 10-12% d) 40-45%

Q 122 Tick the wrong statement about canola ________

a) A variety of rapeseed having very less erucic acid

b) **Developed at USA***

c) Also known as low erucic acid rapeseed (LEAR)

d) Popularly called as Rapeseed 00

* Developed at Canada

Q 123 Match the common name of *Eruca sativa* used at different places

____

A) Punjab	i) Taramira
B) Uttar Pradesh	ii) Tirwa
C) Madhya Pradesh	iii) Sondha
d) Europe	iv) Rocket /Roquuette

a) **A-i,B-ii,C-iii,D-iv** b) A-ii,B-iii,C-iv,D-i

c) A-i,B-iv,C-ii,D-iii d) A-ii,B-iv,C-I,D-iii

Q 124 While going through the literature originally belong to Europe, an Indian student come across the term " Rocket" (*Eruca sativa*) seed meal, he got perplexed and asked you what is it? What do you suggest that it is synonymous with?

a) Rapeseed meal b) Kranjseed meal

c) **Taramira seed meal** d) Matira seed meal

Q 125 The crude protein content of taramira (*Eruca sativa*) cake is around ________

a) **35-40%** b) 20-25%

c) 10-15% d) 55-60%

Q 126 The protein content in hulled sunflower meal is around _____

a) **40-45%** b) 30-35%

c) 20-25% d) 60-65%

Q 127 The byproducts of pulses processing unit having husk and some broken grains in it, is known as _________

a) **Chunnies** b) Groat

c) Draff d) None of these

Q 128 Blood meal is deficient in _________

a) Lysine b) Methionine

c) Arginine d) **Isoleucine**

Q 129 Which of the following meal is unpalatable?

a) **Blood meal** b) Cottonseed meal

c) Fish meal d) Corn gluten meal

Q 130 Crude protein content in meat meal is around _________

a) **50-55%** b) 80-90%

c) 70-80% d) 15-20%

Q 131 Crude protein content in blood meal is around _________

a) **75-80%** b) 55-60%

c) 35-40% d) 25-30%

Q 132 Which of the following is not a non-protein nitrogen (NPN) source for ruminant animal?

a) Biuret b) Amino acid

c) **Polypeptide** d) Amides

Q 133 The nitrogen content in urea is _________

a) **42-46%** b) 30-35%

c) 25-30% d) 55-60%

Q 134 The protein equivalent of urea is _________

a) 112-115% b) **262-281%**

c) 50-75% d) 200-225%

Q 135 The nitrogen content in Biuret is __________

a) **35-45%** b) 25-30%

c) 45-55% d) 15-20%

Q 136 Urea can effectively be used by animal, when it is fed with __________

a) **High TDN (>75%) and 12-13% CP level**

b) Low TDN and 12-13 % CP leve

c) High TDN and High CP (20%)

d) All of these

Q 137 Tick the wrong statement about Biuret __________

a) It is a product formed by heating the urea

b) **Its formula is NH_2CONH_2**

c) Its nitrogen content is around 30-35 %

d) It is an expensive source of NPN

Q 138 The term "Carbamide" can be used for __________

a) **Urea** b) Biuret

c) Both of the above d) None of the above

Q 139 Which of the following is an example of NPN compound?

a) Glutamine b) Histamine

c) Urea d) **All the above**

Q 140 Which of the following is a NPN source for ruminant?

a) Betaine b) Tyramine

c) Ammonia d) **All the above**

Q 141 Which of the following is an NPN source?

a) Cocaine b) Solanin

c) Uric acid d) **All the above**

Q 142 An example of NPN compound is __________

a) Nucleic acid b) Purine

c) Pyrimidines d) **All the above**

Q 143 The most widely used NPN compound in ruminant ration is __________

a) **Urea** b) Biuret
c) Ammonium salt d) Purines

Q 144 Urea used for inclusion in ruminant ration in India is of following type __________

a) **Fertilizer grade urea** b) Feed grade urea*
c) Both a & b type d) None of these

* Feed grade urea is not available in India

Q 145 Tick the wrong statement about urea __________

a) Deficient in all vitamins
b) Deficient in sulphur
c) **It has high energy value***
d) It contains no methionine and cystine

* Urea has no energy value of its own

Q 146 The N:S ratio required in urea supplemented diet is __________

a) **10:1** b) 20:1
c) 5:1 d) 25:1

Q 147 Urea supplemented diet should not be fed to __________

a) Calf b) Pig
c) Horse d) **All the above**

Q 148 Taking Nitrogen percentage at 46%, the one kg urea is equivalent to __________ protein.

a) **2.87 kg** b) 287 kg
c) 0.287 kg d) 4.63 kg

Q 149 As per BIS recommendation, the inclusion level of urea in concentrate mixtue for ruminant is upto __________

a) 2% b) **1%**
c) 3% d) 5%

Q 150 Synonymous of urea is __________

a) Carbamide b) Carbonyldiamide
c) **Both of the above** d) None of the above

Q 151 The concept of feeding of NPN substances to ruminant animals was started in which country?

a) United Kingdom b) **Germany**

c) U.S.A d) Japan

Q 152 Urea was discovered by __________

a) **Rouelle** b) Wohler

c) Prout d) Zuntz

Q 153 The credit of the first synthesis of urea goes to scientist _______

a) Rouelle b) **Wohler**

c) Prout d) Zuntz

Q 154 The first NPN substance reported to be used in ruminant was __________

a) Urea b) Uric acid

c) **Asparagine** d) Ammonium acetate

Q 155 Which of the following factor affects urea utilization in ruminant?

a) Level of protein in ration

b) Level of carbohydrate in ration

c) Age of animal

d) **All the above**

Q 156 For affective utilization of ruminal ammonia by the microflora, the rumen ammonia concentration should be __________

a) **5-8 mg/100ml rumen liquor**

b) 15-20 mg/100ml rumen liquor

c) 21-33 mg/100ml rumen liquor

d) 40-55 mg/100 ml rumen liquor

Q 157 Supplementation of which of the following compound improve the urea utilization in ruminants?

a) Sulphur b) Methionine

c) Molasses d) **All the above**

Q 158 Inclusion level of urea in complete feed is __________

a) **1% of total dry matter fed**

b) 3% of total dry matter fed

c) 4% of total dry matter fed

d) 5% of total dry matter fed

Q 159 Taking urea with 46 % nitrogen and mustard cake with 32 % crude protein, one kg of urea will be able to replace how much of mustard cake on protein equivalent basis?

a) 5 kg b) **9 kg**

c) 15 Kg d) 3 kg.

Q 160 In above question if mustard cake is replaced with groundnut cake having 41 % CP,then how much of groundnut cake will be equal to 1kg urea on protein equivalent basis?

a) 5 kg b) 9 kg

c) **7 kg** d) 11 kg

Q 161 If in a 35 % protein supplement, 12 % protein is from urea. Then, how much percentage of urea is added in it?

a) 3.4% b) **4.3%**

c) 5.3% d) 6.1%

* 12/281x100= 4.3 %

Q 162 If a 40 % protein supplement contain 5% urea,then how much protein in contributed by urea in the supplement?

a) 10% b) 12 %

c) **14 %** d) 18 %

* 5x281/100= 14%

Q 163 Crude protein content in deoiled kranj cake is __________

a) **30%** b) 50%

c) 15 % d) 20%

Q 164 Crude protein content in corn gluten meal is around _______

a) **50-60%** b) 20-30%

c) 10-20% d) None of these

Q 165 Which of the following grain is an example of self balanced concentrate?

a) Oat b) Maize

c) **Gram** d) Barley

* It contains 12.8%DCP and 75 % TDN

Q 166 A protein supplement sample estimation revealed the presence of 35 % protein,less than 1% fat,then the sample is of _______

a) **Plant origin and solvent extracted meal**

b) Plant origin and expeller type meal

c) Animal origin and solvent extracted meal

d) Animal origin and expeller type meal

Q 167 Which of the following grain is added in the poultry ration unground but grinded for use in ruminant ration __________

a) Barley b) **Millet**

c) Sorghum d) Oat

Q 168 Dry matter content in molasses is generally ranged between __________

a) 20-30% b) 10-20%

c) **60-80%** d) 30-40%

Q 169 Tick the wrong statement about molasses __________

a) Its production is about $1/3^{rd}$ of the sugar produced

b) Its production is 3% of sugarcane

c) Both a & b are right

d) **Both a & b are wrong**

Q 170 Fibre percentage in molasses is __________

a) **0%** b) 2%

c) 3% d) 5%

Q 171 Which of the following crop is used as green manure?

a) Sunhemp b) Dhaincha

c) Safflower d) **Both a & b**

Q 172 Grain having highest amount of energy among cereal grains is __________

a) **Maize** b) Sorghum
c) Wheat d) Millet

Q 173 Which of the following cereal grain is more susceptible for mycotoxin infestation?

a) Wheat b) **Maize**
c) Sorghum d) Millet

Q 174 Wheat is a good source of energy next to maize and sorghum. Among wheat and rice bran which has the higher energy?

a) Wheat bran
b) **Rice bran**
c) Both has same
d) Depends upon processing technique

* Rice bran = 2900kcal ME/kg
Wheat bran = 1300kcal ME/kg

Q 175 The another meal of tapioca meal is __________

a) Sal seed meal b) **Cassava meal**
c) Sweet potato tuber meal d) None of these

Q 176 The largest producer of soyabean in world is __________

a) **USA** b) Brazil
c) China d) India

Q 177 Which meal rank first in terms of total world production of protein meals?

a) **Soyabean meal** b) Rapeseed meal
c) Groundnut meal d) Sunflower meal

Q 178 Which meal rank second in terms of total world production of protein meals?

a) Soybean meal b) **Rapeseed meal**
c) Groundnut meal d) Sunflower meal

Q 179 The chemical composition of an ingredient is 13% protein, 13% fat and 13 % fibre. Identify the ingredient ________

a) Maize b) Wheat bran

c) **Rice bran** d) Wheat

Q 180 The nutritionally superior new variety of rapeseed developed in Canada having very less level of glucosinolates and erucic acid is known as ________

a) Duble zero b) Canola

c) None of these d) **Both a & b**

Q 181 Amino acid deficient in soyabean meal is ________

a) Lysine b) Tryptophan

c) Threonine d) **Methionine**

Q 182 Amongst the following protein meals, which is more susceptible for infestation of *Aspergillus flavus* fungus?

a) Soyabean meal b) Rapeseed meal

c) **Groundnut meal** d) Sunflower meal

Q 183 Maximum inclusion level of cottonseed meal in layer ration is ________

a) **0-5%** b) 10-15 %

c) 20-25% d) 30-35%

Q 184 *Phalaris minor* is also known as ________

a) Ghulli- Danda b) Canary grass

c) **Both a & b** d) None of these

Q 185 Canary Grass is a problematic weed in which crop?

a) Rice b) Maize

c) **Wheat** d) Oat

Q 186 "Chhattala" is a common name of which fodder?

a) Lucerne b) Senji

c) **Shaftal*** d) Berseem

* Used mostly in northern states especially in Punjab

Q 187 Sudex is a multicut fodder produced by crossing between __________

a) **Sorghum & Sudan grass** b) Sorghum & Rye grass
c) Sorghum & Napier grass d) Sudan and Rye grass

Q 188 Lopping of trees for animal fodder purpose is called _______

a) Grazing b) **Browsing**
c) Tethering d) Coral feeding
e) None of these

Q 189 Example of perennial fodder crop is _________

a) Maize b) Oat
c) Barley d) **Napier bajra**

Q 190 Example of annual fodder crop is _________

a) Napier Bajra b) Para Grass
c) Guinea Grass d) **Oat**

Q 191 The operation by which the soil is stirs with some implements for the purpose of improving it for the growth of a crop is known as __________

a) **Tillage** b) Soiling
c) Both a & b d) None of these

Q 192 Teosinte was introduced to India in 1881, at which place?

a) Punjab b) UP
c) **Chennai** d) West Bangal

Q 193 Teosinte is a native of _________

a) **Central America** b) Canada
c) Australia d) Germany

Q 194 Which of the following is perennial leguminous fodder crop?

a) Berseem b) **Lucerne**
c) Cluster bean d) Cow pea

Q 195 The term guar phalgati/fati is used in Rajasthan for _______

a) Guar fodder b) **Guar straw**
c) Guar seed d) Both a & c

Q 196 Baru grass (Sorghum halepensis) is also known as ________

a) Johnson grass
b) Banchari grass
c) **Both of these**
d) None of these

Q 197 "Friend of poor" grass is __________

a) Deenanath grass
b) Deenabandhu grass
c) **Both a & b**
d) None of these

Q 198 Finger millet is commonly known as __________

a) **Ragi**
b) Bajra
c) Both of these
d) None of these

Q 199 Leguminous fodder crop that can be used as green manuring as well as for livestock feeding __________

a) Mucuna
b) Lablab
c) **Both a & b**
d) None of these

Q 200 The land management system in which forests are managed for the production of wood as well as for rearing of domesticated animals is known as __________

a) Silvicultural system
b) Agri-silviculture system
c) **Silvipastural system**
d) Agri-silvipastural system

Q 201 The part of tree like tender shoots, twigs, leaves, fruits, pods, etc. when used as feed is known as __________

a) **Browse**
b) Graze
c) Pasturage
d) All the above

Q 202 The term " Top feeds" used by animal nutritionist is related to __________

a) Nutritionally superior feed
b) Total mixed ration
c) **Tree leaves**
d) Novel feed

Q 203 When major branches of the trees are removed for supply of green fodder and firewood, then this type of harvesting is known as __________

a) **Lopping**
b) Prunning
c) Coppicing
d) Pollarding

Q 204 When all the branches including top of the tree are removed, then it is known as __________

a) Lopping
b) Thinning
c) Coppicing
d) **Pollarding**

Q 205 When individual trees are cut at their base,then this type of harvesting is known as __________

a) Lopping
b) Thinning
c) **Coppicing**
d) Pollarding

Q 206 *Leucarna leucocephala* is commonly known as __________

a) Subabul
b) Ipil-pil
c) Wild tamarind
d) **All the above**

Q 207 Which of the following fodder tree is also known as "Miracle tree" due to its multifarious use?

a) **Subabul**
b) Acacia
c) Banyan
d) Fig

Q 208 The per cent protein in detoxified guar meal is around _______

a) **40-45%**
b) 20-25%
c) 10-15%
d) 25-30%

Q 209 *Prosopis cineraria* (loong tree) is commonly known as _______

a) Khejri (Rajasthan)
b) Jand (Punjab)
c) Sami (Maharashtra)
d) Jammi (Tamil Nadu)
d) **All the above**

Q 210 The Crude protein in Khejri (prosopis cineraria) leaves is around __________

a) **12-16 %**
b) 1-5 %
c) 30-36%
d) 40-44%

Q 211 Ficus bengalensis is commonly known as __________

a) **Banyan tree**
b) Peepul tree
c) Both a & b
d) None of these

Q 212 Which of the following meal is used as energy source rather than protein source?

a) Corn gluten meal b) Guar meal
c) Sunflower meal d) **Sal seed meal**

Q 213 The crude protein content in sal seed meal is around _______

a) **7-9%** b) 20-25%
c) 30-32 % d) 35-40%

Q 214 Rubber seed cake is reported to possess which anti-nutritional factor?

a) Nitrate b) Oxalate
c) **Hydrocyanic acid** d) Mowrine

Q 215 "Redgut"- a sudden death syndrome in sheep occur due to prolonged and excessive feeding of _________

a) **Lucerne** b) Maize
c) Rye grass d) None of the above

Q 216 Which of the following is not a byproduct of brewing process?

a) Malt culm b) Spent hops
c) Bewer's yeast d) **Pollard**

Q 217 Sprout of barley are removed during brewing process,they are called as __________

a) **Malt culm/coombs** b) Spent hops
c) Brewers yeast d) Brewers grain

Q 218 The term "Draff" pertain to _________

a) Malt coombs b) Spent hops
c) **Brewers grain** d) Brewer's yeast

Q 219 " Pot ale" is a byproduct of which industry?

a) **Malt distilling industry** b) Pulse milling industry
c) Rice milling industry d) Fruit-juice industry

Q 220 Which of the following protein is present in maize?

a) Zein b) Glutelin
c) Albumen d) **Both a & b**

Q 221 The most abundant amino acid in oat protein is __________

a) Lysine
b) Methionine
c) Arginine
d) **Glutamic acid**

Q 222 " Meal seed" is the byproduct of which industry?

a) **Oat meal milling**
b) Maize-starch manufacturing industry
c) Pulse milling industry
d) Brewers industry

Q 223 Common name of green gram is __________

a) **Moong**
b) Gram
c) Urd
d) Moth

Q 224 Common name of black gram is __________

a) Moong
b) Gram
c) **Urd**
d) Moth

Q 225 Which of the following is known as "Kadbies"?

a) Stover of jowar
b) Stover of maize
c) Millet straw
d) **Both a & b**

Q 226 Crude protein equivalent for pure urea is __________

a) 202.2
b) 260.3
c) **291.6**
d) 300.2

Q 227 Currently, the main cereal component in poultry feed is _____

a) **Maize**
b) Sorghum
c) Rice
d) Pearl millet

Q 228 The waste product of human foods consisting of meat scrap, fish, bones, stale breads, etc. is known as __________

a) **Swill**
b) Chaff
c) Cavings
d) All the above

Q 229 The normal fat content in cereal grain is around __________

a) 10-15%
b) **2-5%**
c) 5-10%
d) 15-20%

Q 230 In India, Opaque-2 variety of maize is also known as _______

a) Shakti ratna
b) Protina
c) Floury-2
d) **Both a & b**

Q 231 The crude protein content of cereal grain is in the range of __________

a) 2-5%
b) **8-12 %**
c) 8-25%
d) 15-25%

Q 232 Debranned and cracked parboiled wheat is known as ______

a) Wheat red dog
b) **Bulgur**
c) Wheat middlings
d) Wheat shorts

Q 233 Which of the following bran is prone to rancidity?

a) Wheat bran
b) Maize bran
c) **Rice bran**
d) All the above

Q 234 The linseed meal can be incorporated in poultry feed upto ________ % without any adverse effect.

a) **Less than 5%**
b) Upto 10%
c) 10-15%
d) 15-20%

Q 235 Out of the common plant protein used in animal feeds, which of the following has highest percentage of essential amino acid as a percent of crude protein?

a) Ground nut cake
b) Canola meal
c) **Soybean meal**
d) Cottonseed meal

Q 236 Cereals are rich in __________

a) Ca
b) Fe
c) Cu
d) **P**

Q 237 The available phosphorus content is present largely in ______

a) Soyabean
b) Groundnut cake
c) **Fishmeal**
d) Maize

Q 238 A pigment present in maize and is precursor of vitamin A _____

a) **Cryptoxanthene**
b) Phytogunine
c) Xanthophyll
d) Chlorophyll

Q 239 Bajra can be fed to ruminants ________

a) As whole grain
b) Alongwith bran
c) **After grinding**
d) Mixing with other cereals

Q 240 Millets are cereal which has higher percentage of ________

a) **Fibre**
b) Protein
c) Fat
d) Minerals

Q 241 Hulls can be used as such for ________

a) Cattle
b) Sheep
c) Pigs
d) **None of the above**

Q 242 Feeding optimum level of molasses to ruminnats leads to _____

a) **Better ruminal activity**
b) Reduces ruminal activity
c) Acidosis
d) Tympany

Q 243 Animal origin protein supplements contain protein level ________

a) **Mostly above 45 %**
b) Mostly below 45%
c) Between 30-40%
d) Between 20-30%

Q 244 Oilseed meals usually have high content of ________

a) P
b) **Ca**
c) Cu
d) I

Q 245 Soyabean meal can be included in the ration of livestock in the range of ________

a) **20-30%**
b) 40-55%
c) 5-10%
d) 10-20%

Q 246 Single cell protein usually contain high level of ________

a) Crude fibre
b) Calcium
c) **Nucleic acid**
d) Iron

Q 247 Fishy smell in yolk of egg can be developed due to feeding of ________

a) Soyabean meal
b) **Mustard/rapeseed meal**
c) Groundnut meal
d) Sunflower meal

Q 248 Structural carbohydrates are made up of __________

a) Cellulose, fructose and saccharin

b) Lignin, sucrose and cellulose

c) Cellulose, hemicellulose and lactose

d) **Cellulose, hemicellulose and lignin**

Q 249 What structural carbohydrate component makes older plants less digestible than younger plants?

a) **Lignin**

b) Cellulose

c) Fructose

d) Sucrose

Q 250 What do non-structural carbohydrates consist of?

a) Proteins, acids and alkalis

b) Plant proteins, pectin and sugar

c) Plant sugars, lactic acid and potassium

d) **Plant starch, pectin and sugar**

❑❑❑

Chapter 12

Digestive System

Q 1 Which of the following part of bird digestive system is not similar to rest three?

a) Esophagus b) Crop
c) **Proventriculus** d) Gizzard

Q 2 Which of the following is known as true stomach of birds?

a) Esophagus b) Crop
c) **Proventriculus** d) Gizzard

Q 3 The part of avian digestive system which act as store house is __________

a) Esophagus b) **Crop**
c) Proventriculus d) Gizzard

Q 4 Which part of avian digestive system is known as muscular stomach?

a) Crop b) Proventriculus
c) **Gizzard** d) Caecum

Q 5 The true sequence of parts of poultry digestive system is ______

a) Esophagus-crop-proventriculus-gizzard
b) Crop-esophagus-proventriculus-gizzard
c) Crop-esophagus- gizzard-proventriculus
d) Esophagus-crop-gizzard-proventriculus

Q 6 Which part of avian digestive system helps in grinding of feed?

a) Esophagus b) Crop
c) Proventriculus d) **Gizard**

Q 7 How many caeca are present in poultry digestive system?

a) **2** b) 4

c) 1 d) 6

Q 8 Ptylin is a synonymous for ________

a) **Salivary amylase** b) Pancreatic amylase

c) Pancreatic lipase d) Enterokinas

Q 9 A week old chicks body contain about ______% water.

a) **85%** b) 75%

c) 65 % d) 55%

Q 10 Percentage of water in adult chicken body is ________

a) 85% b) 75%

c) 65 % d) **55%**

Q 11 The enzyme "ptylin" is absent in the saliva of ________

a) **Ruminants** b) Poultry

c) Pig d) All the above

Q 12 In new born calf, the largest part of stomach is ________

a) Rumen b) Reticulum

c) Omasum d) **Abomasum**

Q 13 In adult ruminant, the largest part of the stomach is ________

a) **Rumen** b) Reticulum

c) Omasum d) Abomasum

Q 14 The percentage share of rumen out of the total stomach in adult cow is ________

a) **80%** b) 8%

c) 55% d) 10%

Q 15 The smallest compartment of the stomach of adult ruminant is ________

a) Rumen b) **Reticulum**

c) Omasum d) Abomasums

Q 16 The percentage wise share of rumen-reticulum-omasum and abomasum in adult ruminant is __________

a) **80-5-8-7**
b) 80 -10-8-2
c) 8-5-7-80
d) 60-20-10-10

Q 17 The pH value of rumen is __________

a) 3-4
b) **6-7**
c) 5-6
d) 8-9

Q 18 Which of the gas is produced in highest amount during ruminal fermentation?

a) **CO_2**
b) CH_4
c) N_2
d) H_2

Q 19 The redox potential of reticulo-rumen is __________

a) **-350 mv (reduced)**
b) -350 mv (oxidized)
c) -100 mv (reduced)
d) -100 mv (oxidized)

Q 20 The most cranial part of ruminant stomach is __________

a) Rumen
b) **Reticulum**
c) Omasum
d) Abomasum

Q 21 "Paunch" is a synonymous term for which part of the ruminant stomach?

a) Rumen
b) Reticulum
c) Omasum
d) Abomasum

Q 22 "Honey comb" pattern is found in which compartment of ruminant stomach?

a) Rumen
b) **Reticulum**
c) Omasum
d) Abomasum

Q 23 "Many Plies" is a synonymous term for which part of the ruminant stomach?

a) Rumen
b) Reticulum
c) Omasum
d) Abomasum

Q 24 An adult cow stomach consists of how many compartments?

a) One
b) Two
c) Three
d) **Four**

Q 25 Among the four compartments of ruminant stomach, which one is the true stomach?

a) Rumen b) Reticulum

c) Omasum d) **Abomasum**

Q 26 Villi movement in Intestine is controlled by hormone _______

a) **Villikinin** b) Gastrin

c) Secretin d) Cholecystokinin

Q 27 In adult cow total volume of saliva secreted/day may range from __________

a) 50-80 litre b) **100-200 litre**

c) 300-400 litre d) 400-500 litre

Q 28 Which of the following is not the function of ruminant saliva?

a) Lubricant b) Surfactant

c) Buffering action d) **Digestion**

Q 29 The largest gland of the body __________

a) **Liver** b) Pancreas

c) Parotid d) Pituitary

Q 30 Which of the following animal does not have gall bladder?

a) **Horse** b) Pig

c) Dog d) Cow

Q 31 Which of the following cell produces HCl in the stomach?

a) Body chief cell b) Neck chief cell

c) **Parietal cell** d) G- cell

Q 32 Pepsinogen is secreted from the cell __________

a) **Body chief cell** b) Neck chief cell

c) Parietal cell d) G–cell

Q 33 Which of the following animal has largest intestine?

a) Cow b) Sheep

c) **Horse** d) Pig

Q 34 Which of the following animal has largest intestine (Small +Large)?

a) Cow b) Sheep
c) **Horse** d) Pig

Q 35 Enzyme "Ptylin" is not present in the saliva of __________

a) Cat b) Dog
c) Horse d) Ruminants
d) **All the above**

Q 36 On normal diet, which of the following Volatile fatty acid predominate in the rumen of cow?

a) **Acetic acid** b) Propionic acid
c) Lactic acid d) Butyric acid

Q 37 Which of the following Volatile Fatty Acid is glucogenic in nature?

a) Acetic acid b) **Propionic acid**
c) Valeric acid d) Butyric acid

Q 38 Which of the following Volatile Fatty Acid is ketogenic in nature?

a) Acetic acid b) Propionic acid
c) Lactic acid d) **Butyric acid**

Q 39 Approximately how much methane is formed after every 100g carbohydrate digested in the rumen?

a) **4.5g** b) 10 g
c) 15 g d) 20 g

Q 40 The acidic digesta that enter into duodenum from the pyloric part of the stomach is known as __________

a) **Chyme** b) Chyle
c) Chylomicron d) Emulsion

Q 41 Feeding the fibrous feed to ruminant animal favours the production of __________

a) **Acetic acid** b) Propionic acid
c) Butyric acid d) Valeric acid

Q 42 Volatile fatty acid produced in higher amount when highly fermentable carbohydrate or high concentrate diet is given to cow __________

a) Acetic acid
b) **Propionic acid**
c) Butyric acid
d) Valeric acid

Q 43 Accumulation of which acid in the rumen lead to condition of acidosis?

a) Acetic acid
b) **Lactic acid**
c) Butyric acid
d) Propionic acid

Q 44 The precursor of glucose needed for the synthesis of lactose in the udder, if the cow is __________

a) Acetic acid
b) **Propionic acid**
c) Butyric acid
d) Valeric acid

Q 45 Which of the following salivary glands of cow is unpaired?

a) Parotid
b) Submaxillary
c) Sublingual
d) **Labial gland**

Q 46 Which of the following salivary gland of ruminant is mucogenic in nature?

a) Parotid gland
b) Inferior molar gland
c) Buccal gland
d) **Submaxillary gland**

Q 47 In camel which of the following compartment of stomach is missing?

a) Rumen
b) Reticulum
c) **Omasum**
d) Abomasum

Q 48 Which of the following animal has three compartmented stomach?

a) Camel
b) Llama
c) Alpaca
d) **All the above**

Q 49 In which of the following animal, reticulum is glandular in nature?

a) **Camel**
b) Cow
c) Buffalo
d) Sheep

Q 50 The pH of ruminant saliva is __________

a) 3 b) 5

c) 7 d) **8**

Q 51 Among the various cations present in the rumen, which of the following is actively transported across the rumen wall?

a) Na^+ b) K^+

c) Ca^{+2} d) All the above

Q 52 Which of the following sugar is known as milk sugar?

a) Glucose b) Galactose

c) Sucrose d) **Lactose**

Q 53 Which of the following volatile fatty acid is related with quantity of milk produced?

a) Acetic acid b) **Propionic acid**

c) Butyric acid d) None of the above

Q 54 Which volatile fatty acid is mainly responsible for milk fat formation in cow?

a) **Acetic acid** b) Propionic acid

c) Butyric acid d) All the above

Q 55 Abomasum in ruminant is different from monogastric stomach in term of its secretion of __________

a) **Lysozyme** b) Hydrochloric acid

c) Pepsin d) Mucous

Q 56 Rumination is also known as __________

a) Cud chewing b) Reverse peristalsis

c) Controlled vomiting d) **All the above**

Q 57 The threshold size of particle in cattle to filter reticulo-omasal orifice lies in the range of __________

a) **3-5 mm** b) 10-15 mm

c) 15-20 mm d) 20-30 mm

Q 58 Which of the following animal is pseudoruminant?

a) **Camel** b) Goat

c) Pig d) Deer

Q 59 The site of microbial digestion in horse is ________

a) Small intestine b) **Large intestine**

c) Stomach d) Rumen

Q 60 Which of the following animal is more capable to utilize the fermentation product occurred in large intestine?

a) Horse b) Pig

c) **Rabbit** d) Poultry

Q 61 The chief prehensile organ in cattle is ________

a) Lips b) **Tongue**

c) Incisor d) Dental pad

Q 62 The chief prehensile organ in horse is ________

a) **Upper lip** b) Lower lip

c) Tongue d) Tongue

Q 63 Principle organ of prehension in pig is ________

a) Upper lip b) **Lower lip**

c) Tongue d) Snout

Q 64 In which of the following animal, percentage crude fibre digested is comparatively higher?

a) **Rabbit** b) Horse

c) Pig d) Dog

Q 65 Which of the following animal practised Caecophagy?

a) **Rabbit** b) Pig

c) Horse d) None of the above

Q 66 Which of the following hexose has the fastest rate of absorption?

a) **Galactose** b) Glucose

c) Fructose d) All have equal absorption

Q 67 Blood glucose level in ruminant is ________

a) **40-60 mg/100ml** b) 80-120 mg/100ml

c) 20-40 mg/dl d) 10-20 mg/dl

Q 68 In the ruminal gaseous portion, which of the following gas predominates the other?

a) **CO_2**
b) CH_4
c) H_2
d) SO_2

Q 69 Theoretically one gram of propionic acid is equal to how much of glucose?

a) 1 gm
b) **1.23 gm**
c) 3 gm
d) 3.23 gm

Q 70 Which of the following is true for rate of absorption from higher to lower?

a) **Tripeptide > Dipeptide > Amino acid**
b) Dipeptide > Tripeptide> Amino acid
c) Amino acid> Dipeptide> Tripeptide
d) Dipeptide> Amino acid > Tripeptide

Q 71 In urea supplemented diet, the N:S ratio should be________ foe effective utilization and microbial protein synthesis.

a) **10:1**
b) 1:10
c) 5:10
d) 10:5

Q 72 The recommended level of urea in the concentrate mixture as per BIS is __________

a) **1%**
b) 2%
c) 3%
d) 4%

Q 73 The term defaunation generally pertains to removal of __________ from the rumen.

a) Fungi
b) **Protozoa**
c) Archaea
d) Bacteriophages

Q 74 Amongst the rumen microbes, which one helps in maintaining the rumen buffer system?

a) Bacteria
b) **Protozoa**
c) Archaea
d) Bacteriophages

Q 75 Which of the following rumen microorganism is known as "Biological Knife"?

a) Bacteria b) Protozoa

c) Archaea d) **Fungi**

Q 76 Which among the following vitamin is synthesized by rumen microbes?

a) Vitamin A b) Vitamin D

c) **Vitamin K** d) Vitamin E

Q 77 Which of the following scientist reported the presence of fungi in the rumne for the first time?

a) **Orpin** b) Gruby & Delafond

c) Parker d) Vansoest

Q 78 Rumen protozoa were first identified by ________

a) Orpin b) **Gruby & Delafond**

c) Parker d) Vansoest

Q 79 Microbes in rumen capable of breaking lignocellulose bond is ________

a) Bacteria b) Protozoa

c) **Fungi** d) Archaea

Q 80 In rumen protease activity is maximum for ________

a) Bacteria b) **Protozoa**

c) Fungi d) Archaea

Q 81 Urea is poorly utilized, when added to concentrate containing more than ________

a) **18% CP** b) 16 % CP

c) 13 % CP d) 10 % CP

Q 82 Urea incorporation is not recommended in complete diet containing more than ________

a) **13 % CP** b) 16 % CP

c) 18 % CP d) 20 % CP

Q 83 " Pigeon milk" in Pigeon comes from which part of the digestive tract?

a) **Crop**
b) Proventriculus
c) Gizzard
d) Beak

Q 84 Oxygen needed to oxidize one gram of starch is __________

a) 0.83 Litre
b) 0.97 Litre
c) 0.56 Litre
d) 2.02 Litre

Q 85 Oxygen needed to oxidize one gram of protein is __________

a) 0.83 Litre
b) **0.97 Litre**
c) 0.56 Litre
d) 2.02 Litre

Q 86 Oxygen needed to oxidize one gram of fat is __________

a) 0.83 Litre
b) 0.97 Litre
c) 0.56 Litre
d) **2.02 Litre**

Q 87 Metabolic water formed, when one gram starch oxidized is __________

a) **0.56 g**
b) 0.40 g
c) 1.07 g
d) 0.83 g

Q 88 Metabolic water formed, when one gram protein oxidized is __________

a) 0.56 g
b) **0.40 g**
c) 1.07 g
d) 0.83 g

Q 89 Metabolic water formed, when one gram fat oxidized is __________

a) 0.56 g
b) 0.40 g
c) **1.07 g**
d) 0.83 g

Q 90 The generally accepted ratio of DMI : Water consumption in adult cattle is __________

a) **1 : 3.5**
b) 1:7.5
c) 1:1
d) 1:10

Q 91 The generally accepted ratio of DMI : Water consumption in sheep/goat is __________

a) **1:4**
b) 1:8
c) 1:1
d) 1:9

Q 92 The generally accepted ratio of DMI : Water consumption in poultry is ________

a) **1:2** b) 1:5
c) 1:7 d) 1:8

Q 93 DMI per unit body weight is higher in which of the following animal?

a) Sheep b) **Goat**
c) Cow d) Buffalo

Q 94 The functional unit of salivary gland is known as ________

a) **Salivon** b) Neuron
c) Nephron d) None of these

Q 95 The nature of saliva in ruminant is ________

a) Highly acidic b) Slightly acidic
c) Neutral d) **Distinctly alkaline**

Q 96 The enzyme "Lingual lipase" in young animal is secreted in which secretion of the GIT?

a) **Salivary** b) Gastric
c) Pancreatic d) Intestinal

Q 97 Which of the following animal is an example of foregut fermentor?

a) **Kangaroo** b) Horse
c) Zebra d) Rabbit

Q 98 Which of the following animal is colon fermentor?

a) Cow b) Rabbit
c) Marsupial d) **Horse**

Q 99 Which of the following animals are caecal fermentor?

a) Cow and buffaloes b) Horse and zebra
c) **Rabbit and hare** d) Kangaroo and hippopotamus

Q 100 The act of swallowing the food is known as ________

a) **Deglutition** b) Eating
c) Both of the above d) None of the above

Q 101 The portion of stomach where oesophagus open is known as __________

a) **Cardia** b) Fundic
c) Pyloric d) Oesophagial

Q 102 Cardiac spinctor is well developed in which animal?

a) Dog b) Cow
c) **Horse** d) Cat

Q 103 "Gastrin" is secreted by which gland?

a) Cardiac b) Fundic
c) **Pyloric** d) Intestinal

Q 104 Parietal cells are present in which gland?

a) Cardiac b) **Fundic**
c) Pyloric d) Intestinal

Q 105 Parietal cells are also known as __________

a) Body chief cell b) Neck chief cell
c) Peptic cell d) **Oxynitic cell**

Q 106 Peptic cells are also known as __________

a) **Body chief cell** b) Neck chief cell
c) Parietal cell d) Oxynitic cell

Q 107 HCL in stomach is secreted by which cells?

a) Body chief cells b) **Parietal cells**
c) Neck chief cells d) Peptic cells

Q 108 Intrinsic factor required for the absorption of vitamin B12 is secreted in which part of GIT?

a) Mouth b) **Stomach**
c) Small intestine d) Large intestine

Q 109 Which of the following hormone inhibit the gastric secretion?

a) Gastric inhibitory peptide b) Secretin
c) Cholecystokinin d) **All the above**

Q 110 The process of rumination consist of how many phases?

a) Two
b) Three
c) **Four ***
d) Five

*Regurgitation-remastication-reinsalivation-redeglutination

Q 111 Which of the following statement in context to rumination is wrong?

a) It increases the surface area for enzymatic digestion
b) It aids in buffering mechanism through saliva production
c) Rumination is proportional to fibre content of the feed
d) **On an average 4-8 hours rumination occur in horse**
e) The control centre for rumination is in medulla oblongata

Q 112 The yellow colour of faeces in human being is due to ________

a) Undigested feedstuff
b) Yellow pigment in feed
c) **Stercobilin**
d) All the above

Q 113 The greenish colour of bile is due to __________

a) Bile salt
b) **Bile pigment**
c) Both of the above
d) None of the above

Q 114 The chief site for absorption of end product of the digestion is __________

a) Stomach
b) **Small intestine**
c) Large Intestine
d) Rectum

Q 115 Pepsinogen is converted into its active form "pepsin" by ______

a) **HCl**
b) Mucous
c) Presence of food
d) Gastrin

Q 116 Gastric mucosa is protected from the action of HCL secreted in the stomach by __________

a) **Mucous**
b) Pepsin
c) Gastrin
d) Salivary amylase

Q 117 The conversion of trypsinogen to trypsin is done by __________

a) **Cholecystokinin** b) Secretin
c) Enterokinase d) Motilin

Q 118 The collagen of meat is mainly digested by __________

a) **Pepsin** b) Trypsin
c) Chymotrypsin d) Elastase

Q 119 Brunner's Gland are present in __________

a) **Small intestine** b) Large intestine
c) Pancreas d) Liver

Q 120 Emulsification of fat occur with the help of __________

a) **Bile salt** b) Bile pigment
c) Both of these d) None of these

Q 121 Cholerectic are substances which __________

a) **Increase bile flow**
b) Decrease bile flow
c) Increase cholesterol formation
d) Decrease cholesterol formation

Q 122 Pancreozymin is also known as __________

a) **Cholecystokinin** b) Secretin
c) Enterokinase d) Motilin

Q 123 Which of the following enzyme involved in luminal phase of digestion?

a) **Amylase** b) Maltase
c) Lactase d) Sucrase

Q 124 Which of the following is not correctly matched?

a) Rumen – papillae b) Omasum- muscular fold
c) Small intestine- villi d) **Large intestine- papillae**

Q 125 Reticulum is also known as __________

a) **Water bag** b) Paunch
c) Manyplies d) True stomach

Q 126 The term "fermentation vat" is given to __________

a) **Rumen** b) Reticulum

c) Omasum d) Abomasum

Q 127 On high concentrate diet, which pathway predominates for propionic acid formation?

a) **Acrylic pathway** b) Succinate pathway

b) Both are equal d) None of these

Q 128 Which pathway predominates for propionic acid formation when cow are kept on fibrous diet?

a) Acrylic pathway b) **Succinate pathway**

b) Both are equal d) None of these

Q 129 Which of the following compartment of ruminant stomach entrapped the irony material?

a) Rumen b) **Reticulum**

c) Omasum d) Abomasum

Q 130 Weight of regurgitated bolus in adult cow lies in the range of __________

a) **90-120 gm** b) 20-30 gm

c) 300-400 gm d) 400-500 gm

Q 131 How many chewing normally occur before the cud is re-swallowed in the cow on normal diet?

a) **50-70** b) 150-200

c) 5-10 d) More than 200

Q 132 The molar proportion of three volatile fatty acid (Acetate: propionate: butyrate) formed in the rumen of cow fed on normal diet __________

a) **7:2:1** b) 5:4:1

c) 2:7:1 d) 4:5:1

Q 133 Total volatile fatty acid concentration in rumen lies in the range of __________

a) **5-15 mg/litre** b) 30-40 mg/litre

c) 50-70 mg/litre d) 80-100 mg/litre

Q 134 Which pathways are employed for the production of propionate, when cow diet consist mainly of fibrous roughage?

a) Acrylate pathways
b) **Succinate pathways**
c) Acrylate pathways
d) None of these

Q 135 Approximately how much energy requirement of ruminants are met by volatile fatty acids?

a) 10-20 %
b) 20-30 %
c) **60-70 %**
d) 100 %

Q 136 In rumen certain branched chain fatty acid are also formed by deamination of amino acids, match the correct sequence _____

A Isobutyric acid — i) Valine
B Valeric acid — ii) Isoleucine
C 2 methyl butyric acid — iii) Proline
D 3-methyl butyric acid — iv) Leucine

a) **A-i,B-iii, C-ii,D-iv**
b) A-iv,B-iii,C-ii,D-i
c) A-ii,B-iv,C-i,D-iii
d) A-iii,B-ii,C-iv,D-i

Q 137 Total weight of volatile fatty acid produced in cow per day is around __________

a) **4 kg**
b) 1 kg
c) 10 kg
d) 8 kg

Q 138 Ruminant animal loses how much food energy as methane?

a) **7%**
b) 10%
c) 2 %
d) > 10%

Q 139 Quick fermentation pattern in rumen inhibit the __________

a) **Cellulose digestion organism**
b) Methanogens
c) Lipid degrader
d) Starch digesting organism

Q 140 How much microbial protein is formed in the rumen on digestion of one Kilogram organic matter?

a) **200 g**
b) 50 g
c) 500 g
d) 750 g

Q 141 The concentration of ammonical nitrogen required in rumen liquor for the optimum growth of rumen bacteria is around __________

a) **2-5 mg NH_3-N/100 ml of rumen liquor**

b) 10-15mg NH_3-N/100 ml of rumen liquor

c) 20-30 mg NH_3-N/100 ml of rumen liquor

d) 40-50 mg NH_3-N/100 ml of rumen liquor

Q 142 Which of the following rumen inhabitator lock up the microbial protein in rumen?

a) Bactria b) **Protozoa**

c) Fungi d) Archaea

Q 143 The number of bacteria in rumen is __________

a) **10^{10}/ml of rumen liquor** b) 10^{5}/ml of rumen liquor

c) 10^{4}/ml of rumen liquor d) 10^{2}/ml of rumen liquor

Q 144 The number of protozoa in rumen is __________

a) 10^{10}/ml of rumen liquor b) **10^{5}/ml of rumen liquor**

c) 10^{8}/ml of rumen liquor d) 10^{2}/ml of rumen liquor

Q 145 Which of the following statement is wrong regarding rumen microorganism?

a) Protozoa number is less than the bacteria

b) Protozoa are bacteria are equal in total mass

c) **Bacteria check the population of protozoa by engulfing them**

d) Protozoa lock up the microbial protein in rumen

Q 146 Which of the following rumen microorganism has the tendency to remain in rumen?

a) Bacteria b) **Protozoa**

c) Fungi d) None of these

Q 147 The first organism presume to invade and commence degrading the structural plant component in rumen is __________

a) Protozoa b) **Fungi**

c) Bacteria d) Bacteriophage

Q 148 Which of the following Volatile fatty acid provides the energy to rumen wall?

a) Acetic acid
b) Propionic Acid
c) **Butyric acid**
d) Lactic acid

Q 149 Which of the following organism in rumen has the highest cellulytic activity?

a) **Neocallimastrix**
b) Piromyces
c) Orpinomyces
d) Spheromonas

Q 150 The major Ketone body is __________

a) **Beta hydroxyl acid**
b) Aceto acetic acid
c) Acetate
d) All are equal

Q 151 In starving animals catabolism of body reserve occur in following order (first to last) __________

a) **Glycogen-Fat-Protein**
b) Fat-Glycogen-Protein
c) Protein-Fat-Glycogen
d) Protein-Glycogen-Fat

Q 152 Which of the following has the higher gross energy?

a) Glucose
b) Cellulose
c) Casein
d) **Fat**

Q 153 Amongst the volatile fatty acids, which one has the highest gross energy value?

a) Acetic acid
b) Propionic acid
c) **Butyric acid**
d) All have the same

Q 154 Which of the following has the highest gross energy value?

a) Carbohydrate
b) Protein
c) Fat
d) **Methane**

Q 155 Which of the following poultry birds does not have crop in its digestive system?

a) Quail
b) Turkey
c) Chick
d) **Emu**

Q 156 Which of the following has the highest dressing percentage?

a) Quail b) **Turkey**

c) Chick d) Emu

Q 157 The largest and most variable loss of consumed energy is in the __________

a) Gaseous eructation b) Urine

c) **Faeces** d) Bile

Q 158 Water in undigested food is digested in __________

a) Stomach b) Small intestine

c) **Large intestine** d) None of these

Q 159 Fat is completely digested in __________

a) Stomach b) Mouth

c) **Small intestine** d) Large intestine

Q 160 Which of the following causes contraction of gall bladder?

a) Secretin b) Gastrin

c) **CCK** d) Enterogastrin

Q 161 Which element is necessary for maintenance of teeth and is generally present in almost all toothpaste?

a) Zn b) Cu

c) **F** d) Mn

Q 162 Substances that give green colour to bile is __________

a) Chlorophyll b) Urochrome from liver

c) **Breakdown product of Hb** d) Urea

Q 163 Stomach of camel does not have __________

a) Rumen b) Reticulum

c) **Omasum** d) Abomasum

Q 164 The digestion by amylase is completed in the __________

a) Mouth b) **Duodenum**

c) Ileum d) Stomach

Q 165 Which of the following prevents the stomach from self digesting?

a) **Mucous** b) Acid

c) Enzymes d) Hormones

Q 166 Which of the following animal is alloenzymatic digester?

a) Pig b) Human

c) Chicken d) **Cow**

Q 167 Which of the following animal is autoenzymatic digester?

a) Sheep b) Cow

c) Deer d) **Chicken**

Q 168 Which of the following is not the category of Hofmann,s ruminant classification system?

a) Concentrate selector (Browsers)

b) Bulk & roughage eater (Grazer)

c) **Specialist feeder**

d) Intermediate feeder

Q 169 Which of the following is not an example of non-ruminant foregut fermentor?

a) Kangaroo b) Hippopotamus

c) Wallaby d) **Moose**

Q 170 Which of the following avian species is caecal fermenter (with enlarged caeca)?

a) Domesticated fowl b) Quails

c) Turkey d) **Ostrich**

Q 171 White substances visible in birds excreta is __________

a) Urea b) **Uric acid**

c) Ammonium Sulphate d) Ornithine

Q 172 Which is the highest energy level you could achieve in a diet?

a) **8500kcal/kg*** b) 11000kcal/kg

c) 12000kcal/kg d) 15000kcal/kg

* The highest energy concentration of any feed stuff is pure fat which contain 9000kcal/kg, so it is impossible to formulate a diet more than this energy.Moreover only fat diet will not be a balanced one.

Q 173 Which of the following animal has the largest small intestine?

a) Cow b) **Horse**

c) Goat d) Dog

Q 174 Which animal has the largest large intestine?

a) Cow b) **Horse**

c) Pig d) Dog

Q 175 Which of the following animal has the largest caeca?

a) Cow b) **Horse**

c) Pig d) Dog

Q 176 Intestine: body length ratio is the highest in __________

a) Cow b) **Goat**

c) Horse d) Dog

Q 177 In ruminants daily saliva production does not depend upon __________

a) Chewing time b) **Rumen acidity**

c) Level of fibre in diet d) Fibre particle size

Q 178 The largest segment of digestive tract of a dog is __________

a) Oesophagus b) **Stomach**

c) Small intestine d) Large intestine

Q 179 The total number of jaw movement/day in cow ruminating an adequate amount of time is estimated to be at least ______

a) 10,000 b) 20,000

c) **40,000** d) 80,000

Q 180 Which of the following is not included in fore-stomach?

a) Rumen b) Reticulum

c) Omasum d) **Abomasum**

Q 181 Buffering capacity of forages is __________

a) Ability to stimulate the cow to produce buffer

b) **Ability of the forages to resist change in pH**

c) Amount of acids relative to protein present in the fermented forages

d) Forages do not have buffering capacity

Q 182 Which of the following feed nutrient fraction is essentially not utilized by rumen bacteria for growth?

a) **Fat** b) Protein

c) Starch d) Cellulose

Q183 The enzymes that can break down cellulose and other sugar locked in plant cell wall are secreted by __________

a) Abomasum

b) Ruminal Wall

c) Pancreas

d) **Rumen & Intestine microbes**

Q 184 Main gases produced by rumen fermentation are __________

a) NH_3& CO_2 b) N_2 and CH_4

c) CH_4& H_2S d) **CH_4& CO_2**

Q 185 Which of the following animal is not a ruminant?

a) Cow b) **Elephant**

c) Giraffe d) Deer

Q186 Which of the following is likely to have the largest digestive tract?

a) **Herbivore** b) Carnivore

c) Omnivore d) Can be any of these

Q 187 The small intestine is the primary site for absorption for which of the following product of digestion in cow?

a) Ammonia and VFA's

b) **Fatty acids & amino acids**

c) VFA's & Fatty acids

d) Ammonia and amino acids

Q 188 The correct sequential order of the small intestine segment is __________

a) Duodenum, Caecum and Jejunum

b) Caecum, Jejunum and Ileum

c) Caecum, Ileum and Jejunum

d) **Duodenum, Ileum and Jejunum**

Q 189 The bicarbonate secreted into the digestive tract of a cow comes from __________

a) Microbes and pancreas

b) Liver and gall bladder

c) Rumen & salivary glands

d) **Salivary glands & pancreas***

* Salivary glands produces saliva having bicarbonate to neutralize the acid produced in rumen, while pancreas produced bicarbonate to neutralize the acid produced in the abomasums.

Q 190 The optimal pH range of pancreatic enzymes is __________

a) 1.5-2.5 b) 3.0-4.0

c) 4.0-5.0 d) **5.0-6.0**

Q 191 Which area of rumen wall has the highest density of papillae?

a) Dorsal b) Anterior

c) Posterior d) **Ventral**

Q 192 What is the primary energy source for ruminants?

a) Glucose b) Protein

c) Lactate d) **VFA's**

Q 193 In ruminants, what digestive structure is the blind sac?

a) **Caecum** b) Rectum

c) Colon d) Jejunum

Q 194 Which of the following animal has the simplest and shortest digestive tract (in relation to body size)?

a) Rabbit b) **Dog**

c) Sheep d) Human

Q 195 Feeding through nasogastric tube is a type of __________

a) **Enteral nutrition** b) Parenteral nutrition

c) Both of these d) None of these

Q 196 When solution containing water, carbohydrates, protein, fat, electrolytes, vitamin and minerals is injected through intravenous route for sustaining the body, it is known as _____

a) Enteral nutrition b) **Parenteral nutrition**
c) Both of these d) None of these

Q 197 When nutrients are supplied in excess of those required for maintenance through parenteral route, it is known as ______

a) **Hyperalimentation** b) Thrombophlebitis
c) Both of these d) None of these

Q 198 Peg teeth(incisor) are present in __________

a) Cow b) Dog
c) Swine d) **Rabbit**

Q 199 Rabbit is a __________

a) Herbivores & foregut fermentor
b) **Herbovores & hindgut fermentor**
c) Omnivores & foregut fermentor
d) Omnivores & hindgut fermentor

Q 200 Caecotropes (soft pellet) is voided from the rabbit body after approximately ____ hours after consumption of meal _______

a) 4 b) **8**
c) 12 d) 15

Q 201 The practices of consuming own faeces by rabbit for better utilization of nutrients is known as __________

a) Coprophagy b) Caecotrophy
c) **Both of these** d) None of these

Q 202 Which of the following is the largest organ in the digestive tract of mature rabbit?

a) **Caecum/colon** b) Small intestine
c) Stomach d) Oesophagus

Q 203 In ruminants lysoenzymes(enzymes that rupture the bacterial cell wall) is produced in the abomasums, while in rabbit it is produced in the __________

a) Stomach b) **Colon**
c) Caecum d) Ileum

Q 204 Fermentative chamber in rabbit is ________

a) Rumen | b) Colon
c) **Caecum** | d) Ileum

Q 205 As compared to rumen Volatile fatty acids (VFA's) pattern (acetic acid, propionic acid and butyric acid on normal diet) the VFA's pattern in rabbit is ________

a) Acetic acid, propionic acid and butyric acid
b) Butyric acid, acetic acid and propionic acid
c) **Acetic acid, butyric acid and propionic acid**
d) Propionic acid,acetic acid and butyric acid

Q 206 Which of the following organ is absent in duck digestive tract?

a) Oesophagus | b) **Crop**
c) Gizzard | d) Proventriculus

Q 207 Which of the following part of cow intestine is similar to our appendix?

a) **Caecum** | b) Colon
c) Ileum | d) Rectum

Q 208 Which of the following cereal grain feeding poses a greater risk of acidosis then others?

a) **Wheat*** | b) Barley
c) Sorghum | d) Corn

* Wheat has high starch content and is highly (app 60%) rumen digestible.

Q 209 Which of the following cereal grain feeding poses least risk of acidosis?

a) Wheat | b) Barley
c) Triticale | d) **Corn***

* Corn and sorghum have lower rumen digestibility (about 30%)

Q 210 Main function of omasum is ________

a) Fermentation | b) **Water absorption**
c) Nutrient absorption | d) Retention of foreign bodies

Q 211 Which of the following does not cause closure of oesophageal groove in cattle?

a) Suckling b) **Copper sulphate***

c) Sodium bicarbonate d) Both b & c

* Copper sulphate work in sheep but not in cattle due to unknown reason

Q 212 The source of rennet required for cheese making is ________

a) A plant b) Sugar beet

c) Insect larvae d) **The abomasums of a milk fed calf**

Q 213 Fats are broken down in which part of the cow digestive system?

a) Rumen b) Pancreas

c) **Small intestine** d) Large intestine

Q 214 Which of the following has buffering action in the rumen?

a) Rumen protozoa b) Saliva

c) Sodium bicarbonate d) **All of these**

Q 215 Rumination starts after ________ hour of ingesting the feed.

a) 5-6 hours b) 8-10 hours

c) Immediately after eating d) **0.5 to 1.5 hours**

Q 216 The cycle of rumination involves how many parts?

a) 1 b) 2

c) 3 d) **4**

Q 217 Which of the following is not a part of rumination cycle*?

a) **Eating (Intake)** b) Regurgitation

c) Chewing d) Salivation

* Rumination cycle: regurgitation, chewing, salivation and swallowing

Q 218 A concentrated form of energy' and 'increases the energy density of the diet so a smaller quantity of food is required'. Which one of the following nutrients is best described by the characteristics above?

a) **Fat** b) Fibre

c) Starch d) Protein

Q 219 The primary acid formed in the abomasums is ________

a) Propionic acid
b) Acetic acid
c) Butyric acid
d) **Hydrochloric acid**

Q 220 The first organ to receive blood from small intestine ________

a) Heart
b) **Liver**
c) Lungs
d) Kidney

Q 221 The most limiting nutrient for a high producing cow is ______

a) Protein
b) Vitamin A
c) **Energy**
d) Calcium

Q 222 Caecotrophy in rabbit starts in the age of ________

a) **3-4 weeks**
b) 5-10 weeks
c) 10-15 weeks
d) 15-20 weeks

Q 223 In rabbit, digestion starts in ________

a) **Mouth**
b) Stomach
c) Small Intestine
d) Caecum

Q 224 The largest part of GIT in rabbit is ________

a) Oesophagus
b) Stomach
c) Caecum
d) Large Intestine

Q 225 Caecum in rabbit constitute about ________________ % of the total volume of GIT.

a) 10-20%
b) 20-30%
c) 5-10%
d) **40-60%**

Q 226 In rabbit, VFA production pattern is ________

a) **Acetic acid > Butyric acid > Propionic acid**
b) Acetic acid > Propionic acid < Butyric acid
c) Propionic acid > Butyric acid > Acetic acid
d) Butyric acid >Acetic acid > Propionic acid

Q 227 The structure "Fusus Coli" is present in the GIT of which animal?

a) Horse
b) Pig
c) **Rabbit**
d) Cow

Q 228 Stomcah oil or milk oil is present in the stomach of ________

a) Horse b) **Rabbit**
c) Pig d) Goat

Q 229 Which of the following animals is the caudal fermentor?

a) Cattle b) Sheep
c) Deer d) **Rabbit**

Q 230 Which of the following is the function of bile?

a) Lower surface tension b) Emulsification of fat
c) Neutralization of acid d) **All the above**

Q 231 Which of the following animal has pioneer role in the discovery of Insulin?

a) **Dog** b) Rat
c) Guinea Pig d) Calf

Q 232 Salivary amylase is absent in saliva of __________

a) **Dog** b) Man
c) Cow d) Both a & b

Q 233 Study on which animal firstly showed that lymph was channel by which fat passed from the intestinal walls into blood?

a) **Dog** b) Horse
c) Man d) Rat

Q 234 Which of the following vitamins is synthesized in dog body?

a) **C** b) A
c) D d) E

Q 235 Absorption of most nutrients occur predominately in _______

a) **Jejunum** b) Ileum
c) Duodenum d) Caecum

Q 236 Absorption of immunoglobulin from clostrum in new born mammals through pinocytosis occur mainly in __________

a) **Ileum** b) Jejunum
c) Duodenum d) Caecum

Q 237 Which of the following is an example of anatagonism?

a) Zn-Cu
b) Ca-Zn
c) Ca-Fe
d) **All the above**

* Other examples are Fe-Cu, Zn-Fe, Ca-P, Lysine-arginine

Q 238 What kind of relationship do cattle and rumen microflora share?

a) Electrostatic
b) Parasitic
c) A-Biotic
d) **Symbiotic**

Q 239 What acid is formed when non-structural carbohydrates are digested in the rumen?

a) Lactic acid
b) Citric acid
c) Acetic acid
d) **Propionic acid**

Q 240 The prehensile organ of the horse is __________

a) Tongue
b) **Upper lip**
c) Lower lip
d) Teeth

Q 241 The average saliva secreted in a horse fed normally is ________

a) 100-150 litre
b) **10-15 litre**
c) 40-50 litre
d) 50-75 litre

Q 242 In which part of the equine digestive system, protein and soluble carbohydrate are mainly digested?

a) Caecum
b) Stomach
c) Large intestine
d) **Small intestine**

Q 243 In horse, which of the following mineral is lost in greater amount in sweat?

a) Na
b) K
c) **Cl**
d) Ca

Q 244 Which of the following animal is less efficient in digesting forages?

a) Cow
b) Buffalo
c) Goat
d) **Horse**

Q 245 "Margo plicatus" structure is found in which animal?

a) Dog
b) Cow
c) Pig
d) **Horse**

Q 246 The junction between glandular and non-glandular stomach of horse is known as ________

a) Saccus caecus
b) **Margo plicatus**
c) Saccus entericus
d) None of the above

Q 247 The largest gland in horse body is ________

a) **Liver**
b) Pancreas
c) Margo plicatus
d) Brunner gland

Q 248 Which of the following is not a macromolecule in living organism?

a) Protein
b) Nucleic acid
c) Polysaccharide
d) **Amino acid**

Q 249 Protein constitutes about ________________ % of the horse body.

a) 10%
b) **18%**
c) 40%
d) 2%

Q 250 Number of essential amino acids required for foal is ________

a) **10**
b) 12
c) 13
d) 7

Q 251 Equine motor neuron disease (EMND) occur due to deficiency of ________

a) Vitamin A
b) **Vitamin E**
c) Vitamin C
d) Vitamin D

Q 252 Equine degenerative myeloencephalopathy (EDM) occur due to deficiency of ________

a) Vitamin A
b) **Vitamin E**
c) Vitamin C
d) Vitamin D

Q 253 The ideal Ca: P ratio for horse is ________

a) 1:1
b) **1.5:1**
c) 3:1
d) 1:2

Q 254 A deficiency or excess of which mineral leads to similar symptoms?

a) Se b) Fe

c) **I** d) Zn

Q 255 The latest NRC edition for horse nutrient requirement was ___

a) **NRC 2007** b) NRC 2010

c) NRC 2001 d) NRC 1992

Q 256 Horse caecum has a capacity of __________

a) **25-35 litre** b) 10-15 litre

c) 100-150 litre d) 80-100 litre

Q 257 Crushed or cracked feed that has been cooked prior to the extrusion process is known as __________

a) **Kibbling** b) Quidding

c) Crumbling d) Middlings

Q 258 Byproduct of the flour milling process that is graded according to the proportion of bran, germ and endosperm is known as __________

a) Kibbling b) Quidding

c) Crumbling d) **Middlings**

Q 259 The dropping of small amount of feed from the horse mouth during chewing (most often as a result of sharp teeth or damage to mouth or tongue) is known as __________

a) **Quidding** b) Kibbling

c) Crib bitting d) Voiding

Q 260 Gall bladder is absent in __________

a) Dog b) Pig

c) Cat d) **Horse**

Q 261 The most popular grain for horse is __________

a) **Oat** b) Corn

c) Sorghum d) Wheat

Q 262 The most common protein supplement for horse is ________

a) **Soyabean meal**
b) Cottonseed meal
c) Peanut meal
d) Maize gluten meal

Q 263 Which is the longest part of the horse digestive system?

a) Large intestine
b) Caecum
c) **Small intestine**
d) Oesophagus

Q 264 Which of the following nutrient is a concentrated form of energy and is used in small quantity to increase the energy density of the diet?

a) **Fat**
b) Starch
c) Protein
d) Minerals

Q 265 Compared to other farm animals, stomach of a horse is ________ in size.

a) Large
b) **Smaller**
c) Relatively same
d) Can be larger or smaller

Q 266 The stomach of the horse make up ________ % of the entire digestive tract.

a) **10**
b) 40
c) 30
d) 60

Q 267 Small intestine of the horse make up ____________% of the entire digestive tract.

a) 10
b) 60
c) **30**
d) 75

Q 268 In the horse ,________________ is the primary site for water absorption.

a) Stomach
b) **Caecum**
c) Small intestine
d) Rectum

Q 269 Nutritional secondary hyperparathyroidism (NSH) in equine is also known as __________

a) Bran disease
b) Millers disease
c) Fibrous osteodystrophy
d) **All the above**

Q 270 Excessive feeding of bran coupled with high oxalate content in the feed of horse can lead to __________

a) Tying up
b) Laminitis
c) **Big head disease**
d) None of these

Q 271 Which of the following animal has more lactose in her milk?

a) Cow
b) Goat
c) Sheep
d) **Mare**

Q 272 Which of the following is not an example of fructans?

a) Inulins
b) Levans
c) Graminan
d) **Galactans**

Q 273 Which of the following straw is generally used for horse feeding?

a) Wheat straw
b) **Oat straw**
c) Rice straw
d) Rye straw

Q 274 The most palatable of all the straw is __________

a) Wheat straw
b) **Oat straw**
c) Rice straw
d) Rye straw

Q 275 Foregut in horse does not include __________

a) Mouth
b) Stomach
c) Small intestine
d) **Caecum**

Q 276 Tick the wrong statement __________

a) Caecum is fully functional in horse at about 2 years of age
b) **Crude fibre is more digestible in horse as compared to ruminants**
c) Gall bladder is absent in horse
d) Caecal fermentation is not as efficient as rumen fermentation

Q 277 Water required per Kg of DMI in horse is __________

a) 5-10 litre
b) 0.5-1.0 litre
c) **2-4 litre**
d) 10-15 litre

Q 278 The most expensive nutrient in horse ration is __________

a) **Protein**
b) Carbohydrate
c) Fat
d) Minerals

Q 279 Feed required by commercial broilers to produce 1 kg of broiler meat is __________

a) 3-4 kg
b) 4-5 kg
c) 0.5- 1.0 kg
d) **1.8- 2.0 kg**

Q 280 Feed required by laying pullet to produce 1 kg of eggs is _____

a) 1-1.5 kg
b) **2.5- 3.0 kg**
c) 0.5-1 kg
d) 4-5.5 kg

Q 281 Which state is known as egg basket of India?

a) Punjab
b) Haryana
c) **A.P.**
d) Maharashtra

Q 282 Drum sticks are the common name of chicken __________

a) **Legs**
b) Ribs
c) Both legs and ribs
d) Claws

Q 283 Crude protein content of dried swine excreta __________

a) 35%
b) 43.88%
c) **18%**
d) 5%

Q 284 Crude protein content in poultry manure (dried poultry dropping) is __________

a) 15%
b) 10%
c) 45%
d) **24%**

Q 285 Which of the following intestinal parameter can not be related with better performance of birds?

a) High villus height (VH)
b) **Larger crypt depth**
c) Thin intestinal wall
d) High villus height: crypt depth ratio

Q 286 Generally maize constitutes how much __________ percentage of broiler/layer feed?

a) **50-60%**
b) 30-35%
c) 20-30%
d) 70-80%

Q 287 Which of the following is an example of protective food*?

a) Milk
b) Eggs
c) Fruits
d) **All the above**

* Protective food are so called because of there ability to balance diets commonly over rich in starch, sugars and fat and all too frequently lacking in balanced protein, minerals and vitamins.

Q 288 Egg is deficient in _________

a) Vitamin A
b) Vitamin D
c) Riboflavin
d) **Vitamin C.**

Q 289 Practically all the Fe content in the egg is localized in _______

a) Albumin
b) **Yolk**
c) Equally distributed
d) Egg don't have any Fe in it

Q 290 Tick the right statement _________

a) **There is no air cell in an egg at the moment it is laid**
b) Air cell is usually at pointed end
c) Air cell size remain the same from laying to until it is broken
d) Air cell is formed from the expired air of chick embryo

Q 291 Which of the following is not a part of egg shell?

a) Mammillary layer
b) Spongy layer
c) Pores
d) **Air cell**

Q 292 Germ spot is present in _________

a) **Every egg**
b) Fertile egg only
c) Brown egg only
d) Albumin of the egg

Q 293 The mean percentage of shell and edible content of the egg is __________

a) 57 & 32
b) **11 & 89**
c) 60 & 40
d) 29 & 71

Q 294 The average percentage of shell, albumin and yolk in normal egg is _________

a) **11, 57 & 32**
b) 57, 11 & 32
c) 32, 11 & 57
d) 57, 32 & 11

Q 295 The average percentage of protein in whole egg is ________

a) 5% b) **12%**

c) 22% d) 32%

Q 296 The average per cent fat content in whole egg is ________

a) 5% b) 20%

c) **10%** d) 17%

Q 297 The per cent water content in whole egg is ________

a) 25.5% b) 35.5%

c) 55.5% d) **65.5%**

Q 298 Which of the following egg part contain higher per cent protein content?

a) Egg white b) **Egg yolk**

c) Both have equal d) Egg shell

Q 299 Which of the following egg part contain higher fat percentage?

a) Shell membrane b) Shell

c) Egg white d) **Egg yolk**

Q 300 Peewee size of the egg refer to ________

a) Extra large size b) Large egg

c) Medium egg d) **Smaller egg**

Q 301 Haugh unit values ranges from ________

a) 0-50 b) **0-110**

c) 0-100 d) 0-140

Q 302 Barley can be added to poultry ration upto ________

a) 40 b) 35

c) **15** d) 50

Q 303 Oat should not constitute more than ________ % of the poultry ration.

a) 40 b) 50

c) **20** d) 60

Q 304 Maize can be incorporated in poultry ration upto __________

a) 20% b) 30%

c) 40% d) **60%**

Q 305 Fletcher scale is used to determine the __________

a) **Yolk colour** b) Yolk quantity

c) Yolk thickness d) All the above

Q 306 Freshly laid egg has a pH of __________

a) **7.6** b) 6.0

c) 5.4 d) 4.5

Q 307 Storing the egg for long time makes its content __________

a) **More alkaline** b) More acidic

c) Neutral d) Depends upon composition of egg

Q 308 Storage of egg for longer period leads to __________

a) **Increase in yolk size** b) Decrease in yolk size

c) No change in yolk sac d) Can increase or decrease

Q 309 Dried poultry litter can be included in the ration of layer at a level of

a) **5-10%** b) 20-25%

c) 12-18% d) 26-28%

Q 310 Rice Polish in poultry ration can be used upto __________%.

a) 10 b) 20

c) 30 d) **50**

Q 311 Which of the following is not a very palatable feedstuff for poultry?

a) Maize b) Rice

c) **Barley** d) Wheat

Q 312 Ground nut meal can be incorporated into poultry ration upto __________ extent.

a) 10% b) 15%

c) 25% d) **35%**

Q 313 The maximum level of mustard meal to be used in poultry ration is __________

a) 20 b) **10**

c) 25 d) 35

Q 314 Blood meal is deficient in __________

a) Arginine b) Lysine

c) **Methionine** d) All the above

Q 315 Phosphorus content of the meat meal should be less than _____

a) 10% b) **4.4 %** *

c) 15% d) 20 %

* If phosphorus content is more than 4.4,then this meat meal should be classed as meat and bone scrap.

Q 316 Blood meal can be incorporated in the poultry ration upto ____

a) 20% b) 25%

c) **10%** d) 35%

Q 317 Magnesium content in limestone should be less than __________

a) 10% b) 15%

c) **5%*** d) 20%

* Limestone's that contain more amount of magnesium are known as Dolomites.

Q 318 One pound is equal to __________

a) **454 gm** b) 28.35 gm

c) 353 gm d) 284 gm

Q 319 One ounce is equal to __________

a) 454 gm b) **28.35 gm**

c) 353 gm d) 284 gm

Q 320 First limiting amino acid in poultry ration is __________

a) **Methionine** b) Lysine

c) Arginine d) Isoleucine

Q 321 In broiler farming, total feed consumed/ total body weight gives the ________

a) Feed efficiency b) Feed conversion efficiency

c) Feed conversion ratio d) **All the above**

Q 322 Formula for protein efficiency ratio is ________

a) Feed intake (g)/ body weight gain (g)

b) **Body weight gain (g)/ total protein consumed (g)**

c) Total protein consumed (g)/ body weight gain (g)

d) Total protein intake (g)/ feed efficiency

Q 323 Tick the wrong statement ________

a) **Higher value of FCR (>2) is desirable**

b) Higher value of BCR(>1) indicates profitability

c) Lower value of FCR indicates better feed efficiency

d) If BCR =1, it indicates no profit no loss

Q 324 Major site of action of pepsinogen in poultry is ________

a) Crop b) **Proventriculus**

c) Gizzard d) Caeca

Q 325 Which of the following cereal grain has the highest amount of metabolisable energy (ME)?

a) **Maize** b) Sorghum

c) Wheat d) Rice

Q 326 Laboratory analysis of a feed ingredient show 13% protein, 13% fat and 13 % fibre, which of the following ingredient it is?

a) Wheat bran b) **Rice bran**

c) Broken rice d) Millet

Q 327 Soyabean meal is deficient in ________

a) Lysine b) Tryptophan

c) Threonine d) **Methionine**

Q 328 In NaCl, the percentage of Na and Cl is ________

a) **39 & 60%** b) 60 & 39%

c) 70 and 30% d) 80 and 20%

Q 329 Calorie protein ratio in broiler starter feed should be (as per BIS 1992) __________

a) 156 b) **122**

c) 170 d) 100

Q 330 Calorie protein ratio in broiler finisher feed should be _______

a) 156 b) **145**

c) 170 d) 180

Q 331 The word "pullet" is used for female of __________

a) **Chicken** b) Turkey

c) Duck d) Quail

Q 332 The calcium content in the plasma of laying hens is around __________

a) 80-120 mg/l b) 150-200mg/l

c) **300-400 mg/l** d) 50-80 mg/l

Q 333 In egg which of the trace minerals is present in greater amount than the others?

a) **Iron** b) Copper

c) Zinc d) Iodine

Q 334 In birds, the main end product of protein metabolism are ____

a) Urea b) **Uric acid**

c) Allantoin d) Creatinine

Q 335 Non-ruminant, omnivorous, animal having a complex foregut and a reletively simple intestine tract is __________

a) Pig b) **Poultry**

c) Cow d) Rabbit

Q 336 An oesophageal out pocketing present in most of the birds is __________

a) **Crop** b) Gizzard

c) Proventriculus d) Pancreas

Interesting Knowledge

Whale, horse, zebra, rat, dear, mouse, rhinoceros, giraffe, camel, elephant, pigeon and dove do not have gall bladder.

❑❑❑

Chapter 13

Experimental Nutrition

Q 1 Proximate system of analysis is also known as __________

a) Van soest system of analysis

b) **Weende system of analysis**

c) Both a & b

d) None of these

Q 2 The scheme of "proximate analysis" was devised by ________

a) **Henneberg & Stohmann**

b) Crampton & Maynard

c) Vansoest

d) Fonnesbeck & Harris

Q 3 The Weende system of analysis was developed at Weende experiment station. This station is located at v

a) **Germany** b) Japan

c) Holland d) USA

Q 4 Henneberg and Stohmann devised the scheme of proximate analysis in the year __________

a) **1865** b) 1870

c) 1845 d) 1896

Q 5 How many proximate principles are there in the proximate system of analysis?

a) 10 b) **6**

c) 3 d) 8

Q 6 Toluene distillation method is used to estimate the moisture content of __________

a) Concentrate feed b) **Silage**

c) Cake d) Cakes

Q 7 The commonly used technique to estimate dry matter in silage, haylage and molasses is __________

a) High temperature drying

b) **Toluene distillation method**

c) Freeze drying

d) Infrared moisture meter

Q 8 Which statement is wrong regarding estimation of crude protein (CP) in feed stuff by Kjeldahl method?

a) All protein contain 16 % Nitrogen

b) **Nitrogen comes from true protein only**

c) CP is calculated by multiplying a factor 6.25 with nitrogen content

d) $CuSO_4$ is used as catalyst

Q 9 Digestion mixture used in CP estimation consists of ________

a) **$CuSO_4$ and K_2SO_4** b) $CuSO_4$ and $MgSO_4$

c) $MgSO_4$ and K_2SO_4 d) K_2SO_4 and $FeSO_4$

Q 10 The role of K_2SO_4 in above mixture is _________

a) To act as catalyst b) **To raise the boiling point**

c) Both a & b d) None of these

Q 11 In the digestion step of Crude protein estimation, the heating is done till the solution become clean blue in colour. This blue colour is due to __________

a) **$CuSO_4$** b) K_2SO_4

c) Nitrogen of feed d) None of these

Q 12 The pungent smell in the digestion step of CP estimation is of __________

a) **SO_2** b) NO_2

c) Chlorine d) None of these

Q 13 What thing is in excess in ether extract estimated in proximate system?

a) Fat b) Oil

c) Fatty acid d) **Waxes**

Q 14 Which of the following thing is missing in ether extract?

a) Fat b) Chlorophyll

c) **Protein bound lipid** d) Carotenoids

Q 15 Which of the following thing is missing in crude fibre fraction estimated in proximate system of feed analysis?

a) Cellulose b) **Hemicellulose**

c) Lignin d) None of the above

Q 16 Which of the following scientist (s) portioned the carbohydrate into hemicellulose, cellulose, lignin and silica?

a) Henneberg & Stohmann b) **Vansoest**

c) Crampton & Maynard d) None of these

Q 17 Arrange the following method of feed analysis from oldest to latest __________

i) Proximate system of feed analysis

ii) Crampton and Maynard method of analysis

iii) Vansoest method of feed analysis

iv) Fonnesbeck and Harris method of analysis

a) **i-ii-iii-iv** b) ii-i-iii-iv

d) iv-ii-i-iii d) iv-i-ii-iii

Q 18 In Vansoest method of analysis, NDF- ADF will give you __________

a) Cellulose b) **Hemicellulose**

c) Insoluble ash d) Lignin

Q 19 Vansoest method of feed analysis was developed in the year __________

a) **1963** b) 1971

c) 1957 d) 1966

Q 20 Tick the right sequence of crude protein estimation by kjeldahl method __________

a) Ashing- digestion- distillation – titration
b) Distillation- digestion- titration
c) **Digestion-distillation-titration**
d) Digestion-titration-distillation

Q 21 Crude protein estimation is done by determining the per cent nitrogen first and then multiplying it with the following factor __________

a) 6.20
b) **6.25**
c) 6.15
d) 6.35

Q 22 Tick the wrong statement __________

a) NDF of a given feed is always greater than Crude fibre
b) Crude protein of a given feed is always greater than true protein
c) **In proximate system of analysis, ether extract is underestimated**
d) Crude fibre estimation in proximate system is simulation of monogastric digestion

Q 23 Which of the following factor is used for converting milk nitrogen to crude protein?

a) 5.30
b) 6.25
c) 5.71
d) **6.38**

Q 24 Factor required to convert meat nitrogen to crude protein is __________

a) 5.30
b) **6.25**
c) 5.71
d) 6.38

Q 25 Estimation of which parameter will help to know the level of contamination/adulteration of the feedstuff __________

a) Total ash
b) Nitrogen free extract (NFE)
c) **Acid insoluble ash**
d) None of the above

Q 26 The ashless filter paper are made up of ________

a) **Organic cellulose**
b) Ordinary paper
c) Dacron
d) None of the above

Q 27 The method in which digestibility is studied by inoculating the test feed with rumen microorganism under controlled condition in the laboratory is known as ________

a) Insacco method
b) In situ method
c) **In vitro method**
d) In vivo method

Q 28 The method is which digestibility is studied by suspending the test feed in the rumen of live animal is known as ________

a) In sacco method
b) In vivo method
c) In situ method
d) **Both a & c**

Q 29 The method in which digestibility is studied by taking the difference between nutrient intake and nutrient voided in faeces and urine of an animal is known as ________

a) In sacco
b) In situ
c) **In vivo**
d) In vitro

Q 30 The widely adopted in vitro method was developed by ________

a) **Tilley & Terry**
b) Menke et al
c) Quin et al
d) Orskov & Mcdonald

Q 31 Which of the following material is not suitable for rumen bag used in insacco method?

a) Dacron
b) Nylon
c) Both a & b
d) **Cotton**

Q 32 The optimum pore size of ruminal bag used for in sacco study is ________

a) 10-20 μ
b) 20-30 μ
c) 30-40 m
d) **40-60** μ

Q 33 In in-sacco method, how many bags/cattle are optimum for incubation in the rumen without interfering rumen fill and digestion?

a) **30-50 bags/300-500kg B wt**
b) 50-80 bags/300-500kg B wt
c) 80-100 bags/300-500kg B wt
d) 130-150 bags/300-500kg B wt

Q 34 Optimum number of ruminal bags in 40 kg Goat is ________

a) 10 b) **6**
c) 15 d) 20

Q 35 In vitro gas production method for feed evaluation was developed in which country?

a) USA b) Holland
c) **Germany** d) Japan

Q 36 In vitro gas production method was developed by ________

a) Tilley and Terry b) Quin et al
c) Sniffen et al d) **Menke et al**

Q 37 The rumen simulation technique(rusitec) was given by _____

a) Chalupa Sniffen
b) **Czerkawski & Breckenridge**
c) Tilley and Terry
d) Erwin and Elliston

Q 38 Markham apparatus is used in the estimation of which parameter?

a) **VFA of rumen** b) Rumen microbial enzyme
c) Lactic acid in silage d) None of the above

Q 39 Which of the following thing is in excess in NFE(nitrogen free extract) estimated by deducting total value of crude protein, crude fat, crude fibre and ash from 100?

a) Starch b) Sugar
c) **Hemicellulose** d) None of these

Q 40 In Weende system of analysis, carbohydrate is divided into how many fraction?

a) One b) **Two***

c) Three d) Four

* CF and NFE

Q 41 Which of the following represents the semi-normal solution?

a) **N/2** b) N/5

c) N/10 d) N/100

Q 42 Which of the following represents pentinormal solution?

a) 0.5N b) **0.2 N***

c) 0.1N d) 0.01N

*0.2N= N/5

Q 43 In Vansoest Method of analysis, sodium lauryl sulpahte is used to __________

a) Dissolve cellulose b) **Dissolve cell contents**

c) Dissolve lignin d) Dissolve hemicellulose

Q 44 In Vansoest method, CTAB (Cetyl trimethyl ammonium bromide) is used to solublize __________

a) Cell content b) **Hemicellulose**

c) Cellulose d) None of the above

Q 45 Crude fibre estimation in proximate analysis is the simulation of digestion of which animal?

a) Cattle b) Sheep

c) Goat d) **Horse***

* It simulates monogastric digestion

Q 46 Which of the following is a misnomer?

a) Milk fever b) Bypass protein

c) Bypass fat d) **All the above**

Q 47 RDP and UDP concept was first proposed by __________

a) **ARC (1980)** b) ARC (1989)

c) NRC (1980) d) NRC (1989)

Q 48 Cornell net carbohydrate and protein (CNCP) of analysis was given by __________

a) **Sinffen et al** b) Orskov & Mcdonald
c) Menke et al d) Quin et al

Q 49 In CNCP system of analysis, protein is divided into how many fractions?

a) 2 b) **5**
c) 7 d) 8

Q 50 In above system of analysis, non-protein nitrogen was represented by which fraction?

a) **A** b) B_1
c) B_2 d) C

Q 51 In CNCP system of analysis, which fraction represents the true protein?

a) A b) **B**
c) C d) None of these

Q 52 Nitrogen free extract (NFE) represents the __________

a) **Soluble carbohydrate** b) Insoluble carbohydrate
c) Soluble protein d) Soluble Vitamin

Q 53 PPM (parts per million) is __________

a) **mg per Kg** b) gm per Kg
c) 10 gm per Kg d) None of the above

Q 54 Which of the following fraction is not included in ADF (Acid detergent fibre)?

a) **Hemicellulose** b) Cellulose
c) Lignin d) Silica

Q 55 The study of energy change accompanying the biochemical reaction is called __________

a) **Biochemical thermodynamic**
b) Thermogenic effect
c) Specific dynamic reaction
d) Transformation

Q 56 The study of energy and its metabolism is called __________

a) Bioenergetic

b) Biochemcal thermodynamic

c) **Both a & b**

d) None of the above

Q 57 The amount of heat required to raise the temperature of 1 kilogram water by 1°C is known as __________

a) **Kilocalorie** b) Calorie

c) British Thermal Unit d) None of the above

Q 58 The amount of heat required to raise the temperature of 1 lb water by 1°F is known as __________

a) Kilocalorie b) Calorie

c) **British Thermal Unit** d) None of the above

Q 59 One Kcal is equal to __________

a) 1 British Thermal Unit b) 2 British Thermal Unit

c) 3 British Thermal Unit d) **4 British Thermal Unit**

Q 60 One Kcal is equal to __________

a) **4.184 KJ** b) 4.184 J

c) 41.84 KJ d) 41.84 J

Q 61 Heat Increment (HI) is also known as __________

a) Specific dynamic action b) Work of digestion

c) Thermogenic effect d) Calorigenic effect

d) **All the above**

Q 62 Essential Amino acids are also known as __________

a) **Indispensible amino acids** b) Dispensible amino acids

c) Limiting amino acids d) Critical amino acids

Q 63 One Kilojoule is equal to __________

a) **0.239Kcal** b) 2.39 Kcal

c) 0.239 cal d) 2.39 cal

Q 64 The heat of combustion of feed is also known as __________

a) **Gross energy** b) Digestible energy
c) Metabolic energy d) Net energy

Q 65 Gross energy value for carbohydrate is __________

a) **4.1 Kcal/g** b) 5.7 Kcal/g
c) 9.4 Kcal/g d) 7.0 Kcal/g

Q 66 Gross energy value for protein is __________

a) 4.1 Kcal/g b) **5.7 Kcal/g**
c) 9.4 Kcal/g d) 7.0 Kcal/g

Q 67 Gross energy value for fat is __________

a) 4.1 Kcal/g b) 5.7 Kcal/g
c) **9.4 Kcal/g** d) 7.0 Kcal/g

Q 68 In ruminants the portion of gross energy lost as methane is to the tune of __________

a) 1-2 % b) **7-9%**
c) 15-20% d) 30-32%

Q 69 Metabolic energy is equal to __________

a) **0.82 x Digestible energy (DE)**
b) 10.5 x DE
c) 1.82 x DE
d) 3.6 x DE

Q 70 Which of the following is considered as tax on energy of the food?

a) **Heat increment** b) Digestible energy
c) Metabolic energy d) Urinary energy

Q 71 Which one of the following four has the higher heat increment?

a) **Fibre** b) Protein
c) Starch d) Fat

Q 72 Which one of the following has least heat increment?

a) Fibre
b) Protein
c) Starch
d) **Fat**

Q 73 Descending order of heat increment in the following substances is __________

a) **Cellulose > Protein > Starch > Fat**
b) Protein > Cellulose > Fat > Starch
c) Fat > Cellulose > Starch > Protein
d) Starch > Cellulose > Fat > Protein

Q 74 In the calculation of TDN, which of the following factor is multiplied by the factor 2.25?

a) DCP
b) DNFE
c) DCF
d) **DEE**

Q 75 The ratio of sum of digestible carbohydrate and fat,later being multiplied by 2.25 to digestible protein represent the ________

a) **Nutritive ratio**
b) Physiological fuel value
c) Biological value
d) Gross protein value

Q 76 Amount of heat produced when carbohydrate or glucose or fats are oxidized in the body per litre of oxygen is known as __________

a) **Thermal equivalent of oxygen**
b) Respiratory quotient
c) Chemical score
d) Protein efficiency ratio

Q 77 The ratio of volume of carbon dioxide produced by the animal to volume of oxygen used under the same temperature and pressure is known as __________

a) Thermal equivalent
b) **Respiratory quotient**
c) Chemical score
d) Protein efficiency ratio

Q 78 Respiratory quotient(RQ) for glucose is __________

a) **1**
b) 6
c) 0.7
d) 0.8

Q 79 RQ for Fat is ________

a) 1 b) 5

c) **0.7** d) 0.8

Q 80 RQ for protein is ________

a) 1 b) 5

c) 0.7 d) **0.8**

Q 81 RQ in fattening animal is ________

a) **1.4 and above** b) 1 and less

c) 0.7 d) 0.8

Q 82 RQ in fasting or hibernating animal is ________

a) Above 1.0 b) Above 1.5

c) **Below 0.7** d) None of these

Q 83 How many amino acid are included in essential amino acids?

a) **10** b) 5

c) 7 d) 15

Q 84 Which of the following reagent can be used to separate the true protein fraction of feed from NPN Fraction?

a) **Stutzer reagent** b) Digestion mixture

c) Both of these d) None of these

Q 85 Which of the following method can not be used to evaluate the protein quality?

a) Protein efficiency ratio b) **Albuminoid ratio**

c) Biological value d) Chemical score

Q 86 The product of biological value and digestibility of protein gives the ________

a) **Net protein value** b) Protein replacement value

c) Protein efficiency ratio d) Net protein retention

Q 87 The ideal protein concept was given by ________

a) **Mitchell** b) Oser

c) Murlin d) Black and Mitchell

Q 88 In modified Ideal protein concept, the requirement of all the essential amino acids are set on the basis of which amino acid?

a) **Lysine** b) Methionine

c) Tryptophan d) Arginine

Q 89 The arithmetic mean of percent DCP and DTP is known as __________

a) **Protein equivalent** b) Starch equivalent

c) Thermal equivalent d) Ideal protein

Q 90 Pilot experiment is synonymous with __________

a) Comparative feeding trial

b) **Feeding experiment with lab animal**

c) Purified diet method

d) Pair feeding method

Q 91 Before conducting a digestion trial animal should be fed on test feed for a particular time to make the GIT free from indigestible material or from previous feed. This time period is known as __________.

a) **Preliminary period** b) Adaptation period

c) Collection period d) Feeding period

Q 92 The optimum preliminary period for conducting a digestion trial in ruminant is __________

a) 1-2 days b) 2-3 days

c) **8-10 days** d) 30 days

Q 93 The optimum preliminary period for conducting a digestion trial in pigs is __________

a) **3-5 days** b) 15 days

c) 20 days d) 25-30 Day

Q 94 The optimum collection period for conducting a digestion study in ruminants is __________

a) **7 days** b) 2 days

c) 3 days d) 1 day

Q 95 The optimum collection period for conducting a digestion study in pig and poultry is _________

a) **3-4 days** b) 7-10 day

c) 1-2 days d) None of the above

Q 96 The term metabolic trial is used for the digestion study for which animal?

a) Cow b) Buffalo

c) Goat d) **Poultry**

Q 97 For calculating the digestibility of non-maintenance type straw which method is generally used?

a) **Digestibility by difference method**

b) By conducting digestion trial directly on the animal with straw

c) Both can be used

d) None of the above

Q 98 When Natural compounds are used in indicator method of determining digestibility, then these compounds are known as __________

a) Internal indicator b) External indicator

c) Natural indicator d) **Both a & c**

Q 99 When an unnatural or a non-component of feed is used as indicator, then this indicator is known as _________

a) Internal indicator b) **External indicator**

c) Natural indicator d) None of these

Q 100 Which of the following is not an example of internal indicator?

a) Lignin b) Silica

c) Acid insoluble ash d) **Carmine red**

Q 101 Which of the following is not an example of external indicator?

a) **Silica** b) Magnesium ferrite

c) Cerium d) Carmine red

Q 102 Which of the following is an example of internal indicator?

a) **Chromogen** b) Ferric oxide

c) Chromic oxide d) Cromium EDTA

Q 103 For determining the digestibility of range fodder/pasture the best method is __________

a) **Indicator method**
b) Digestion trial with cut pasture grass
c) Both of the above
d) None of the above

Q 104 The optimum sample size to bag surface area ratio in calculating the degradability of substances in in-sacco technique should be __________

a) **10-20 mg/cm²** b) 20-40 mg/cm²
c) 40-60 mg/cm² d) 60-80mg/cm²

Q 105 The body surface area per unit weight is __________

a) **More in smaller animal**
b) More in larger animal
c) Depends upon weight of animal
d) None of the above

Q 106 1 Kg TDN is equal to __________

a) **4.409 Mcal DE** b) 0.4409Mcal DE
c) 44.09Mcal DE d) 440.9 Mcal DE

Q 107 Normally, In Fat corrected milk, fat percentage is adjusted at __________

a) **4 %** b) 5%
c) 6% d) 7%

Q 108 The formula used for fat corrected milk (4%) is __________

a) **FCM (kg)= 0.4(kg milk)+ 15 (kg fat)**
b) FCM (kg) = 4 (kg Milk) + 1.5 (kg Fat)
c) FCM (kg) = 15 (kg milk)+ 0.4 (kg fat)
d) FCM (kg) = 1.5 (kg Milk) + 4 (kg Fat)

Q 109 The net energy content of 1 KG of Fat corrected milk is ______

a) 650 Kcal b) **750 Kcal**
c) 850 Kcal d) 950 Kcal

Q 110 Which of the following is not a method for calculation protein requirement of maintenance?

a) Factorial method b) Feeding trial

c) Nitrogen balance d) **Adlib feeding**

Q 111 Which of the following is not a component of metabolic faecal nitrogen (MFN)?

a) Sloughed off cells

b) Digestive enzyme and juice

c) Microorganism of GIT

d) **Dietary nitrogen**

Q 112 The metabolic faecal Nitrogen (MFN) value determined in Indian cattle/buffalo was __________

a) **3.4-3.5 g/kg DMI** b) 6.5-7.5 g/kg DMI

c) 7.5-8.5 g/Kg DMI d) 0.5-1.0 g/Kg DMI

Q 113 The main component of endogenous urinary nitrogen (EUN) in mammal is __________

a) Uric acid b) **Urea**

c) Amino acid d) Ammines

Q 114 The relationship between endogenous urinary nitrogen and metabolic body size is __________

a) **EUN g/day = 0.146$W^{0.75}$** b) EUN g/day = 1.46 $W^{0.75}$

c) EUN g/day = 0.156 $W^{0.75}$ d) EUN g/day = 1.56 $W^{0.75}$

Q 115 Which of the following is not a characteristic of a marker?

a) **Digestible** b) Unabsorable

c) Inert to digestive system d) Easily detectable

Q 116 In Insacco technique, the optimum particle size should be

a) **1-2 mm** b) 3-5 mm

c) 6-9 mm d) 10-15 mm

Q 117 Apparent digestibility of feed stuff is _____________ than the true digestibility.

a) **Less** b) Equal

c) Higher d) May be on any side

Q 118 According to associative effect, the effect of one feed on the other feed is __________

a) Always positive

b) Always negative

c) **May be positive or negative**

d) No effect

Q 119 To measure the digestibility of test feed in different section of GIT, which of the following technique is used?

a) In vitro

b) **Mobile nylon bag technique**

c) Gas production technique

d) All the above

Q 120 To measure the " ileal digestibility" which of the following technique is used?

a) **Mobile nylon bag technique**

b) In Sacco method

c) In Vitro method

d) Gas production technique

Q 121 Semi in vivo technique is also known as __________

a) **In Sacco**

b) In Vivo

c) In Vitro

d) None of these

Q 122 While doing calcium estimation by Talpatra method, which of the following parameter should not be estimated in the same lab at the same time?

a) Crude fat

b) Crude Fibre

c) **Crude protein**

d) NDF

Q 123 Thimble used in fat estimation are made up of __________

a) **Cellulose**

b) Teflon

c) Decron

d) Nylon

Q 124 Tick the wrong statement __________

a) Never pour water in the acid

b) In colourless solution, read the lower level of meniscus from burette.

c) **Bottle containing ammonium solution should be kept in hot water before opening**

d) Primary standard are used for the standarization of secondary standard.

Q 125 Tick the write answer __________

Chemical	Equivalent weight
i) Sodium hydroxide	A) 40.0
ii) Sulphuric acid	B) 49.0
iii) Sodium carbonate	C) 53.0
iv) Hydrocholric acid	D) 36.5

a) **i-A,ii-B,iii-C,iv-D** b) i-B,ii-A,iii-C,iv-D

c) i-D,ii-B,iii-C,iv-A d) i-C,ii-B,iii-A,iv-D

Q 126 If a feed sample has 16% CP on as such basis and has 90% DM, then CP percentage on DM basis is __________

a) **17.78%*** b) 18.40%

c) 14.40% d) 21.56%

* %CP on DM basis = 16/0.90 = 17.78

Q 127 Phosphorus percentage in a poultry feed is found to be 0.41% on as such basis. Its DM content is 88 %, then phosphorus percentage on DM basis is __________

a) **0.47** b) 0.57

c) 0.67 d) 0.77

Q 128 Suppose a feed contain 10% CP on a fresh basis and has 10% moisture, then the CP content on DM basis is __________

a) 10.4% b) 10.9%

c) **11.11%** d) 11.89%

Q129 A feed having 90% DM reported to possess 16% CP on DM basis. Then, the CP percentage on as such basis (ASB) is ______

a) 16.9
b) **14.4***
c) 15.4
d) 20.9

* % CP on ASB = 16 x .90 = 14.4

Q 130 "Wet Ashing" method is used for ashing, then which of the following mineral (s) is/are to be estimated?

a) Se
b) Cd
c) Pb
d) **All the above**

* These mineral may be volatilized by high temperature ashing.

Q 131 A test sample has 3% nitrogen in it and has 90% DM, then the CP percentage in it is __________

a) 10.40%
b) 27%
c) **18.75%**
d) 30%

Q132 Tick the wrong statement __________

a) Litmus is a water soluble mixture of different dyes extracted from lichens
b) **Under acidic condition red litmus turn blue**
c) In alkaline condition, red litmus paper turn blue
d) Litmus was used for the first time by Arnaldus de villa Nova.

Q 133 Which of the following Indian scientist developed a method for the estimation of phosphorus used widely in India?

a) Dr ND Kehar
b) **Dr SK Talapatra**
c) Dr KC Sen
d) Dr SN Ray

Q 134 Till the year 2013, the latest NRC for poultry is __________

a) **NRC (1994)**
b) NRC (2001)
c) NRC (2006)
d) NRC (1998)

Q 135 The latest NRC for swine is (till 2013) __________

a) NRC (1994)
b) NRC (2001)
c) **NRC (1998)**
d) NRC (2006)

Q 136 The latest NRC for dairy cattle in India is ________

a) NRC (1998) b) **NRC (2001)**

c) NRC (2006) d) NRC (2013)

Q 137 The latest NRC for DOG is ________

a) NRC (1994) b) NRC (1998)

c) **NRC (2006)** d) NRC (2001)

Q 138 The acid used to estimate the acid insoluble ash (AIA) is ______

a) **Hydrochloric acid** b) Sulphuric acid

c) Nitric acid d) Perchloric acid

Q 139 The first chemical used for treatment of straw is ________

a) **NaOH** b) O_3

c) H_2O_2 d) Urea

Q 140 Ammonia treatment of straw was started in ________

a) **Norway** b) Newzeland

c) Germany d) Japan

Q 141 For conducting a metabolic trail the minimum age of ________ weeks is necessary in poultry and pig.

a) 1 week b) 2 week

c) **3 week** d) 6 week

Q 142 Tick the wrong statement for conducting digestion/metabolic trial.

a) **Calves under 6 months of age are preferred**

b) Male animals are preferred in ruminants

c) Equal sex ratio is maintained in pig and poultry

d) Animals of same body weight are choosen.

Q 143 Which of the following factor affects the digestibility of feed ________ stuffs?

a) Animal factor b) Plant factor

c) Feed processing factor d) **All the above**

Q 144 Tick the wrong statement __________

a) Buffaloes are superior to cattle in digesting organic nutrients

b) **Young chicks have higher fat digestibility as compared to adult**

c) Ruminants are more efficient in digesting the fibre portion than the non-ruminants

d) High level of feeding depress the digestibility

Q 145 Tick the wrong statement __________

a) Soaking increases the digestibility of nutrients

b) **Cooking decreases the digestibility of nutrients**

c) High fat in rumen diet reduces the digestibility of other nutrients

d) Adequate salt improves the digestibility of nutrients

Q 146 Which of the following is not an example of liquid phase marker in ruminants?

a) Polyethylene glycol b) Chromium EDTA

c) Cobalt EDTA d) **Cr_2O_3**

Q 147 The most accurate method of determining digestibility of pasture grass is by __________

a) Calculating digestibility by difference method

b) **Calculating digestibility by indicator method**

c) By cutting and feeding the pasture grass to the animals

d) All the above

Q 148 Effect of one type of feed on the digestibility of other feed is known as __________

a) Digestion effect b) Digestion kinetic

c) **Associative effect** d) Supplementary effect

Q 149 If 50 Kg dry matter of a feed is to be added in a ration mix and feed has a dry matter percentage of 50%. Then, the total weight of the feed to be added in Ration mix is __________

a) 50 kg b) 250 kg

c) **100 kg** d) 150 kg

Q 150 To calculate the total amount of crude protein as gram per kilogram of dry matter in the feed. The percentage figure is multiplied with _________

a) **10**
b) 100
c) 1000
d) 1

Q 151 As per vansoest method, which of the following is not considered as structural carbohydrate?

a) Cellulose
b) Hemicellulose
c) Lignin
d) **Pectin**

Q 152 How much percentage of metabolisable protein formed from the dietary protein in?

a) 60%
b) 55%
c) **75%**
d) 955

Q 153 Propionic acid is a _________

a) One of the VFA produced in the rumen
b) Fungal inhibitor
c) Glucogenic in ruminant
d) **All the above**

Q 154 Which of the following is not an indicator of negative energy balance in cow after calving?

a) Elevated level of serum NEFA
b) Increased plasma concentration of Beta- hydroxyl butyrate
c) **Increased plasma glucose level**
d) Fatty liver syndrome

Q 155 Periparturient period is the period _________

a) 1-2 weeks after calving
b) **3 weeks before and after calving**
c) 1-2 weeks before calving
d) 3 months before calving

Q 156 Which of the following level of NEFA represent that cow is in positive energy balance?

a) **Less than 0.2 mM** b) 0.5m M

c) 0.5 to 0.7mM d) 1.0 mM

Q 157 Metabolizable protein is ________ % of the dietary protein.

a) 60% b) **75%**

c) 50% d) 95%

Q 158 True protein can be separated from the NPN compounds by precipitation with __________

a) Sulphuric acid

b) **Alkaline cupric hydroxide**

c) Hydrochloric acid

d) Nitric acid

Q 159 Digestible crude protein is equal to __________

a) **CP x Digestible coefficient**

b) Biological Value x Digestibility

c) Weight gain/protein consumed

d) All the above

Q 160 Which of the following method is used to measure the protein quality for monogastric animal?

a) Protein efficiency ration b) Chemical score

c) Essential amino acid index d) **All the above**

Q 161 Which of the following methods used for measuring protein quality is not based on weight gain method?

a) Protein efficiency ratio b) Net protein retention

c) Gross protein value d) **Biological value**

Q 162 Which of the following methods used for measuring protein quality is not based on nitrogen balance?

a) **Protein efficiency ratio** b) Net protein utilization

c) Protein replacement value d) Biological value

Q 163 The value of protein efficiency ratio can be influenced by _____

a) Palatability
b) Age
c) Level of protein
d) **All the above**

Q 164 Weight gain on test protein- weight loss on protein free diet/ protein intake gives the _________

a) PER
b) **Net protein retention**
c) Gross protein value
d) Biological value

Q 165 Weight gain per unit weight of protein consumed gives the value of _________

a) **PER**
b) CCR
c) FCR
d) BV

Q 166 Ratio of weight gain per unit of test protein to that of weight gain per unit of standard protein is known as _________

a) PER
b) **Gross protein value**
c) Biological value
d) Feed conversion ratio

Q 167 Percentage of absorbed nitrogen retained by body for repair or synthesis of nitrogen tissue is known as _________

a) **Biological value**
b) Protein efficiency ratio
c) Feed conversion ratio
d) Gross protein value

Q 168 Metabolic faecal nitrogen (MFN) consists of _________

a) Spent digestive enzymes
b) Abraded mucosa
c) Bacterial nitrogen
d) **All the above**

Q 169 Which of the following ingredients has the highest biological value of protein?

a) Soybean meal
b) Fish meal
c) **Egg**
d) Wheat

Q 170 Biological value X digestibility gives the _________

a) Protein replacement value
b) **Net protein utilization**
c) Protein efficiency ratio
d) Gross protein value

Q 171 "Chemical score method" for estimation of protein quality in monogastric was devised by __________

a) Murlin
b) **Black & Mitchell**
c) Oser
d) Mitchell

Q 172 Lysine was found to be 63 % deficit in wheat protein as compared to egg protein. Then, the chemical score for wheat is __________

a) 63
b) 36
c) **37**
d) 73

Q 173 Essential amino acid index (EAAI) was given by __________

a) Murlin
b) Black and Mitchell
c) **Oser**
d) Mitchell

Q 174 Which of the following methods for estimation of protein quality in monogastric was based on amino acid composition?

a) Protein efficiency ratio
b) Biological value
c) **Essential amino acid index**
d) Gross protein value

Q 175 Ideal protein concept for measuring protein quality was proposed by __________

a) **Mitchell**
b) Oser
c) Murlin
d) Black and Mitchell

Q 176 In Ideal protein concept which amino acid is taken as base for setting the concentration of other amino acids?

a) **Lysine**
b) Methionine
c) Tryptophan
d) Glycine

Q 177 Arithmetic mean of the percentage of digestible crude protein and digestible true protein is known as __________

a) **Protein equivalent**
b) Protein efficiency ratio
c) Biological value
d) Net protein value

Q 178 Which of the following methods of measuring protein quality does not apply to ruminants?

a) Protein equivalent
b) Digestible crude protein
c) **Biological value**
d) In vivo method

Q 179 Study of energy and its metabolism is known as __________

a) Bioenergetics

b) Biochemical thermodynamic

c) **Both a & b**

d) None of the above

Q 180 Term "Specific dynamic effect" was coined by __________

a) Mitchell b) **Rubner**

c) Oser d) Black & Mitchell

Q 181 Heat Increment is synonymous with __________

a) Specific dynamic action b) Calorigenic effect

c) Thermogenic action d) **All the above**

Q 182 Heat Increment includes __________

a) Heat of fermentation b) Heat of digestion

c) Heat of product formation d) **All the above**

Q 183 Heat produced following consumption of feed by animal in a thermo- neutral environment is known as __________

a) **Heat increment** b) Gross energy

c) Digestible energy d) Metabolizable energy

Q 184 ME-HI =

a) **NE** b) DE

c) FE d) UE

Q 185 Fill right answer in the blank space __________

TDN = DCP + DNFE + DCF + DEE x ______

a) 4.4 b) **2.25**

c) 6.25 d) 1.0

Q 186 If a cow ate 9 kg of feed having 8 kg of DM and excreted 3 kg of DM in faeces, then digestibility coefficient of dry matter is __________

a) **62.5 %** b) 43.6%

c) 25.7% d) 88.7%

Q 187 Physiological fuel value (PFV) was given by __________

a) **Atwater** b) Lavoisier and Laplace

c) Murlin d) Black and Mitchell

Q 188 Physiological fuel value of carbohydrate is ________

a) **4.0 kcal/g**
b) 5.0 Kcal/g
c) 10.0 Kcal/g
d) 15.0 Kcal/g

Q 189 Gross energy X digestible coefficient gives the value of ______

a) Chemical score
b) **Physiological fuel value**
c) Biological value
d) Nutritive ratio

Q 190 Albuminoid ratio is also known as ________

a) **Nutritive ratio**
b) Biological value
c) Protein efficiency ratio
d) Chemical score

Q 191 Ration with narrow (1:0.7) nutritive ratio is suitable for ________

a) Lactating animal
b) **Young stock**
c) Cattle
d) Horse

Q 192 Which of the following statement is wrong in pretext to animal just before calving?

a) Mammary uptake of glucose increase
b) **Dry matter intake start increasing**
c) Blood flow to mammary gland increases
d) Acetate uptake by mammary gland increases

Q 193 Animal is in comfort zone when Temperature Humidity Index (THI) is ________

a) **Below 72**
b) 72-79
c) 80-88
d) >90

Q 194 Maximum safe limit of urea /adult animal/day is ________

a) **136 g**
b) 200 g
c) 250 g
d) 336 g

□□□

Chapter 14

Feed Additives

Q 1 Antibiotic growth promoters enhance the performance of the animal by __________

a) Suppressing the microbial load in the gut

b) Thinning of the intestinal wall

c) Improving the absorption of nutrients

d) **All the above**

Q 2 Which of the following feed additive can be used to prevent the oxidative rancidity of high fat containing feeds?

a) Flavomycin b) **Ethoxyquin**

c) Salinomycin d) Bentonites

Q 3 Which of the following is not a synthetic antioxidant?

a) Butylated hydroxyl toluene (BHT)

b) Butylated hydroxyl anisol (BHA)

c) Ethoxyquin

d) **Ascorbic acid**

Q 4 Feed additive used to scavenge the free radicals is known as __________

a) **Antioxidants** b) Emulsifier

c) Anticoccidials d) Adsorbents

Q 5 Feed additives used to increase the surface area of fat for digestion and absorption by dispersing it as droplets in water is known as __________

a) Antioxidants b) **Emulsifier**

c) Adsorbents d) All the above

Q 6 Which of the following is an example of emulsifier?

a) Ethoxyquin b) **Lecithin**

c) Bentonite d) Arsenicals

Q 7 Bentonite is a __________

a) Anticoccidial b) **Pellet binder**

c) Antioxidants d) Enzyme

Q 8 Which of the following feed additives is not a binder?

a) Bentonite b) Lignin sulphonate

c) Attapulgite d) **Monensin**

Q 9 Direct fed microbials are also known as __________

a) **Probiotics** b) Prebiotics

c) Synbiotics d) Xenobiotics

Q 10 Stone grits or shell grit is generally added to which of the following animal's diet?

a) Cow b) Dog

c) Horse d) **Layer**

Q 11 Which of the following can be used to improve the yellow colour of egg yolk, body fat and shank of the birds?

a) Copper sulphate b) **Merigold petal meal**

c) Shrimp meal d) Mannan oligosaccharides

Q 12 Adsorbents is added in feed as they __________

a) **Adsorb mycotoxin**

b) Adsorb antinutritional factor like HCN, nitrate etc

c) Help in absorption of nutrient by acting as carrier

d) Adsorb water and act as binder

Q 13 Which of the following is not an example of adsorbents?

a) Charcoal b) Zeolites

c) Aluminium silicate d) **Sodium arsenate**

Q 14 The most commonly used commercial adsorbent is ________

a) Charcoal
b) Zeolites
c) Bentonite
d) **HSCAS***

* HSCAS- Hydrated sodium calcium aluminium silicate

Q 15 HSCAS adsorbent is useful in binding ________

a) **Aflatoxin**
b) Ochratoxin
c) Citrinin
d) Pesticide residue

Q 16 Which of the following feed additive can be used as prebiotic as well as adsorbent?

a) Activated charcoal
b) Zeolites
c) Bentonite
d) **MOS**

Q 17 Probiotic exert their effect by ________

a) Competitive exclusion of pathogens from gut
b) Neutralization of enterotoxin produced by pathogenic bacteria
c) Bactericidal activity on pathogen
d) **All the above**

Q 18 The substances which are used to enhance the population of beneficial bacteria are known as ________

a) Probiotic
b) **Prebiotic**
c) Synbiotic
d) Xenobiotic

Q 19 Example of prebiotic is ________

a) Galacto oligosaccharides
b) Fructo oligosaccharides
c) Mannan oilgosaccharides
d) **All the above**

Q 20 When Direct fed microbials and Mannan oligosacsharides are collectively fed to animals, they are known as ________

a) Probiotics
b) Prebiotics
c) **Synbiotics**
d) Xenobiotics

Q 21 Enzyme Phytase is generally used in the diet of ________

a) Cow
b) Buffalo
c) Sheep
d) **Poultry birds**

Q 22 Betaine is a (tick the right answer) __________

a) Methyl group donor

b) Derivative of choline

c) Improve the production performance through methionine sparing effect

d) **All the above**

Q 23 The term probiotic was coined by __________

a) **D.M. Lilly and R.H. Stillwell**

b) R.B. Parke

c) R. Fuller

d) V. Bottazzi

Q 24 The term prebiotic was coined by __________

a) Lilly and Stillwell

b) **Gibson and Roberfroid**

c) A.Lee

d) R.B Parker

Q 25 A non-digestible food ingredients that beneficially affects the host by selectively stimulating the growth and or activity of one or a limited number of bacteria in colon is known as _____

a) Probiotic

b) **Prebiotic**

c) Synbiotic

d) Xenobiotic

Q 26 If a poultry ration is containing a high NSP content, which of the following feed additive is most useful for it?

a) **Enzymes**

b) Antioxidants

c) Probiotics

d) Adsorbents

Q 27 Which of the following is a anti-caking agent?

a) Kaolin

b) Lignin sulfonate

c) **Iron ammonium citrate**

d) Bentonite

Q 28 Which of the following antibiotic is commonly known as terramycin?

a) Chlortetracycline

b) **Oxytetracylcine**

c) Bacitracin

d) Streptomycin

Q 29 Which of the following is not an ionophore antibiotic?

a) Monensin
b) Lasalocid
c) Salinomycin
d) **Flavomycin**

Q 30 Mode of action of ionophore antibiotic is ________

a) Interfering with the synthesis of material forming the bacterial cell wall
b) Inhibition of bacterial protein synthesis
c) Inhibition of bacterial DNA synthesis
d) **Interfere with electrolyte balance (Na/K) of the bacterial cell**

Q 31 Which of the following feed additive cause the redening of combs and wattle?

a) **Arsenicals**
b) Copper sulphate
c) Monensin
d) All the above

Q 32 Example of catabolic hormone is ________

a) Somatotropin
b) Thyroxine
c) Androgen
d) **Estrogen**

Q 33 Certain metals like Fe and Cu act as catalyst in oxidation process, to prevent this oxidation, these need to be eliminated/ immobilized. Substances added in feed to scavenge these free metals are known as ________

a) Antioxidants
b) Prooxidants
c) **Sequestrants**
d) Emulsifier

Q 34 Which of the following is not an example of sequestrants?

a) CaEDTA
b) Polyphosphate
c) Citric acid
d) **Calcium formate**

Q 35 Lignosulphonates are the byproducts from ________

a) Sugar industry
b) Fruit processing industry
c) Wine industry
c) **Wood pulp manufacturing Industry**

Q 36 Which of the following pellet binder is not used in pelleting of diet for rabbit as it causes ulceration of colon?

a) **Lignosulphonates** b) Molasses

c) Bentonite d) Guar meal

Q 37 Which of the following is not an artificial sweetner?

a) Saccharine

b) Glycyrrhicine

c) Neohesperidine dihydrochalcone

d) **Betafin**

Q 38 The substances which have ability to attract and hold water in a formulation is known as __________

a) Emulsifier b) Surfectant

c) **Humectants** d) Sequestrants

Q 39 Which of the following is an example of humectant?

a) Glycerol b) Mannitol

c) Sorbitol d) **All the above**

Q 40 Example of anticaking agent is __________

a) **Sodium aluminosilicate** b) Sodium ferrocyanide

c) Calcium carbonate d) Sodium sesquicarbonate

Q 41 Which of the following is the original rumen buffer?

a) **Sodium bicarbonate** b) Magnesium oxide

c) Calcium carbonate d) Sodium sesquicarbonate

Q 42 Which of the following is not a true buffer?

a) Sodium bicarbonate b) Sesquicarbonate

c) Limestone d) **Magnesium oxide***

** MgO is an alkalizer which neutralize the acidity while true buffer prevents increase in acidity.*

Q 43 Use of buffer is not required when __________

a) Grain exceeds 50% of ration dry matter

b) High starch feedstuff is fed

c) **High fibre diet is fed**

d) Corn silage make up more than 50% of forage dry matter

Q 44 Example of true buffer is __________

a) Bicarbonate
b) Sesquicarbonate
c) Bentonite
d) **All the above**

Q 45 Which of the following organic acid has the highest bactericidal effect?

a) **Benzoic acid**
b) Fumaric acid
c) Formic acid
d) Propionic acid

* Benzoic acid > fumaric acid > lactic acid > Butyric acid > formic acid > propionic acid

Q 46 Milliequivalent of 1.0M HCl required to acidify 1 kg of material to pH 3-5 is known as __________

a) **B-value**
b) D-value
c) Pka value
d) All the above

Q 47 Tick the wrong statement regarding B-value __________

a) Cereal has low B-value
b) **Protein sources have low B- value**
c) Mineral sources have high B-value
d) Limestone has a very high B-value

Q 48 Acidifier in poultry feed __________

a) **Lower the pH and inhibit the growth of pathogens**
b) Increase the palatability
c) Decrease the protein and energy digestibilities
d) All the above

Q 49 The hormone "Leptin" was discovered by __________

a) **Zhang *et al* (1994)**
b) Kojima *et al* (1999)
c) Kline *et al* (1997)
d) Banks *et al* (1996)

Q 50 The hormone "Ghrelin" was discovered by __________

a) Zhang *et al* (1994)
b) **Kojima *et al* (1999)**
c) Kline *et al* (1997)
d) Banks *et al* (1996)

Q 51 Which of the following substance is used as metabolic modifiers in swine?

a) **Ractopamine hydrochloride**
b) Sodium ferrocyanide
c) Sodium propionate
d) Sorbic acid

Q 52 Which of the following animal has the highest number of taste buds?

a) Chicken b) Cat
c) Dog d) **Calf**

Q 53 Which of the following animal has the lowest number of taste buds?

a) **Chicken** b) Calf
c) Rabbit d) Goat

Q 54 The recommended inclusion level of sodium bicarbonate in ruminant diet is __________

a) **1.0-1.5% of concentrate mixture**
b) 2.0-3.5% of concentrate mixture
c) 3.0-4.0 % of concentrate mixture
d) 4.0-5.0% of concentrate mixture

Q 55 If sodium bicarbonate and magnesium oxide to be used collectively as buffer, then their optimum ratio should be _____

a) 1:1 b) **3:1**
c) 7:1 d) 11:1

Q 56 Any substance that may be considered as a food or part of a food which provide health benefits including the prevention and treatment of disease is known as __________

a) Drug b) Botanicals
c) **Nutraceuticals** d) Essential oil

Q 57 Use of alpha-lipoic acid (ALA) in animal feed is done as ______

a) Acidifier b) **Antioxidants**
c) Pellet binder d) Adsorbents

Q 58 The most common yeast used in animal feed industry is _____

a) ***Saccharomyces cerevisiae*** b) *Candida albicans*

c) *Saccharomyces telluris* d) Torulopsis

Q 59 Which of the following is a non-nutritive feed additive in poultry?

a) Enzyme b) Carotenoids

c) Antioxidants d) **All the above**

Q 60 Roche Scale is used to measure __________

a) Albumin quality b) **Yolk colour**

c) Shell quality d) All the above

Q 61 Which of the following has zero protein equivalency?

a) L - lysine

b) L - arginine

c) **Methionine hydroxyl analogue**

d) Glutamic acid

Q 62 500 Units of phytase activity are equivalent to how many gram of phosphorus?

a) **1** b) 3

c) 5 d) 7

Q 63 Which of the following feed has high phytase activity?

a) Maize b) Sorghum

c) **Wheat** d) Pea nut meal

Q 64 Which of the following fodder has the highest phytoestrogenic content?

a) Lucerne b) **Berseem**

c) Shaftal d) Maize

Q 65 Phytase is generally added in the ration of __________

a) Cow b) Buffalo

c) Sheep d) **Swine**

Q 66 Acrolein and methyl mercaptan are the starting material for the most common process to synthesize which amino acid?

a) **DL-methionine** b) L-lysine

c) L-Threonine d) L-Arginine

Q 67 Commercially phytase can be produced from ________

a) *Aspergillus niger* b) *E. coli*

c) *Penicillium funiculosum* d) **All the above**

Q 68 Which of the following feed additive is used to produce high percentage lean muscle in meat animal?

a) Antioxidant

b) **β-agonists**

c) Antibiotic growth promoters

d) Cytokinin

Q 69 Betaine- a feed additive used in animal feed is a ________

a) **Oxidative product of choline**

b) Oxidative product of methionine

c) Oxidative product of lysine

d) Oxidative product of arginine

Q 70 Betaine - a feed additive is a ________

a) Heptaoprotective b) Methyl donor

c) Osmolytes d) **All the above**

Q 71 Animal protein factor is present in ________

a) Ground nut cake b) **Fish meal**

c) Soyabean meal d) Meat meal

Q 72 Anti-metabolite is a compound that ________

a) Interfere in physiological function

b) Interfere in digestion

c) Improve the growth rate

d) **Both a & b**

Q 73 Saccharin __________

a) Is a energy source b) Is a protein source

c) Is a fat source d) **Improves the palatability**

Q 74 Shell grit in layer ration is a source of __________

a) Energy b) **Calcium**

c) Phosphorus and calcium d) Magnesium

Q 75 Fuller's earth is synonymous to __________

a) **Bentonite** b) Calcium carbonate

c) Creatine d) Saccharin

Q 76 Which of the following feed additive increases the surface area of fat for digestion and absorption by dispersing it as droplets in water?

a) Anti-oxidants b) **Emulsifier**

c) Adsorbents d) Arsenicals

Q 77 Which of the following is an example of emulsifier?

a) **Lecithin** b) Bentonite

c) Attapulgite d) Copper sulphate

Q 78 Anti-coccidials feed additive is used in __________

a) Poultry b) Swine

c) Calf d) **All the above**

Q 79 The chemical substances which are man made and are foreign to animal body are known as __________

a) Prebiotic b) Probiotic

c) Synbiotic d) **Xenobiotic**

Q 80 Which of the following is an example of carcass modifier?

a) Nystatin b) Copper sulphate

c) Citric acid d) **Carnitine**

Q 81 Which of the following feed additive is not an example of carcass modifier used in swine?

a) Betaine b) Conjugated linolinic acid

c) Ractopamine d) **Phosphoric acid**

Q 82 Which of the following is an example of inorganic acidifier?

a) Citric acid b) **Phosphoric acid**

c) Fumaric acid d) Propionic acid

Q 83 Substances added to feed to improve the pourabaility and storage stability is known as ________

a) **Free flowing agents** b) Antioxidants

c) Binder d) Surfactants

Q 84 Example of free flowing agent is ________

a) **Hydated sodium aluminium silicate**

b) Carcoal

c) Calcium carbonate

d) Sodium chloride

Q 85 Which of the following is not an example of coccidiostats?

a) Amprolium b) Diclazuril

c) Monensin d) **Copper sulphate**

Q 86 The substance/chemical derived from plants or part of plants, which can be used as feed additive is known as ________

a) Phytogenic b) Phytobiotic

c) Phytochemicals d) **All the above**

Q 87 Largest user of commercial enzyme (exogenous) is ________

a) Dairy industry b) **Poultry industry**

c) Pig industry d) Value addition of live stock product

Q 88 The most commonly used buffer in ruminant animal is ____

a) Magnesium bicarbonate b) Potassium bicarbonate

c) **Sodium bicarbonate** d) Sodium bentonite

Q 89 Sialagogues stimulate the production and secretion of ______

a) **Saliva** b) Gastric juice

c) Mucous in digestive tract d) Intestinal juice

Q 90 Ionophore are not used in feed of which animal ______________ because they are toxic to them.

a) Poultry
b) Pig
c) Cattle
d) **Horse**

Q 91 An example of repartitioning agent (which increases lipolysis and stimulate protein synthesis) is __________

a) Monensin
b) **Ractopamine HCl**
c) Lysocelin
d) Lasalocid

Q 92 Antibiotic growth promoters should not be used in the diet of

____

a) Chicks
b) Pigs
c) Calves
d) **Cow***

* Antibiotic growth promoters suppress the rumen bug activities.

Q 93 Which of the following feed additive get lodged in gizzard of poultry and help in grinding?

a) **Grit**
b) Bentonnite
c) Zeolites
d) Enzymes

Q 94 Which of the following feed additive uses in poultry industry was banned in many developed countries, as it assumes to poses serious threat to mankind through development of resistant bugs?

a) **Antibiotic growth promoters**
b) Immunomodulators
c) Anthelmentics
d) Acidifiers

❑❑❑

Chapter 15

Feeding Standards

Q 1 Feeding standards are __________

a) Quantitative description of the amounts of one or more nutrients needed by animals

b) Tabulation of nutrient requirement of farm animals for various physiological satges

c) **Both a & b**

d) None of the above

Q 2 Hay feeding standard was given by __________

a) **Albrecht Thaer**

b) Bohimia

c) Emil Von Wolff

d) Haecker

Q 3 In which feeding standard meadow hay was used as a unit to compare other feeds?

a) Wolffs feeding standard

b) Kellner's feeding standard

c) Armsby feeding standard

d) **Thaer's feeding standard**

Q 4 Broadly feeding standard can be classified into how many types?

a) Two

b) **Three***

c) Four

d) Five

* Comparative, digestible nutrient type and productive type

Q 5 Scandinavian feeding standard was given by __________

a) Albrecht Thaer

b) **Fzord**

c) Grouven

d) Frap

Q 6 In which feeding standard grains were used as a unit for comparison?

a) Thaer feeding standard

b) **Scandinavian feeding standard**

c) Savage feeding standard

d) Morrison feeding standard

Q 7 Which of the following is an example of comparative type feeding standard?

a) **Thaers feeding standard**

b) Morrison feeding standard

c) Kellner feeding standard

d) Wolff's feeding standard

Q 8 Which of the following is not an example of digestible nutrient type feeding standard?

a) Hacker's feeding standard b) Savage feeding standard

c) NRC feeding standard d) **Kellner feeding standard**

Q 9 Development of feeding standard was initiated in which country?

a) Australia b) USA

c) **Germany** d) India

Q 10 The first feeding standard which took the crude protein, carbohydrate and fat in the feed as the base of standard formulation was prepared by __________

a) Frap b) **Grouven**

c) Kellner d) Haecker

Q 11 Which of the following is an example of productive type feeding standard?

a) Grouven feeding standard b) Wolffs feeding standard

c) **Kellner feeding standard** d) Scandinavian feeding standard

Q 12 Which of the following feeding standard was based on the concept of digestible protein, fat and carbohydrates derived from feeding trial?

a) **Wolffs feeding standard** b) Hacker's feeding standard

c) Kellners feeding standard d) Thaer feeding standard

Q 13 Which of the following standard considered the quantity and quality (fat percentage) of milk produced in formulating the standard along with digestible nutrients requirements of animals?

a) Kellners feeding standard b) **Haecker feeding standard**

c) Grouven feeding standard d) Wolffs feeding standard

Q 14 In savage feeding standard,the protein requirement was incresead about ________ percent above the Haecker feeding standard.

a) 10% b) **20%**

c) 40% d) 50%

Q 15 Which of the following scientist proposed that about 2/3rd of the dry matter should be from the roughage and 1/3rd from the concentrate?

a) Haecker b) **Savage**

c) Morrison d) Kellner

Q 16 As per NRC feeding standard which of the following energy parameter is not used in poultry?

a) TDN b) GE (Gross energy)

c) DE (Digestible energy) d) **All the above**

Q 17 Which of the following feeding standard first time proposed the separate requirement for maintenance and production?

a) **Hackers feeding standard** b) Savage feeding standard

c) Morrison feeding standard d) NRC

Q 18 According to NRC, which of the following parameter is used to express the energy requirement in swine and horse?

a) TDN b) Gross energy

c) **Digestible energy** d) Net energy

Q 19 As per NRC feeing standard, energy requirement in poultry is expressed as __________

a) Gross energy b) **Metabolizable energy**

c) Net energy d) All the above

Q 20 Who is the first director of NDRI(National Dairy Research Institute), Karnal?

a) Dr N.D. Kehar b) **Dr K.C. Sen**

c) Dr K. Prodhan d) Dr S.K. Ranjhan

Q 21 The concept of starch equivalent was given by __________

a) **Kellner** b) Armsby

c) Morrison d) None of the above

Q 22 Starch equivalent system was investigated by Kellner in the year of __________

a) 1917 b) **1907**

c) 1943 d) 1960

Q23 Armsby feeding standard is based on __________

a) Starch equivalent

b) **True protein & Net energy value**

c) Mid Morrison value

d) Fuel value of food

Q 24 Factor required to convert digestible carbohydrate to starch equivalent is __________

a) 1.0 b) 2.4

c) 2.1 d) **0.94**

Q 25 ARC (Agricultural Research Council) belongs to __________

a) USA b) Denmark

c) **UK** d) Germany

Q 26 NORFOR feeding standard is prevalent in __________

a) Denmark b) Norway

c) Sweden d) Finland

e) **All the above***

* Nordic countries- Denmark, Norway, Sweden, Finland and Iceland

Q 27 Bureau of Indian Standard(BIS) is working under the aegis of __________

a) **Ministry of consumer affairs, food and public distribution**
b) Ministry of food processing
c) Department of industries and supplies
d) None of these

Q 28 BIS came into existence in the year __________

a) 1992 b) **1986**
c) 1860 d) 1971

Q 29 ICAR (Indian Council of Agricultural Research) first time published the feeding standard for Indian livestock and poultry in the year of __________

a) 1977 b) **1987**
c) 1992 d) 1993

Q 30 Which of the following scientist proposed the mid Morrison value for adoption in India as Indian feeding standard?

a) Dr K. Pradhan b) Dr S.K. Ranjhan
c) **Dr K.C. Sen** d) Dr N.D. Kehar

Q 31 Tick the wrong statement regarding morriosn feeding standard __________

a) Standards were expressed in term of DM,DCP and TDN
b) **Requirement of animals was indicated in a one figure**
c) Allowances for Ca,P, carotene, DCP and NE were included in revised edition
d) The average value of this standard was used for Indian standard.

Q 32 ME (Metabolic energy) system was devised by __________

a) Kellner in Germany b) Kellner in United States
c) **Blaxter in UK** d) Blaxter in Germany

Q33 NRC 2001 is the ________ edition of nutrient requirement of dairy cattle published by National Research council.

a) Fifth b) Sixth
c) **Seventh** d) Eighth

❐❐❐

Chapter 16

Anti-Nutritional Factors

Q 1 Anti-nutritional factor present in mustard cake is __________

a) **Gluconsinolate** b) Gossypol

c) Phtohaemagglutinin d) Linamarin

Q 2 Which of the following contain Trypsin Inhibitor?

a) Mustard cake b) **Soybean**

c) Cottonseed cake d) Linseed

Q 3 ANF present in cottonseed is __________

a) **Gossypol** b) Glucosonilate

c) Linamarin d) Sinapine

Q 4 Which of the following ANF does not interfere with mineral utilization?

a) Phytic acid b) Oxalic acid

c) Glucosinolates d) **Lectin**

Q 5 Which of the following ANF does not interfere /depress digestion of protein?

a) Protease inhibitor b) Lectins

c) Tannins d) **Gossypol**

Q 6 Which of the following protease inhibitor is/are found in soyabean?

a) Kunitz inhibitor b) Bowman Birk

c) **Both a & b** d) None of the above

Q 7 Kunitz inhibitor has specificity for inhibiting the __________

a) **Trypsin** b) Chemotrypsin

c) Ptylin d) None of the above

Q 8 ANF present in castor bean cake is __________

a) **Ricin** b) Tannin

c) Oxalic acid d) Gossypol

Q 9 Excessive feeding of lucerne may lead to bloat, it may be due to __________

a) **High saponin content** b) High protein content

c) High nutritive value d) None of these

Q 10 Dry sensation in the mouth after taking tea/coffee is due to high __________

a) Saponin b) Lignin

c) **Tannin** d) Caffeine

Q 11 How many phosphorus molecules are there in phytic acid?

a) 2 b) 4

c) **6** d) 7

Q 12 Paddy straw contain __________

a) High oxalic acid b) High selenium

c) **Both a & b** d) None of the above

Q 13 Anti-nutritive effect of oxalic acid is mainly due to occurance of

a) **Hypocalcemia** b) Hypercalcemic

c) Hypomagnesmia d) Hypermagnesmia

Q 14 ANF present in Rapeseed is __________

a) **Glucosinolate** b) Prussic acid

c) Phytic acid d) Tannin

Q 15 Increasing order of gossypol tolerance is __________

a) **Pig <poultry < horse < cattle***

b) Cattle < pig < horse < poultry

c) Cattle < horse < poultry < pig

d) Horse < cattle < poultry < pig

* Pig is more sensitive while cattle is resistant.

Q 16 Toxic effect of gossypol can be ameliorated by supplementing the feed with __________

a) Copper b) Cobalt

c) **Iron** d) Sodium

Q 17 Raw soyabean has following activity __________

a) Antivitamin A b) Antivitamin D

c) **Antivitamin E** d) Antivitamin K

Q 18 Sweet clover disease exhibit its effect through __________

a) Lowering Vitamin A utilization

b) Lowering Vitamin D utilization

c) Lowering Vitamin E utilization

d) **Lowering Vitamin K utilization**

Q 19 The ANF "Linatine" found in linseed has __________

a) **Antipyidoxine activity** b) Anti-vitamin D activity

c) Anti-vitamin E activity d) Anti-vitamin A activity

Q 20 ANF present in Subabul is __________

a) **Mimosine** b) Linamarin

c) Dicoumarol d) Dhurrin

Q 21 Mimosine exhibit its effect through inhibiting the __________

a) **Thyroxine synthesis** b) Protease action

c) Vitamin A synthesis d) Sex hormone

Q 22 Which of the following ANF is not a cyanogen?

a) Amygdalin b) Dhurrin

c) Linamarin d) **Mimosine**

Q 23 ANF in Jowar is __________

a) Amygdalin b) **Dhurrin**

c) Linamarin d) Mimosine

Q 24 Feeding of drought affected sorghum to animals can prone them for __________

a) **Cyanide toxicity** b) Nitrate toxicity

c) Oxalate toxicity d) Phytate toxicity

Q 25 Feeding of frost damaged grasses to animal can prone them for ________

a) **Cyanide toxicity** b) Oxalate toxicity

c) Nitrate toxicity d) Phytate toxicity

Q 26 Which of the following animal is more susceptible for cyanide poisoning?

a) **Ruminants** b) Horse

c) Pig d) All are equal

Q 27 Excessive use of nitrogen fertilizer in the fodder may cause the following toxicity in the animal ________

a) Cyanide toxicity b) **Nitrate toxicity**

c) Oxalate toxicity d) Selenium toxicity

Q 28 Excessive supplementation of nitrogenous fertilizers in the fodder crops followed by abundent rainfall may increase the chances of following poisoning ________

a) Nitrate b) **Cyanide**

c) Fluorine d) Selenium

Q 29 Zearalenone- a mycotoxin is produced by which of the following fungi?

a) ***Fusarium* spp** b) *Aspergillus* spp

c) *Penicillium* spp d) *Claviceps* spp

Q 30 Castor cake contain ANF known as ________

a) **Ricin** b) Strychnine

c) Dicoumarol d) Linamarin

Q 31 Feeding of Sudan grass after rainy season may cause ________

a) **Cyanide toxicity** b) Nitrate toxicity

c) Oxalate toxicity d) Selenium toxicity

Q 32 Feeding rice straw exclusively to the animal can cause ________

a) **Degnalla disease** b) Nitrate toxicity

c) Fluorine toxicity d) None of the above

Q 33 ANF present in linseed is __________

a) **Linamarin** b) Lasctrile

c) Tropane d) Ricin

Q 34 Due to lipoxygenase enzyme soyabean has following properties __________

a) Anti-vitamin A b) Anti-vitamin D

c) **Anti-vitamin E** d) Anti-vitamin K

Q 35 ANF in Neem seed cake is __________

a) Erucic acid b) Phytate

c) Oxalate d) **Nimbidins**

Q 36 ANF erucic acid is generally found in __________

a) **Rapeseed** b) Cotton seed

c) Soybean d) Linseed

Q 37 Feeding of *Argemone maxicana* oil in human being can lead to disease known as __________

a) Hypothyroidism b) **Dropsy**

c) Stomatitis d) Gingivitis

Q 38 Olive green discolouration of yolk can occur if layers are fed on __________

a) **Cottonseed meal** b) Soybean meal

c) Mustard cake d) Ground nut cake

Q 39 Which of the following is not the soluble form of oxalate?

a) Sodium oxalate b) Potassium oxalate

c) **Calcium oxalate** d) All the above

Q 40 Genistein-an estrogenic compound is generally found in ______

a) **Soybean** b) Mustard

c) Cassava d) Canola

Q 41 Mycotoxicosis (aflatoxicosis) is generally encountered with the feeding of __________

a) **Ground nut cake** b) Mustard cake

c) Soyabean d) Cotton seed cake

Q 42 Sesame meal have following ANF __________

a) **Oxalic acid** b) Cyanogen

c) Glucosinolates d) None of the above

Q 43 ANF in Karanj meal is __________

a) **Karanjine** b) Linatine

c) Linamarin d) Mimosine

Q 44 ANF in Mahua seed meal is __________

a) **Mowrine** b) Linatine

c) Linamarin d) Mimosine

Q 45 Which of the following ANF is not protein in nature?

a) Lectin b) Mimosine

c) Lathyrogens d) **Gossypol**

Q 46 Lectin is synonymous with __________

a) **Haemagglutinin** b) Saponin

c) Lathyrogen d) Mimosine

Q 47 ANF " Haemagglutinin" was first isolated from __________

a) Soybean b) Moong bean

c) **Castor bean** d) Kidney bean

Q 48 The disease "lathyrism" in human occur due to consumption of __________

a) **Chick pea** b) Subabul

c) Soyabean d) Kidney bean

Q 49 Tick the wrong statement about gossypol __________

a) **It occurs in three forms***

b) All gossypol in unprocessed seed is in free from

c) Free gossypol lead to toxicities.

d) Bound form of gossypol not readily absorbed

* occur in two form : bound and free

Q 50 Which of the following condition (s) favour the cyanide toxicity?

a) Freezing b) Plant injury

c) High nitrogen and low P d) **All the above**

Q 51 Which of the following method is useful in detoxification of mimosine in Subabul?

a) Sun drying b) Soaking

c) Ensiling d) **All the above**

Q 52 Conditions like draught, cloudy weather and spray of Insecticide (like 2,4-D) increase the accumulation of which of the following in the fodder crop?

a) Oxalate b) **Nitrate**

c) Phytate d) None of the above

Q 53 Tick the wrong statement __________

a) Bound gossypol is non-toxic

b) Solvent extracted cottonseed meal has the higher amount of free gossypol

c) Gossypol in cottonseed is located in glands

d) **Free form of gossypol is not toxic**

Q 54 Which of the following can induce the deficiency of Vitamin K?

a) **Coumarin** b) Gossypol

c) Dhurin d) Ricin

Q 55 Excessive feeding of which can lead to external and internal haemorrhage?

a) Sorghum b) **Sweat clover**

c) Turnip d) Cabbage

Q 56 Anti-nutritional factor in Sugarcane top is __________

a) Phytic acid b) Nitrate

c) **Oxalic acid** d) HCN

Q 57 Match column I with column II __________

Column I	Column II
i Anti-Niacin	A. Maize
ii Anti-Vitamin A	B. Soyabean

iii Anti-vitamin E — C. Kidney bean

iv Anti-Pyridoxine — D. Linseed

a) **i-A, ii-B, iii-C, iv-D** b) i-B, ii-D, iii-C, iv-A

c) i-D, ii-B, iii-C, iv-A d) i-C, ii-B, iii-A, iv-D

Q 58 Feeding of raw eggs to animals or human being can lead to deficiency of __________

a) **Biotin** b) Niacin

c) Choline d) None of these

Q 59 One molecule of 'Avidin' binds with how many molecule of biotin?

a) 2 b) 6

c) **4** d) 8

Q 60 The toxicant present in '*Cassia Tora*' is __________

a) Chemotrypsin b) **Chrysophanic acid**

c) Cyanogens d) Erucic acid

Q 61 Gizzzerosine is a toxic substance found in __________

a) **Fish** b) Maize gluten

c) Mustard seed d) Cotton seed

Q 62 Which of the following compound is not an example of glucosinolate?

a) Sinigrin b) Sinapine

c) Myrosine d) **Prunasin**

Q 63 Which of the following ANF has goitrogenic activity?

a) **Glucosinolate** b) Gossypol

c) Cynogenic glycoside d) Gums

Q 64 ANF present in guar meal/korma __________

a) Gums b) Trypsin inhibitors

c) **Both a and b** d) None of these

Q 65 "Leucenine" is synonymous with the __________

a) **Mimosine** b) Protectins
c) Mowrin d) Amygdalin

Q 66 Anti-metabolite reported to be present in Maize and wheat bran having anti-niaicn activity __________

a) **Niacytin** b) Nimbidine
c) Nitrate d) Phlorizin

Q 67 ANF present in apple leaves __________

a) **Phlorizin** b) Nimbidin
c) Mowrin d) None of these

Q 68 Formation of layer of precipitation on tongue on drinking tea or eating Jamun (blue berry)/banana is due to presence of __________

a) **Tannin** b) Phytic acid
c) Saponin d) Caffeine

Q 69 ANF present in young shoot of bamboo is __________

a) **Hydrocyanic acid** b) Tannin
c) Protease inhibitor d) Gum

Q 70 Formation of layer of precipitation on tongue on during cleaning the teeth with thin branch of Acacia tree (Commonly known as Datun/meswak) is due to presence of __________

a) **Tannin** b) Oxalate
c) Gum d) Goitrogens

Q 71 The ANF present in mango seed kernals is __________

a) **Tannin and HCN** b) Oxalate
c) Protease inhibitor d) None of these

Q 72 Anti-nutritional factors present in Jatropha kernal meal _____

a) Trypsin inhibitor b) Lectins
c) Phytate d) **All the above**

Q 73 ANF present in Babul (*Acacia*) pod is __________

a) **Tannin** b) Hydrocynic acid
c) Nitrate d) Oxalate

Q 74 An estrogenic compound namely 'Genistein' is reported to present in __________

a) **Soyabean meal** b) Neem seed meal

c) Linseed meal d) Rapeseed meal

Q 75 Low erucic acid and low glucosinolate variety of rapeseed is known as __________

a) Toria b) Taramira

c) **Canola** d) Mustard

Q 76 3,4dihydroxy pyridine is the break down product of which anti nutritional factor?

a) **Mimosine** b) Phytic acid

c) Oxalic acid d) All the above

Q 77 The ANF present in almond and apricot is __________

a) Avidin b) **Amygdalin**

c) Linnamarin d) Dhurrin

Q 78 Adulterant usually added in green fodder kept for sale purpose is __________

a) Saw dust b) Cobs dust

c) **Water** d) Sand

Q 79 Which of the following can be used as adulterant in fish meal?

a) Salt b) Urea

c) Leather meal d) **All the above**

Q 80 *Argimona maxicana* seed can be used as adulterant in which of the following?

a) **Mustard cake** b) Ground nut cake

c) Cotton seed cake d) Soyabean meal

Q 81 Toxic effect of gossypol can be ameliorated by supplementing the diet with __________

a) Copper sulphate b) **Ferrous sulphate**

c) Zinc sulphate d) Manganese sulphate

Q 82 Which of the following feed ingredients are not recommended for breeding bull?

a) **Cottonseed** b) Fish meal

c) Mustard d) Soyabean

Anti-nutritional Factors (ANF)

Anti-nutritional Factors (ANF) arethose substances present in the feed/diet which by themselves or their metabolic products arising in the system interfere with the feed utilization, reduce production or affect the health of the animal. These ANF are also known as toxic factor because of their deleterious effect they produce, when eaten by animals..They can be classified as under-

1. Depending upon the chemical properties the ANF's are classified as :

Group-I	Protein	1.Protease inhibitor
		2.Heamagglutinins (Lectin)
		3. Mimosine
		4. Lathyrogens
Group-II	Glycosides	1.Saponins
		2. Cyanogens
		3.Goiterogen or glucosinolate
Group-III	Phenols	1.Gossypol
		2.Tannins
Group-IV	Miscellaneous	1.Antimatal
		2.Antivitamins

2. On the basis of nutrient they affect directly or indirectly

a) Substances depressing digestion or metabolic utilization of protein __________

i) Protease inhibitors ii) Haemagglutinins

iii) Saponin iv) Polyphenolic components

b) Substances interfering with the utilization of minerals ______
  i) Phytic acid ii) Glucosinolate
  iii) Oxalic acid iv) Gossypol

c) Substances increasing the requirement of certain vitamins ____
  i) Anti-vitamins-A,D,E,K
  ii) Anti-vitamin-B_1,B_6,B_{12}&Nicotinic acid

d) Substances with a negative effect on the digestion of carbohydrate __________
  i) Amylase inhibitor ii) phenolic compounds
  iii) Flatulence factor

Common adulterants in feed and fodders

Adulteration is defined as the intentional admixture of pure substances with some cheaper and low quantity substances to make money. Costly feed ingredients like oil cakes and feed products from animal origin like fish meal are adulterated.

S.No.	Feed ingredients	Adulterants
1.	GN cake	Groundnut husk, urea, non-edible oilcakes.
2.	Mustard cake	Argimonamaxicana seed, urea
3.	Soyabean meal	Urea
4.	DORB	Ground rice hulls, saw dust.
5.	Wheat bran	Ground rice hulls, saw dust.
6.	Fish meal	Common salt, urea
7.	Mineral mixture	Common salt, marble powder, sand, limestone
8.	Molasses	Water
9.	Fodder	Water
10.	Rice polish	Rise husk

❑❑❑

Chapter 17

Feed Technology

Q 1 The Association of American Feed Control Official (AAFCO) was established in __________

a) **1909** b) 1911

c) 1961 d) 1985

Q 2 Compound Livestock Feed Manufacturer Association (CLFMA) came into existence in __________

a) 1961 b) 1948

c) **1967** d) 1998

Q 3 American Feed Industry Association (AFIA) earlier known as American Feed Manufacturer Association (AFMA) was found in __________

a) 1961 b) **1909**

c) 1985 d) 1971

Q 4 "Linear Programming" was developed by __________

a) **George B. Dantzig** b) W.V. Waugh

c) G.A. Karstins d) None of the above

Q 5 Pulses milling byproducts are commonly known as __________

a) **Chunnies** b) Glutens

c) Brans d) Husks

Q 6 The era of compound livestock feed in India was started with the establishment of first feed mill at __________

a) **Ludhiana (Punjab)** b) Brailly (UP)

c) Bikaner (Rajasthan) d) Karnal (Haryana)

Q 7 Permissible limit of toxic seed in edible cereal grain is _______

a) **Less than 0.05%** b) 1-2 %

c) 2-5% d) 5-10%

Q 8 Tick the right statement regarding method of oil extraction ___

a) Solvent extraction method is most efficient

b) Generally Ghani pressed cake are more palatable

c) Ghani and expeller pressed cakes are lustrous as compare to solvent extracted

d) **All are correct**

Q 9 For making cattle and buffalo feed, the soundness of grain must be __________

a) **> 70%** b) 55-70%

c) 30-35 % d) < 30%

Q 10 How many minimum bags are to be sampled in order to get the accurate sample from a lot of 50 bags of feed?

a) 50 b) **5**

c) 15 d) 20

Q 11 Dry rolling is also known as __________

a) **Cracking** b) Crimping

c) Crumbling d) All the above

Q 12 The process of disintegration of kernels into particle with the use of corrugated roller is known as __________

a) Cracking b) Dry rolling

c) **Crimping** d) Both a & b

Q 13 Grinding of pelleted feed to produce granular particle is known as __________

a) Cracking b) Crimping

c) **Crumbling** d) All the above

Q 14 The process in which application of dry heat cause a sudden expansion of grain due to rupture of endosperm is known as __________

a) Popping b) Puffing

c) Micronizing d) **Both a & b**

Q 15 In above question ,if infrered heat energy is used, then the process is known as __________

a) **Micronizing** b) Roasting
c) Puffing d) Baking

Q 16 Which of the following statement is wrong regarding popping?

a) It increases palatability
b) It improves digestibility
c) **It increases the density of grain**
d) Popped grain are good molasses carrier

Q 17 Conditioning of grains by addition of water to raise the moisture content is called as __________

a) **Reconstitution** b) Sprouting
c) Extrusion d) Exploding

Q 18 The treatment of grains with hot steam for 3-5 minute followed by rolling is known as __________

a) Dry rolling b) **Steam rolling**
c) Steam flaking d) Extrusion

Q 19 Which of the following process increases the density of feed?

a) Popping b) Micronizing
c) **Pelleting** d) Sprouting

Q 20 The process in which grains are subjected to high pressure steam (205 psi) for about 20 sec followed by sudden decrease to atmosphere pressure is known as __________

a) **Exploding** b) Steam rolling
c) Pressure cooking d) Extrusion

Q 21 Which of the following is roughage processing method?

a) Dry rolling b) Extruding
c) **Balling** d) Micronizing

Q 22 "Shearing" is a combination of __________

a) Cutting and grinding b) **Cutting and crushing**
c) Cutting and bailing d) Crushing and bailing

Q 23 Which of the following is a wet method of grains processing?

a) Crimping
b) Micronizing
c) **Extrusion**
d) Roasting

Q 24 Which of the following is a dry method of grain processing?

a) Extrusion
b) Gelatinization
c) Exploding
d) **Pelleting**

Q 25 Which of the following is a hot method of grain processing?

a) Dry rolling
b) Crumbling
c) Crimping
d) **Popping**

Q 26 Which of the following is a cold method of grain processing?

a) Steam rolling
b) Exploding
c) Micronizing
d) **Extrusion**

Q 27 Modulus of uniformity and fineness is used to determine the feed ___________

a) **Particle size**
b) Particle shape
c) Both a and b
d) None of the above

Q 28 While measuring particle size using seven sieve system (0.375,4,8,14,28,48,100 mesh size), which statement is wrong?

a) Particle remaining on 0.375, 4 and 8 are coarse particles
b) **Particle remaining on 0.375, 4 and 8 are fine particles**
c) Particle remaining on 48 and 100 are fine particles
d) Particle remaining on 14 and 28 are medium particles

Q 29 The triangular shaped compressed feed is known as _______

a) **Prism**
b) Wafer
c) Brick
d) Briquette

Q 30 The small size square and rectangular compressed is known as ___________

a) Prism
b) **Wafer**
c) Brick
d) Briquette

Q 31 Soft pellet generally have __________

a) No Molasses
b) 5 % Molasses
c) 5-10 % Molasses
d) **30-40 % Molasses**

Q 32 Time between the emptying and reloading of the feed mixer is known as __________

a) Loading time
b) Emptying time
c) **Dead time**
d) All the above

Q 33 Pelleting is also known as __________

a) **Agglomeration**
b) Impact grinding
c) Both of the above
d) None of the above

Q 34 The structure used for storage of grain is known as __________

a) Ghada (pitcher)
b) Bhandari
c) Bukhari
d) **All the above**

Q 35 Which of the following is used for fumigation of grain for increasing their shelf life?

a) Malathion
b) Dichlorovos
c) Pyrethrum
d) **Ethylene dibromide**

Q 36 A lot of feed prepared at one time at processing unit is known as __________

a) **Batch**
b) Barrel
c) Bale
d) Capacity

Q 37 The edible ingredient used for the uniform mixing of micro ingredients in the feed to prepare compound feed is known as __________

a) Additives
b) **Carriers**
c) Supplement
d) All the above

Q 38 The process of particle reduction by combined action of breaking and crushing of feed ingredients is known as __________

a) **Cracking**
b) Crimping
c) Both of the above
d) None of the above

Q 39 AOAC (Association of Official Analytical Chemist) originally belong to which country?

a) Canada
b) Britain
c) **USA**
d) Holland

Q 40 AOAC was founded at Philadelphia, USA in the year _______

a) 1864
b) 1874
c) **1884**
d) 1894

Q 41 The concept to prepare complete feed block in India emerged from which institute?

a) **NDRI, Karnal**
b) IARI, New Delhi
c) PAU, Ludhiana
d) None of these

Q 42 An edible material to which ingredients are added to facilitate uniform incorporation of latter into feed is known as _______

a) **Carriers**
b) Scratch
c) Kibbled
d) All the above

Q 43 The process of treatment of straw with NaOH was first used in which country?

a) USA
b) **Germany**
c) India
d) Denmark

Q 44 "Modulus of uniformity and fineness" for determining the particle size was developed by which country?

a) **America**
b) Germany
c) Denmark
d) New Zealand

Q 45 "Animal Nutrition and Feed Technology" journal is publishing from which of the following centre?

a) **IVRI, Izzatnagar**
b) NDRI, Karnal
c) GADVASU, Ludhiana
d) TANUVAS, Chennai

Q 46 Ingredeints can account for how much cost of producing feeds?

a) 40-50%
b) **70-90%**
c) 10-40%
d) 20-50%

Q 47 The first seminar of CLFMA was held at _________

a) **Hyderabad**
b) Ludhiana
c) Mumbai
d) Bangalore

Q 48 Among the following methods of densification of roughage, which one result in product of bigger size?

a) **Baling**
b) Block making
c) Pelleting
d) Wafering

Q 49 The acceptable coefficient of variation in the composition of mixed feed ins in the range of ________

a) 10-20 %
b) 20-30%
c) **5-10 %**
d) 5-15 %

* Preferably less than 5%

Q 50 ANA (Animal Nutrition Association), India was formed at ____

a) **Deptt. of Animal Nutrition, IVRI, Izzatnagar**
b) Division of Catlle Nutrition, NDRI, Karnal
c) Deptt. of Animal Nutrition, PAU, Ludhiana
d) Deptt. of Animal Nutrition, Bikaner

Q 51 Animal Nutrition Society of India was formed at ________

a) IVRI, Izzatnagar
b) GADVASU, Ludhiana
c) **NDRI, Karnal**
d) TANUVAS, Chennai

Q 52 An edible material or natural substances mixed in a feed to decrease the concentration of a nutrient is known as ________

a) Carriers
b) **Diluent**
c) Additive
d) Supplement

Q 53 Weight of 100 kg is known as ________

a) Ton
b) **Quintal**
c) Both of the above
d) None of the above

Q 54 Which of the following method causes the gelatinization of starch?

a) Steam flaking
b) Popping
c) Extruding
d) **All the above**

Q 55 "Codex Alimentarius" structure comprise of how many volumes?

a) 10
b) 11
c) 12
d) **13**

Q 56 How many minimum bags are to be sampled in order to get the accurate sample from a lot of 500 bags of feed ingredients?

a) **5 % of the total bags** b) 15% of the total bags

c) 20 % of the totals bags d) 30 % of the total bags

Q 57 India's first commercial densified feed project was established at (in 1944) __________

a) **Bulandshahar (UP)** b) Ludhiana, Punjab

c) Karnal (Haryana) d) Hissar (Haryana)

Q 58 The optimum pellet durability index is __________

a) 70-75 b) 80-83

c) **90-93** d) 60-65

Q 59 Which of the following is the major factor influencing the pellet quality?

a) **Mash formulation** b) Cooling

c) Pellet die d) Conditioning

Q 60 Which of the following is not a buffer?

a) Sodium bicarbonate b) Sodium sesquicarbonate

c) **Zinc oxide** d) None of these

Q 61 The ratio of sodium bicarbonate to Magnesium oxide in buffer is generally __________

a) **2-3:1** b) 5-6:1

c) 8-10:1 d) 1:1

Q 62 Sodium sesquicarbonate contain a mixture of __________

a) **Sodium bicarbonate and sodium carbonate**

b) Sodium bicarbonate and NaCl

c) Sodium bicarbonate and MgO

d) None of these

Q 63 Sodium carbonate is a __________

a) Buffer b) **Alkalinizer**

c) Acid d) Anti-oxidants

Q 64 Which of the following is not a buffering agent?

a) Sodium bicarbonate
b) Sodium sesquicarbonate
c) **Calcium carbonate**
d) Potassium carbonate

Q 65 Which of the following first time proposed the formalin treatment for protein protection from rumen degradation?

a) **INRA***
b) CSIRO
c) NRC
d) ARC

* INRA- Instit National de la Recherche Agronomique (French Institute of National Agriculture Research)

Q 66 The main mechanism by which formalin act in protecting the protein from rumen degradation is through formation of __________

a) Peptide linkage with amino acid
b) Co-ordinate covalent bond
c) **Methylene bridge**
d) Mallard product

❑❑❑

Chapter 18

Silage and Hay

Q 1 Silage is generally prepared from the crop having high content of __________

a) **Carbohydrate** b) Protein

c) Fat d) Water

Q 2 The chief acid formed in silage process which is responsible for good quality silage is __________

a) **Lactic acid** b) Acetic acid

c) Butyric acid d) Valeric acid

Q 3 Very good quality silage must have pH in the range of ______

a) **3.5-4.2** b) 4.5-5.0

c) 5.0-6.0 d) 6.0-7.0

Q 4 During silage formation upto what extent DM can be lost?

a) 10 b) **20**

c) 40 d) 50

Q 5 The process of making the silage of grass is known as ________

a) Haylage b) Wastelage

c) **Ensiling** d) None of the above

Q 6 The process of silage making is known as __________

a) Soiling b) **Ensiling/siloling**

c) Both of the above d) None of the above

Q 7 The minimum dry matter required in the crop for making good quality silage is __________

a) **35 %** b) 45%

c) 15% d) 25%

Q 8 Which of the following is mainly responsible for the creation of favourable condition for the preservation of silage?

a) **Lactic acid bacteria** b) Clostridium

c) Listeria d) *E. coli*

Q 9 The gross energy of the well preserved silage is generally ______ than those of parent material.

a) **Higher** b) Lower

c) Equal d) None of the above

Q 10 In AIV process of silage making, following combination is used __________

a) **Sulphuric acid & hydrochloric acid**

b) Sulphuric acid & Formic acid

c) Sulphuric acid & Formalin

d) Formalin & Formic acid

Q 11 One cubic metre space of silo pit is sufficient for following amount of chaffed green fodder __________

a) **5-6 quintal** b) 10-15 quintal

c) 1-2 quital d) 15-20 quintal

Q 12 The optimum size of chaffing for preparing the good quality silage is __________

a) **5-8 cm** b) 10-15 cm

c) 15-20 cm d) 20-25 cm

Q 13 Silo filler disease was caused by __________

a) **Oxides of nitrogen** b) Oxides of sulphur

d) Oxides of zinc d) Oxides of copper

Q 14 In badly formed silage, which of the following acid is formed in higher amount?

a) Acetic acid b) **Butyric acid**

c) Lactic acid d) Valeric acid

Q 15 In good quality silage, Ammoniacal nitrogen will be ________

a) **Less than 10% of the total nitrogen**

b) Between 10-15%

c) Between 15-20%

d) More than 20%

Q 16 Removal of nutrient through running water is known as _____

a) Bleaching b) Drainage

c) **Leaching** d) Effluent loss

Q 17 Bleaching while hay making generally reduced the following contents __________

a) **Carotene** b) Carbohydrate

c) Minerals d) Amino acids

Q 18 The best method of hay making in excessive rainfall area is ___

a) Spreading in the filed b) Windows method

c) **Tripod method** d) None of the above

Q 19 Poola system of hay making is very much common in the following state __________

a) Punjab b) Haryana

c) **Uttar Pradesh** d) Rajasthan

Q 20 The typical light brown colour or golden yellow colour of the silage is due to the following pigment __________

a) Chlorophyll b) **Phacophytin**

c) Xanthophill d) None of the above

Q 21 Which of the following microorganism is not used in the silage production as additive?

a) *Lactobacillus acidophilus* b) *Torulopsis* sp.

c) *Bacillus subtilis* d) ***Clostridium* sp.**

Q 22 In good quality hay, moisture content should be in the range of __________

a) **15-20 %** b) 30-35%

c) 20-30% d) 40-45%

Q 23 DCP% is highest for ________

a) **Lucerne hay** b) Barseem hay

c) Oat hay d) Wheat straw

Q 24 Hay is generally prepared from the fodder high in ________

a) **Protein** b) Carbohydrate

c) Fat d) Mineral contents

Q 25 Which of the following ANF is reduced to almost negligible amounts through silage making?

a) **Prussic acid** b) Oxalate

c) Selenium d) Nitrate

Q 26 The average weight of one cublic feet silage in a pit silos ______

a) 10-15 kg b) **28 kg**

c) 18-20 kg d) 38 kg

Q 27 The average weight of one cubic feet silage in a trench silo is __

a) **15-16 kg** b) 35-36 kg

c) 25-26 kg d) 45-46 kgs

Q 28 Which crop is more suitable for silage making?

a) **Sorghum** b) Guar

c) Barseem d) Senji

Q 29 Which of the following is not required for making good quality silage?

a) High water soluble carbohydrate

b) Low buffering capacity

c) Optimum moisture content

d) **High protein level**

Q 30 Fleig index is a commonly used method for evaluation of _____

a) **Silage quality** b) Hay quality

c) Fresh fodder quality d) Straw quality

Q 31 In Haylage, the forage crop is dried to a moisture level of about __________

a) 25-35 % b) **45-55 %**
c) 15-20% d) None of the above

Q 32 The suitable moisture in fodder crop content for the silage making is __________

a) **60-70 %** b) 75-80%
c) 80-85% d) 85-90%

Q 33 Loss of nutrient along with running water (rain etc.) in silage making is known as __________

a) Bleaching b) Drainage
c) **Leaching** d) Effluent loss

Q 34 Bleaching while hay making generally reduced the following content of the fodder __________

a) **Carotene** b) Sugar
c) Minerals d) Amino acid

Q 35 Farmers lung disease in man was caused by handling of _____

a) **Actinomycetis affected mouldy hay**
b) Cow dung
c) Wheat straw
d) Smoke

Q 36 The origin of silage making reported to be occur in __________

a) **Germany** b) Japan
c) New Zealand d) USA

Q 37 Toulene distillation method is used to measure the ________

a) **Dry matter of silage**
b) Acid content in silage
c) VFA in rumen
d) Ammoniacal Nitrogen in the rumen

Q 38 The origin of silage making was reported to be occur in ______

a) **Germany** b) Japan
c) Newzealand d) Greenland

Q 39 Fleig's value/index for grading of silage belongs to ________

a) USA b) Australia

c) Holland d) **Germany**

Q 40 For very good quality silage, the Fleigs value range between ________

a) **44-50** b) 10-19

c) 30-36 d) 20-29

Q 41 Silage that undergo excessive heating due to yeast or bacillus growth has following odour __________

a) Earthy b) **Tobacco/burnt**

c) Musty d) Vinegar

Q 42 Clostridial dominant silage will give __________

a) **Putrid smell** b) Earthy smell

c) Sweet smell d) Vinegar smell

Q 43 Rancid milk odour from silage point toward __________

a) Excessive heated silage

b) **Clostridial fermentation**

c) High lactic acid fermentation

d) Mold infestation

Q 44 In India, (especially Northern) lean period pertain to _______

a) May –June b) Oct-November

c) **Both of these** d) None of these

Q 45 Optimum stage of maize to be ensiled is __________

a) **Dent stage** b) Ear formation stage

c) 1.5 feet hight d) Can be cut at any stage

Q 46 Grab/squeeze test in silage making is used to measure ______

a) **Moisture content in chopped fodder before ensiling**

b) Moisture content in silage

c) Both of the above

d) Seepage rate in silage

Q 47 Low moisture silage of grasses and legumes is known as _____

a) Balage b) **Haylage**

c) Haysel d) None of these

Q 48 High moisture (40-60%) forage rolled up in big round bales and then wrapped in plastic for preservation is known as _________

a) Balage b) Big bale haylage

c) Round bale silage d) **All the above**

Q 49 Oatlage is silage made from _________

a) **Oat** b) Berseem + oat

c) Maize + oat d) Oat + mustard

Q 50 Baled silage is known as _________

a) **Balage** b) Tube silage

c) Both of the above d) None of these

Q 51 Match the crop with their proper stage of harvesting for silage making _________

A) Maize i) Late dent stage

B) Sorghum ii) Early dent stage

C) Oat iii) Flower formation

D) Napier bajra iv) One metre height

a) **A-ii,B-i,C-iii,D-iv**

b) A-iv, B-i,C-iii,D-i

c) A-iv,B-ii,C-iv,D-iii

d) A-ii,B-iv,C-i,D-iii

Q 52 Haysel is _________

a) Process of hay making on barbed wire

b) **Hay making season**

c) Making hay from non leguminous crops

d) None of the above

Q 53 AIV silage originated in which country?

a) Newzealand b) **Finland**

c) Greenland d) Canada

Q 54 Silage is __________

a) Preserved dry fodder b) **Fermented fodder**

c) Succulent fodder d) None of these

Q 55 When grass and legumes generally meant for hay are ensiled, then it is known as __________

a) **Haylage** b) Wastelage

c) Shredlage d) Earlage

Q 56 When animal organic waste is incorporated in silage, then it becomes __________

a) Haylage b) **Wastelage**

c) Shredlage d) Balage

Q 57 When corn grain, cobs and in some cases husk and a proportion of stalk is ensiled, then it is known as __________

a) Haylage b) **Earlage**

c) Shredlage d) Balage

Q 58 When maize is chopped and shredded before ensiling, then product formed is known as __________

a) **Shredlage** b) Snaplage

c) Haylage d) Earlage

Q 59 Urea can be safely incorporated in silage at level of ________

a) **0.5%** b) 5%

c) 10% d) 15%

Q 60 A preserved fodder having characteristics between those of hay and silage is known as __________

a) **Haylage** b) Tillage

c) Earlage d) Balage

Q 61 In good quality silage, which types of fermentation predominates?

a) **Lactic acid type** b) Butyric acid type

c) Both are equally present d) None of these

Q 62 About lactic acid type fermentation of silage ,which statement is true?

a) Homofermentative and hetrofermentative types of bacteria involved

b) 2 moles of lactic acid are formed/glucose in homofermentive type

c) Hetrofermentative type is less efficient as compared to homofermentative in terms of lactic acid production.

d) **All are true**

Q 63 If hay is stored with high moisture, then fermentation occur and heat so produces causes the breakdown of sugar to alcohol, such type of hay is known as __________

a) Cocking of hay b) Mow-burnt hay

c) Brown hay d) **Both b & c**

Q 64 In the process of hay making, which vitamin content is increased?

a) A b) C

c) **D** d) E

Q 65 The correct sequence from starting to end of the ensiling process is __________

a) **Aerobic phase - fermentation phase-stable phase- feed out phase**

b) Aerobic spoilage phase-stable phase-fermentation phase-aerobic phase

c) Stable phase-aerobic phase-fermentation phase-feed out phase

d) Fermentative phase-stable phase-aerobic phase-feed out phase

* Feed out phase is also known as aerobic spoilage phase

Q 66 The desirable microorganism in ensiling process is ________

a) Yeast b) Enterobacter

c) **Lactic acid bacteria** d) Acetic acid bacteria

Q 67 The undesirable microorganism in silage microflora is ______

a) Yeast
b) Clostridia
c) Acetic acid bacteria
d) Bacilli
e) **All the above**

Q 68 The most nutritious hay is __________

a) **Alfalfa hay**
b) Cow pea hay
c) Ground nut hay
d) Oat hay

Q 69 Which of the following is a good source of calcium?

a) **Lucerne hay**
b) Berseem forages
c) Oat Straw
d) Wheat bran

Q 70 What is the effect of silage with extremely high ethanol content on the animal?

a) Lower milk production
b) Lower milk component
c) **Off flavoured milk**
d) No effect

Q 71 When lactic acid dominates the acid profile of silage, what level of quality do you have?

a) Very low
b) Low
c) Moderate
d) **High**

Q 72 What is the ideal ranking from highest to lowest for the acid profile for silage?

a) **Lactic acid, acetic acid and butyric acid**
b) Butyric acid, acetic acid, and lactic acid
c) Acetic acid, butyric acid and lactic acid
d) Acetic acid, lactic acid and butyric acid

Q 73 Addition of urea to corn silage meant for dairy cow is generally done to __________

a) Inhibit the overgrowth of bacteria in the cow digestive tract by decreasing the pH of the gastric juices.
b) **Increase the nitrogen available to the bacteria that synthesize amino acid in the cow rumen**
c) Prevent the growth of molds and fungi that may make silage unpalatable
d) Add high quality carbohydrate to the silage to increase the amount of digestible energy in the feed.

Q 74 Tick the right statement __________

a) Hay and silage contain higher amount of NPN, then the same feed because of proteolysis that occur during wilting and fermentation

b) Fermented forages have higher concentration of free amino acid, ammonia, amine and lower concentration of peptides and nitrates

c) In fresh forage, NPN content composed largely of peptide, free amino acid and nitrates.

d) **All the above**

Q 75 Which of the following option represents the silage quality?

a) **70 % water & 30% DM** b) 50 % water & 50% DM

c) 20% water & 80% DM d) All the above

Q 76 Which of the following option describe the hay parameters?

a) 70 % water & 30% DM b) 50 % water & 50% DM

c) **15% water & 85% DM** d) All the above

Q 77 Which of the following option describe the haylage

a) 70 % water & 30% DM b) **50 % water & 50% DM**

c) 20% water & 80% DM d) All the above

Q 78 Paddy straw has __________

a) High digestibility b) Optimum digestibility

c) **Poor digestibility** d) High nutritive value

Q 79 Paddy straw is rich in __________

a) Keratin b) **Lignin**

c) Carbohydrate d) Protein

Q 80 What is buffering capacity of forages?

a) Ability to stimulate the cow to produce buffer

b) **Ability of forages to resist changes in rumen pH**

c) Amount of acid relative to protein present in the fermented forages

d) Forages does not have buffering capacity

Q 81 When lactic acid dominate the acid profile of silage, what level of quality do you have?

a) Very low
b) Low
c) Moderate
d) **High**

Q 82 What is the effect of silage with extensively high ethanol content on the animal?

a) Lower milk production
b) Lower milk components
c) **Off flavoured milk**
d) No effect

Q 83 Presence of classic smell of mouse dropping indicate that silage is putrefied by ________

a) **Clostridium**
b) Yeast
c) Bacillus
d) Mould

Q 84 Presence of bread odour in the silage indicate the ________

a) Clostridium growth
b) **Yeast growth**
c) Bacillus growth
d) Mould growth

Q 85 Heating of silage (> 120^{0}F) can occur by ________

a) Slow filling
b) Structure air leaks
c) Poor compaction
d) **All the above**

Q 86 Out of the following acids present in the silage, which one is stronger than other?

a) Acetic acid
b) **Lactic acid**
c) Butyric acid
d) Propionic acid

Q 87 Which type of fermentation in silage result in the lowest losses of DM?

a) **Lactic acid bacterial fermentation**
b) Enetrobacterial fermentation
c) Clostridial fermentation
d) Can be any of these

Q 88 High Butyric acid in silage indicates that silage has undergone ________

a) Lactic acid bacterial fermentation
b) Enterobacterial fermentation
c) **Clostridial fermentation**
d) None of these

Q 89 High content of which acid in the silage can sometime lead to ketosis in lactating cow?

a) Lactic acid
b) Acetic acid
c) **Butyric acid**
d) Propionic acid

Q 90 Which of the following fermentation produces the good quality silage?

a) **Lactic acid bacterial fermentation**
b) Enterobacterial fermentation
c) Clostridial fermentation
d) All of these

Q 91 Which type of the fermentation in silage result in the lowest losses of DM?

a) **Lactic acid bacterial fermentation**
b) Enterobacterial fermentation
c) Clostridial fermentation
d) Can be any of these

Q 92 High butyric acid in silage indicate that silage has undergone __________

a) Lactic acid bacterial fermentation
b) Enterobacterial fermentation
c) **Clostridial fermentation**
d) None of these

Q 93 Generally, silage fermentation can be divided into how many phase?

a) 4
b) 5
c) **6**
d) 8

❑❑❑

C. NUTRIENT REQUIREMENT AND FEEDING OF DIFFERENT ANIMALS

by Dr Jaspal Singh Hundal

Chapter 19

Nutrients Requirements and Feeding of Cattle and Buffaloes

Q 1 Latest feeding standard available for dairy cows ________

a) NRC (1992)
b) NRC (1994)
c) **NRC (2001)**
d) NRC (2007)

Q 2 Latest Indian feeding standard available for dairy cows ________

a) ICAR (2001)
b) **ICAR (2013)**
c) BIS (1998)
d) BIS (2007)

Q 3 NE requirement for maintenance of cattle is sum of the NE required for ________

a) Basal metabolism
b) Activity increment
c) Body temperature regulation
d) **All**

Q 4 Metabolic faecal nitrogen consists of ________

a) Residual bile
b) Digestive enzymes
c) Epithelial cell
d) **All the above**

Q 5 The conditions of animals which are not essential for measuring metabolic rate are ________

a) Good nutritive condition
b) Environmental temperature
c) Rest
d) **Productive status**

Q 6 The energy requirement for basal metabolism and activity factor is called as __________

a) **Maintenance requirement**

b) Growth requirement

c) Production requirement

d) Basal requirement

Q 7 Loss of protein through urine is called as __________

a) **Endogenous Urinary Nitrogen**

b) Exogenous Urinary Nitrogen

c) NPN

d) Undigested protein

Q 8 The nutrient allowance is ___________ than the nutrient requirement.

a) **Lower** b) Higher

c) Same d) None

Q 9 Which is not related with the continuously loss of protein from body.

a) Wear and tear of body tissues

b) Renewal of feathers

c) Renewal of nails/hoof

d) **None**

Q 10 Faecal nitrogen of a cow consists of undigested nitrogen from feed and __________

a) Keratin

b) Uric acid

c) **Metabolic faecal nitrogen**

d) NPN

Q 11 The most common limiting factor in ruminant nutrition __________

a) Protein b) **Energy**

c) Fat d) Water

Q 12 The accurate method of estimating the protein requirement is by ________

a) Age
b) Weight gain
c) **N-balance study**
d) Digestion trial

Q 13 The amount of protein to be supplied through diet should be the sum of protein deposited in tissues plus EUN and ________

a) Extra 10%
b) Extra 20%
c) Extra 30%
d) **MFN**

Q 14 The DCP required for milk production compared to maintenance is ________

a) Same
b) 25% more
c) 50% more
d) **100% more**

Q 15 Weight gained during pregnancy is ________

a) **Reduces**
b) Retained
c) Not altered
d) Increases

Q 16 Pregnancy anabolism in dam ________

a) **Helps in lactation**
b) Does not help in lactation
c) Helps in calving
d) Problematic

Q 17 Lactation requirement for minerals is defined as the concentration the mineral in ________ multiplied by the 4 per cent FCM milk yield.

a) **Milk**
b) Blood
c) Ruminal fluid
d) Feed

Q 18 'Requirement for absorbed mineral' for diary animal means sum of ________ requirement of the tissues for the mineral.

a) Maintenance
b) Lactation
c) Pregnancy and growth
d) **All**

Q 19 An animal obtaining all its energy by the oxidation of glucose will result in the release of ________

a) **5.007 Kcal of Heat**
b) 6.007 Kcal of Heat
c) 4.007 Kcal of Heat
d) 5.63 Kcal of Heat

Q 20 Net energy value of the feed is __________ % of the digestible energy.

a) 65% b) 82%

c) **70%** d) 96%

Q 21 One kilogram of TDN is equal to __________ Mcal DE.

a) 5.63 b) **4.4**

c) 3.6 d) 4.0

Q 22 Young calves require protein in the form of __________

a) NPN b) Keratine

c) Creatinine d) **Oil seed cakes**

Q 23 Biological value of protein for cattle is __________

a) 50% b) 65%

c) **70%** d) 100%

Q 24 Biological value of protein for body building activity in growing animals is only __________

a) 50% b) **65%**

c) 70% d) 100%

Q 25 The animal body ultimately derives all of its energy through __________

a) **Oxidation** b) Fermentation

c) Environment d) Anabolism

Q 26 Water intake is stimulated by diets with high __________

a) Salt b) Sodium bicarbonate

c) Protien d) **All**

Q 27 The fat which is not meant for animal feeding __________

a) Vegetable oils b) Protected fats

c) Dry-granular fats d) **None**

Q 28 Dry-granular fats are often referred as __________

a) **Ruminally inert fats** b) Unpalatable fats

c) 'D' Fats d) None

Q 29 With increase in degree of unsaturation, the digestibility of fatty acids __________

a) **Increases** b) Decreases

c) Remains unaffected d) None

Q 30 The total dietary fat should not exceed___________percent of dietary dry matter.

a) 9% b) **7%**

c) 1% d) 3%

Q 31 Amount of fat to be included in ration of dairy cattle does not depends upon.

a) Type of fat

b) Feed making up the basal diet

c) Environment

d) **None**

Q 32 In general, mixtures of cereal grains and forages usually forms ___________ percent fat of dairy animal ration.

a) 1% b) 0.5%

c) **3%** d) 5%

Q 33 Feeding supplemental fat to ruminants may reduce the digestibility of __________

a) Calcium b) Magnesium

c) **Both** d) None

Q 34 Carbohydrates are the major source of energy for dairy animals and it usually forms ___________ % of their total diet.

a) 45% b) **60-70%**

c) 25-35% d) 90%

Q 35 Ruminal fermentation of non-structured carbohydrates does not vary greatly with __________

a) Type of feed b) Conservation of fodder

c) Processing methods d) **None**

Q 36 Trace minerals do not serve as components of __________

a) Metalloenzymes b) Enzyme cofactors

c) Hormones **d) None**

Q 37 Nutrients requirements of calcium (%) for dairy cows (NRC, 2001) __________

a) 0.67 b) 0.36

c) 0.20 d) 0.22

Q 38 Nutrients requirements of phosphorus (%) for dairy cows (NRC, 2001) __________

a) 0.67 **b) 0.36**

c) 0.20 d) 0.22

Q 39 Nutrients requirements of magnesium/sulfur (%) for dairy cows (NRC, 2001) __________

a) 0.67 b) 0.36

c) 0.20 d) 0.22

Q 40 Nutrients requirements of sodium (%) for high yielding dairy cows (NRC, 2001) __________

a) 0.67 b) 0.36

c) 0.20 **d) 0.22**

Q 41 Dairy cattle require absolute dietary requirement of the vitamins __________

a) A, D and E b) A, D, E and K

c) A and E d) A, D, K

Q 42 The vitamin which can be synthesized by ruminal and intestinal bacteria __________

a) A **b) K**

c) D d) E

Q 43 The vitamins which can be synthesized by ruminal microorganism __________

a) A, B and K b) K and E

c) K, B and C d) A and C

Q 44 Nutrients requirements of vitamin A (IU/kg) for high yielding dairy cattle (NRC, 2001) __________

a) **2800** b) 760

c) 20 d) 1900

Q 45 Nutrients requirements of vitamin E (IU/kg) for high yielding dairy cattle (NRC, 2001) __________

a) 2800 b) **760**

c) 20 d) 1900

Q 46 Nutrients requirements of vitamin D (IU/kg) for high yielding dairy cattle (NRC, 2001) __________

a) 2800 b) 760

c) **20** d) 1900

Q 47 Overfeeding of nutrients results in __________

a) Increase in feed cost

b) Excessive of excretion of nutrients

c) Environment pollution

d) **All**

Q 48 The factors affecting dry matter intake of animals __________

a) Plant factors b) Animal factors

c) Environmental factors d) **All**

Q 49 Which plant factor is not related with dry matter intake?

a) Physical form of fodder b) Processing of fodder

c) Nutritive value d) **None**

Q 50 Which animal factor is not related with dry matter intake?

a) Type of animal b) Stage of production

c) Social behavior d) **None**

Q 51 Which environmental factor is not related with dry matter intake?

a) Temperature b) Humidity

c) Both d) **None**

Q 52 The dry matter requirement for maintenance in cattle is __________

a) **80 g/$W^{0.75}$** b) 50 g/$W^{0.75}$

c) 110 g/$W^{0.75}$ d) 25 g/$W^{0.75}$

Q 53 Dairy cattle consume dry matter __________% of their body weight to fulfill maintenance requirements.

a) **2.0-2.5%** b) 5-7%

c) 1.0-1.5% d) 3.0-3.8%

Q 54 Dairy cattle consume dry matter __________% of their body weight to fulfill growth requirements.

a) 2.0-2.5% b) 5-7%

c) **2.5-3.0%** d) 3.0-3.8%

Q 55 Average energy requirement (TDN) for maintenance of dairy cattle __________

a) **31-48 g/$W^{0.75}$** b) 50 g/$W^{0.75}$

c) 110 g/$W^{0.75}$ d) 25 g/$W^{0.75}$

Q 56 Average energy requirement (Kcal ME/$W^{0.75}$ Kg/d) for maintenance of dairy cattle __________

a) 101 b) 98

c) 106 d) **142**

Q 57 Crude protein maintenance requirement for dairy cattle __________

a) 3.1-4.8 g/$W^{0.75}$ b) 40-50 g/$W^{0.75}$

c) **5.28-7.5 g/$W^{0.75}$** d) 2.0-3.5 g/$W^{0.75}$

Q 58 Average digestible crude protein maintenance requirement for dairy cattle __________

a) **7.12 g/$W^{0.75}$** b) 4.50 g/$W^{0.75}$

c) 5.28 g/$W^{0.75}$ d) 3.50 g/$W^{0.75}$

Q 59 Digestible crude protein maintenance requirement (g/g of body weight gain) for dairy cattle __________

a) 0.10 b) **0.19**

c) 0.5 d) 2.5

Q 60 Salt should be included in the concentrate mixture of ruminants __________

a) **1%** b) 2.5%
c) 0.5% d) 3.5%

Q 61 Molasses can be used upto __________ % in dairy ration.

a) 5% b) **10%**
c) 3% d) 13%

Q 62 Feed the calf with colostrums __________ of their body weight for first three weeks.

a) **1/10th** b) 1/15th
c) 1/20th d) 1/5th

Q 63 Feed the calf with colostrums with in _______ hrs of their birth.

a) **2** b) 12
c) 8 d) 24

Q 64 Milk replacer should be fed at the age of __________

a) 5 days b) 20 days
c) **10 days** d) 15 days

Q 65 Milk replacer can be given to calves upto __________ of age.

a) **One month** b) Two month
c) Three month d) Four month

Q 66 Calf starter rations should contain __________

a) 14-16% DCP and 72% TDN
b) 18-20% DCP and 72% TDN
c) **20-23% DCP and 65-70% TDN**
d) 18-20% DCP and 65% TDN

Q 67 In general, best roughage to concentrate ratio for dairy animals __________

a) 80:20 b) 50:50
c) **70:30** d) 30:70

Q 68 Dry matter requirement for maintenance in buffaloes is __________

a) **60-80 g/$W^{0.75}$** b) 50-55 g/$W^{0.75}$
c) 100-110 g/$W^{0.75}$ d) 25-30 g/$W^{0.75}$

Q 69 Buffaloes consume dry matter __________ % of their body weight to fulfill maintenance requirements.

a) 2.0-2.2% b) **2.4-2.9%**

c) 1.15-1.5% d) 3.0-3.8%

Q 70 Dry matter requirement for growth (g/g body weight gain) in buffaloes is __________

a) 1.7-2.0 b) 3.0-3.5

c) 1.0-1.5 d) **2.1-2.5**

Q 71 Average energy requirement (TDN) for maintenance of buffaloes __________

a) **29-47 g/$W^{0.75}$** b) 50 g/$W^{0.75}$

c) 110 g/$W^{0.75}$ d) 25-30 g/$W^{0.75}$

Q 72 Average energy requirement (Kcal ME/$W^{0.75}$ Kg/d) for maintenance of buffaloes __________

a) 101 b) 98

c) 106 d) **142**

Q 73 Crude protein maintenance requirement for buffaloes __________

a) 3.1-4.8 g/$W^{0.75}$ b) 40-50 g/$W^{0.75}$

c) **5.15-7.64 g/$W^{0.75}$** d) 2.0-3.5 g/$W^{0.75}$

Q 74 Digestible crude protein maintenance requirement for buffaloes __________

a) **2.50-5.05g/$W^{0.75}$** b) 2.0-3.50 g/$W^{0.75}$

c) 5.28-7.21 g/$W^{0.75}$ d) 3.50-6.0 g/$W^{0.75}$

Q 75 Digestible crude protein maintenance requirement (g/g of body weight gain) for buffaloes __________

a) 0.10-0.19 b) **0.27-0.32**

c) 0.5-0.7 d) 2.5-3.5

Q 76 Riboflavin deficiency during pregnancy causes __________

a) Over growth b) **Hairlessness**

c) Stunted growth d) Blindness

Q 77 In vitamin A deficiency in the dam, mainly affects the new borns __________

a) **Eyes** b) Bones
c) Weight d) No affect

Q 78 The commonly used green fodder in our country is __________

a) Barley b) **Bajra**
c) Sorghum d) Lucerne

Q 79 Liberal feeding is over feeding __________

a) Agreed b) **Not agreed**
c) No relation d) Can't say

Q 80 The bulkiness of dairy cattle ration is provided by __________

a) **Roughage** b) Mill byproducts
c) Grains d) Mustard cake

Q 81 Including varieties in ration helps in balancing __________

a) Only proteins b) Only carbohydrates
c) **All nutrients** d) All trace minerals

Q 82 A palatable ration will be __________

a) Fowl smelling b) Acidic
c) Mouldy d) **Pleasant smell**

Q 83 The chief difference between Colostrum and milk is that it contains __________

a) Water b) Fat
c) **Immunoglobulins** d) Casein

Q 84 After one year of age for calves concentrate can be given upto __________

a) 500g b) **1500-2000g**
c) 1000g d) Not required

Q 85 The commonly used animal protein in calf starter is __________

a) **Fish meal** b) Meat meal
c) Cotton seed meal d) Liver meal

Q 86 The following is not a legume _________

a) Lucerne b) **Guinea grass**

c) Stylo d) Cowpea

Q 87 Which is not a cereal grain?

a) Wheat b) Rice

c) **Tapoica** d) Barley

Q 88 Concentrate mixture contains _________

a) Grains b) Oil seed cakes

c) Bran d) **All the above**

Q 89 Mineral mixture contains _________

a) Calcium b) Phosphorus

c) Trace minerals d) **All the above**

Q 90 For non-working bullocks, the ration should contain _________

a) Extra concentrate b) Extra Oilseed cakes

c) **Maintenance ration** d) None of above

Q 91 Which is not a NPN compound?

a) Urea b) Glycine

c) Biuret d) **None of above**

Q 92 NPN compounds can be used in ruminant ration upto _________

a) **1%** b) 0.5%

c) 3% d) 3.5%

Q 93 Urea contains nitrogen _________

a) 52.5% b) 16.0%

c) **46.7%** d) 35.6%

Q 94 One kilogram of pure urea furnishes as much as _______ kg of protein.

a) 1.0kg b) 1.6 kg

c) **2.92 kg** d) 3.5 kg

Q 95 By addition of 1 kg of urea, __________ kg of mustard cake can be replaced in concentrate mixture.

a) 4 b) 2
c) 10 d) **7**

Q 96 Urobran contains __________

a) **36% DCP and 70%TDN** b) 18% DCP and 65%TDN
c) 36% DCP and 65%TDN d) 18% DCP and 70%TDN

Q 97 To combat negative energy balance during early lactation, if we increase energy of diet by using cereal grains, it decreases __________

a) Dry matter intake b) Fiber digestion
c) Milk fat d) **All**

Q 98 Nutrients which escape rumen degradation and get digested and absorbed in the lower gastrointestinal tract are called __________

a) Bypass nutrients
b) Protected nutrients
c) Rumen undegradable proteins
d) **Both A and B**

Q 99 Bypass nutrients which can be used in dairy animal nutrition __________

a) Fat and proteins
b) Fat, proteins and starch
c) **Fat, proteins, starch and choline**
d) None

Q 100 Bypass proteins are beneficial for __________

a) Fast growing animals b) High yielders
c) Transition cows d) **All**

Q 101 During early lactation, __________ of total dietary proteins should be bypass protein.

a) **35-38%** b) 5-8%
c) 15-20% d) 50%

Q 102 Bypass proteins are important because a large portion of rumen degradable proteins is converted into __________ in rumen.

a) **Ammonia** b) Nitrogen

c) Urea d) NPN substances

Q 103 In forages,__________ % of the protein taken in by the animal is bypassed to the intestines.

a) 35-38% b) **20-30%**

c) 5-8% d) 50%

Q 104 The protein supplements could be categorized as bypass sources.

a) High (70-90%), intermediate (40-70%) and low (10-40%)

b) High (50-60%), intermediate (40-50%) and low (30-40%)

c) **High (60-80%), intermediate (30-60%) and low (10-30%)**

d) None

Q 105 Which is poor source of bypass proteins?

a) **Soyabean meal** b) Maize gluten

c) Meat meal d) Linseed meal

Q 106 Which is rich source of bypass proteins?

a) Soyabean meal b) **Maize gluten**

c) Groundnut cake d) Sunflower cake

Q 107 Which is medium source of bypass proteins?

a) Soyabean meal b) **Dehydrated alfalfa**

c) Groundnut cake d) Sunflower cake

Q 108 Which of following is not related with bypass proteins?

a) Heat treatment

b) Encapsulation

c) Oesophegeal groove closure

d) **None**

Q 109 Roasting of soybean at ________ C for______ minutes protect its protein from ruminal degradation.

a) **140°C for 30 minutes** b) 140°C for 60 minutes

c) 120°C for 30 minutes d) 120°C for 60 minutes

Q 110 Chemicals used to make the proteins bypass in ruminants.

a) Formaldehyde b) Tannic acid

c) Glyoxal d) **All**

Q 111 Optimum level of formaldehyde (40%) recommended is different for different sources __________

a) **Protein supplement (1-1.5%), for hay (1.5-2.0%) and for silage (3-5%)**

b) Protein supplement (1-1.5%), for hay (3.0 %) and for silage (4-5%)

c) Protein supplement (1-1.5%), for hay (1.5-2.0%) and not for silage

d) None

Q 112 Dietary fat, that resist lipolysis and biohydrogenation in rumen by rumen microorganisms, but gets digested in lower digestive tract.

a) **Bypass fat** b) Unsaturated fats

c) Saturated fats d) All

Q 113 The deleterious effects of fats on rumen activity can be overcome with the use of __________

a) Buffers in ration

b) **Bypass fat**

c) Antioxidant in ration

d) Protein for synchronization in ration

Q 114 Methods used to make the fats bypass __________

a) Crystalline or prilled fatty acids

b) Formaldehyde treated protein encapsulated fatty acids

c) Calcium salts of long chain fatty acids (Ca-LCFA)

d) **All**

Q 115 Feeding bypass fat at the rate of __________ g/day to high yielders during the transition period helps to improve their productive and reproduction efficiency.

a) 50-100g b) 400-500g

c) **150-200g** d) 300-400g

Q 116 On the basis of dry matter intake, lactating cow require bypass fat supplementation @ __________

a) **2.5%** b) 4.0%

c) 1.0% d) 6%

Q 117 On the basis of dry matter intake, lactating buffalo require bypass fat supplementation @ __________

a) 2.5% b) **4.0%**

c) 1.0% d) 6%

Q 118 Based on the milk production, use bypass fat supplements @__________ g per kg milk production in lactating cows.

a) 20g b) 5g

c) **10g** d) 50g

Q 119 Based on the milk production, use bypass fat supplements @__________ g per kg milk production in lactating buffaloes.

a) **20g** b) 5g

c) 10g d) 50g

Q 120 Bypass fat supplements can be used @ __________ % in concentrate mixture of high yielder dairy animals.

a) **2%** b) 5%

c) 1% d) 4%

Q 121 Dry matter intake is reduced upto __________ percent in early lactation.

a) 5% b) 10%

c) **18%** d) 40%

Q 122 Which is not a true buffer?

a) Sodium bicarbonate b) **Magnesium oxide**

c) Sodium bentonite d) None

Q 123 Sodium bicarbonate used as buffer in concentrate mixrure @ __________

a) 2% b) 5%

c) **1%** d) 4%

Q 124 Anionic salt used in animal feed to prevent milk fever _______

a) $MgSO_4$ b) $CaCl_2$

c) NH_4Cl d) **All**

Q 125 In dairy animals, effectiveness of feeding of the anionic salts can be monitored from __________

a) Rumen pH b) **Urine pH**

c) Blood pH d) Dry matter intake

Q 126 In dairy animals, in order to monitor the effectiveness of the anionic ration, urine pH should be between __________

a) **5.5-6.5** b) 4.0-5.2

c) 6.5-6.9 d) Not monitored

Q 127 Ammonium chloride used as anionic salt in animal feed@ __________ g/day 2-3 weeks prior to calving.

a) **50-100g** b) 30-50g

c) 15-20g d) 150-200g

Q 128 Feed a diet with a negative dietary electrolyte balance to alleviate milk fever problems __________

a) -20 to -30 mEQ/100g DM b) -5 to -7 mEQ/100g DM

c) **-10 to -15 mEQ/100g DM** d) -50 to -65 mEQ/100g DM

Q 129 Drenching of propylene glycol to dry cows one week prior to calving helps to __________

a) Reduce fat liver formation

b) Raise circulating blood glucose levels

c) Minimize ketosis risk

d) **All**

Q 130 Drench propylene glycol to dry cows @ __________ kg/day one week prior to calving to prevent ketosis.

a) 0.05 b) **0.5**

c) 0.1 d) 1.0

Q 131 Feeding higher levels of vitamin E (1000 I.U. per day) to dry cows may results in __________

a) Reduce somatic cell counts and mastitis risk

b) Higher blood levels of vitamin E in the unborn calf

c) Higher colostrum levels of vitamin E

d) **All**

Q 132 Feeding of cows during first 10 weeks of lactation ________

a) **Challenge feeding** b) Lead feedings

c) Both a and b d) None

Q 133 Lead feeding is feeding of animal __________

a) **3 weeks before calving** b) First 10 weeks of lactation

c) Birth to Weaning d) Mid to late lactation

Q 134 Feeding of cows prior to three weeks of calving __________

a) Challenge feeding b) **Lead feedings**

c) Both a and b d) None

Q 135 Cows are _______ efficient in replacing body tissue while lactating than during the dry period.

a) Less b) **More**

c) Equally d) None

Q 136 The risk of milk fever immediately after calving can minimize by feeding of __________

a) Anionic salts

b) **Niacin**

c) Zinc

d) High Ca diets before calving

Q 137 During lead feeding, rumen papillae elongated from 0.5 to 1.2 cm in size in order to __________

a) Increase surface area of the rumen

b) Absorb more volatile fatty acids

c) Reduce acid load in the rumen

d) **All**

Q 138 Which is essential for successful feeding of total mixed ration?

a) Good quality fodder

b. Proper moisture determination of feeds

c) Accurate weighing and feed intake monitoring

d) **All**

Q 139 Densified TMR block is also known as __________

a) **Complete feed block** b) Bale block

c) Urea mineral block d) None

Q 140 Animals consume TMR Blocks @ _________ of its body weight.

a) 2-2.5% b) **3-3.5%**

c) 4-4.5% d) 1.0-1.5%

Q 141 To maximize ___________ the ration in 4 to 5 portions over the day.

a) Milk fat b) Reproductive efficiency

c) **Dry matter intake** d) None

Q 142 Non-structural carbohydrates in diet should range from ___________ to ___________ % of the DM for optimal rumen fermentation.

a) 20-25% b) **38-40%**

c) 45-48% d) 18%

Q 143 Feed ___________ % more total mixed ration than the cow is expected to eat.

a) **5-10%** b) 3.8-4.0%

c) 2% d) 10%

Q 144 Which is not an advantage of TMR feeding?

a) Stabilize rumen environment

b) Control and accuracy of the feed amounts fed

c) Reduction in feed cost

d) **Single ration for all animals**

Q 145 Which is not true regarding TMR feeding?

a) Non-economical for small herds

b) Mixing or blending devices needed

c) Over mixing or under mixing

d) **Easily adopted in existing sheds**

Q 146 Acute state that responds dramatically to the systematic administration of the needed metabolites although the animal may require subsequent dietary supplementation to avoid reoccurrence is called __________

a) Disorder

b) Nutritional deficiency disease

c) **Metabolic disease**

d) Systematic disease

Q 147 Aureomycin hychloride is fed to young calves 80mg/calf/day because __________

a) It treats calf scours

b) **It increases growth from 10 to 30%**

c) It helps to develop rumen

d) It helps in digestion of milk

Q 148 Feeding cow with cottonseed cake __________

a) **Increases mlik fat content**

b) Decreases fat globule size

c) Increase sugar content

d) Decreases milk fat content

Q 149 In calculation of TDN, which nutrient is multiplied by 2.25?

a) **Digestible fat extract**

b) Digestible crude protein

c) Digestible crude fibre

d) Digestible NFE

Q 150 Calcium to phosphorus ratio for the maximum reproductive efficiency in cattle should be between __________

a) **1:2 and 2:1**

b) 1:3 and 2:1

c) 1:2 and 3:1

d) 1:1 and 2:1

Q 151 Which of following is not a metabolic disease?

a) Milk fever b) **Degnala**

c) Downer cow syndrome d) Grass tetany

Q 152 Milk fever occurs due to decline in blood level of ________

a) **Calcium** b) Potassium

c) Sodium d) Magnesium

Q 153 Age increases the risk of milk fever by approximately _____per lactation.

a) 15% b) 25%

c) 3% d) **9%**

Q 154 Elevated level of acetoacetic acid, â -hydroxybutyric acid and acetone in body tissues and fluids observed in ________

a) Milk fever b) **Ketosis**

c) Downer cow syndrome d) Grass tetany

Q 155 Grass tetany is also known as ________

a) Lactation tetany b) Grass staggers

c) Hypomagnesemic tetany d) **All**

Q 156 Lactation tetany is caused by a metabolic deficiency of ________

a) **Mg and Ca** b) Mg

c) Ca d) Ca, Mg and K

Q 157 Plasma non-esterified fatty acid (NEFA) concentrations are high in fat cow is due to ________

a) Depressed feed intake b) Altered endocrine status

c) **Both A and B** d) None

Q 158 Ingestion of large quantity of grains may lead to ________

a) **Ruminal acidosis** B) Poisoning

c) Bloat d) None

Q 159 The condition leads to Downer cow syndrome ________

a) Hypoclacemia b) Trauma

c) Hypokalemia d) **All**

Q 160 Slow-release insulin compound (single 100 IU IM dose) immediately after calving may be used as prophylactic to prevent __________

a) Milk fever
b) Ketosis
c) **Fat cow syndrome**
d) Grass tetany

Q 161 Nutritional prevention of milk fever includes __________

a) Oral drenching of $CaCl_2$ around calving
b) Feeding of acidifying rations
c) Prepartum administration of vitamin D
d) Increasing Mg supplementation
e. **All the above**

Q 162 The main precursor of glucose in ruminants __________

a) Acetic acid
b) **Propionic acid**
c) Butyric acid
d) Glycol

Q 163 Acid in silage which increase the risk of ketosis in dairy animals __________

a) Acetic acid
b) Propionic acid
c) **Butyric acid**
d) Lactic acid

Q 164 Nutritional prevention of ketosis does not include __________

a) Balanced ration feeding
b) 6-8g/cow/day niacin orally starting 20 days prior to expected calving
c) Sodium propionate (100g daily for 6 weeks) arround calving
d) **High grain diet**

Q 165 Low concentrations of Mg in the forage/pasture predispose the animals to lactation tetany __________

a) **<0.2 % DM**
b) <0.8 % DM
c) <0.02 % DM
d) <1.2 % DM

Q 166 Nutritional prevention of lactation tetany does not include __________

a) Balanced feeding and adequate mineral intake
b) Application of fertilizers high in N and K should be avoided to fodder/pasture
c) Feeding of common salt along with MgO
d) **None of above**

Q 167 Colostrum coagulates on heating because of presence of __________

a) Saturated fat
b) **Albumin and globulins**
c) Lactose
d) High minerals and lactose

Q 168 Optimum ratio of nitrogen to sulphur in dairy animal ration should be __________

a) 1:10
b) 20:1
c) **10:1**
d) 1:20

Q 169 Less degraded protein supplement in ruminant ration _______

a) Fish meal
b) **Urea**
c) Barley
d) Mustard meal

Q 170 Cereal grain by products are __________

a) Rich in proteins
b) **Low in P and Rich in Ca**
c) Rich in P and low in Ca
d) None of above

Q 171 Bone meal is a good source of __________ for ruminants.

a) Carbohydrates
b) **Phosphorus and calcium**
c) Fat
d) Phosphorus

Q 172 For ruminants, urea is __________

a) Energy concentrate
b) True protein source
c) **NPN**
d) Best protein source

Q 173 Molasses contains __________

a) 30-35% DM, 20% proteins and 3-7% fibre
b) 0% DM, 10% proteins and 13% fibre
c) **60-70% DM, less than 7% proteins and 0% fibre**
d) 10% DM, 2% proteins and 3% fibre

Q 174 For successful management of pasture, one should recommend __________

a) Annual pasture
b) **Rotational grazing**
c) Short rotation
d) Alternate grazing

Q 175 For good quality silage, pH, lactic acid and butyric acid content should be __________

a) 3.5-4.2, >3% and <0.5%
b) 3.5-4.2, <4% and >0.1%
c) 3.5-4.2, >3% and <1%
d) **3.5-4.2, >4% and <0.1%**

Q 176 As a thumb rule, animal require green fodder __________ % of their body weight.

a) **10%** b) 5%
c) 3% d) 15%

Q 177 Calf for excellent quality veal must be reared exclusively on __________

a) Hay b) Milk
c) **Cereal grains** d) None

Q 178 Feeding of following helpful in production of granular ghee __________

a) **Cotton seed cake** b) Soybean cake
c) Mustard cake d) Linseed cake

Q 179 The fodder suitable for getting more milk from cows __________

a) Sorghum b) **Cowpea**
c) Maize d) Napier bajra

Q 180 Average weight of one cubic feet silage in a silo pit __________

a) **15-16 kg** b) 30-32 kg
c) 10-13 kg d) 40 kg

Q 181 Moisture content of good quality silage __________

a) 30-35% b) 10%
c) **60-70%** d) 45-50%

Q 182 Moisture content of good quality hay __________

a) 20% b) **10%**
c) 18% d) 25%

Q 183 The calf rearing system is __________

a) Liberal feeding system
b) Limited milk feeding plus calf starter
c) Using milk replacers
d) **All**

Q 184 Generally, calf starter contains __________

a) Fish meal b) Cereal grains
c) Iodized salt and probiotics d) **All**

Q 185 Calf started eating grass after ________

a) One week of birth
b) **Two weeks of birth**
c) Four weeks of birth
d) Six weeks of birth

Q 186 How much total digestible crude protein and TDN are required by a draft bullock weighing 400kg for normal work?

a) 0.55 kg crude protein and 4.0 kg TDN
b) 0.45 kg crude protein and 5.0 kg TDN
c) **0.45 kg crude protein and 4.0 kg TDN**
d) 0.55 kg crude protein and 5.0 kg TDN

Q 187 Silo-fillers disease is an illness of farm workers that is caused by inhalation of the oxides of ________

a) **Nitrogen**
b) Carbon
c) Nitrate
d) HCN

Q 188 Beneficial effect of condensed tannin in legumes is attributed to their ability to ________

a) Degrade starch
b) Increase digestibility
c) Increase availability of minerals
d) **Protect protein**

Q 189 Maximum permitted level of aflatoxin in animal feeds (as per Prevention of food adulteration act) is ________

a) **0.03 ppm**
b) 0.03ppb
c) 0.30ppm
d) 0.30ppb

Q 190 If no green grass is fed to ruminants, the concentrate mixture should have Vitamin A at the rate of ________

a) **5000IU/kg**
b) 7000IU/kg
c) 3200IU/kg
d) 2500IU/kg

Q 191 Chief acid of silage is ________

a) **Lactic acid**
b) Acetic acid
c) Butyric acid
d) All the above

Q 192 Efficiency of conversion of ß carotene to vitamin A is in the order __________

a) Rat > Ruminants > Pig > Poultry

b) Rat > Poultry > Pig > Ruminants

c) **Rat > Poultry > Ruminants > Pig**

d) Pig > Poultry > Ruminants > Rat

Q 193 Rumen degradable protein content is the highest for __________

a) Soybean meal b) Coconut cake

c) **Groundnut cake** d) Fish meal

Q 194 The feed which is fed "whole" to poultry but "crushed" to cattle and pig __________

a) **Pearl millet** b) Great millet

c) Barley d) Jowar

Q 195 DCP% is the highest for __________

a) **Lucerne hay** b) Berseem hay

c) Oat hay d) Wheat straw

Q 196 The order of toxicity is __________

a) Tyrosin > Threonine > Methionine

b) Methionine > Threonine > Tyrosine

c) Threonine > Tyrosine > Methionine

d) **Methionine > Tyrosine > Threonine**

Q 197 Which of the following is most important in inhibiting the digestibility of paddy straw?

a) Lignin b) **Silica**

c) Hemicellulose d) Oxalate

Q 198 Most promising initial symptom of Vitamin A deficiency in cows and horses?

a) **Copius lacrymation** b) Copius salivation

c) Xeropthalmia d) Night blindness

Q 199 __________ % NDF in total ration is critical for maintenance of normal milk fat.

a) 66%
b) 18%
c) 73%
d) **36%**

Q 200 Urea treatment of straw increases __________

a) CP and DCP
b) TDN
c) Dry matter digestibility and feed intake
d) **All the above**

Q 201 The order of salt tolerance __________

a) **Sheep > Cattle > Pig > Poultry**
b) Sheep > Pig > Cattle > Poultry
c) Cattle > Sheep > Pig > Poultry
d) Pig > Cattle > Sheep > Poultry

Q 202 Urea supplementation is not recommended, if CP content of ruminant diet is above __________

a) 18%
b) 25%
c) 7%
D) **13%**

Q 203 Which of the following deficiency contribute to perosis?

a) Manganese and Choline
b) Biotin and Folic acid
c) Thiamine, Manganese, Choline, Biotin and Folic acid
d) **Vitamin B_{12}, Manganese, Choline, Biotin and Folic acid**

Q 204 Arrange the susceptibility to aflatoxin by domestic animals in descending order __________

a) **Rabbit > Pig > Cattle > Sheep > Chicken**
b) Pig > Rabbit > Sheep > Chicken > Cattle
c) Chicken > Rabbit > Pig > Sheep > Cattle
d) Cattle > Sheep > Rabbit > Pig > Chicken

Q 205 Which of the following is used as energy source (not protein source)?

a) Linseed meal b) **Salseed meal**

c) Mustard cake d) Sunflower cake

Q 206 Which of the following cereal has more lysine content?

a) Rice b) Wheat

c) Corn d) **Oats**

Q 207 Silo with minimum spoilage is ________

a) **Upright silo** b) Tube silo

c) Stack Silo d) Bunker silo

Q 208 More than 10% dietary carbohydrates fed in ruminant diet ________

a) Reduce microbial activity

b) **Enhance microbial activity**

c) No effect on microbial activity

d) None

Q 209 Extra feeding of pregnant animal recommended during last ________ months of their pregnancy.

a) **2 months** b) 3 months

c) 1 month d) No need

Q 210 Dry matter requirement for a 400kg buffalo is ________

a) 10 kg b) 8 kg

c) **12 kg** d) 15 kg

Q 211 Voluntary intake of protein is ________ than of maize.

a) **More** b) Less

c) Same d) No relation

Q 212 Dry milk replacer powder is mixed in boiled water in the ratio of ________

a) 1:4 b) 1:5

c) 1:2 d) **Both a and b**

Q 213 Of the total digestible energy, the amount used up by an animal on maintenance is __________

a) 10%
b) 20%
c) **30%**
d) 40%

Q 214 A bullock of 500kg while pulling a load on a plain road for 15 kms, perform mechanical work equivalent to 3421 kcal. Taking net efficiency of bullock for draft as 31.3%, the net energy needed for the work of draft would be __________

a) 9.93 Mcal
b) **10.93 Mcal**
c) 11.93 Mcal
d) 12.93 Mcal

Q 215 Excess feeding of grass causes deficiency of __________

a) Ca
b) P
c) **Mg**
d) Cu

Q 216 Water requirement for adult cattle is __________

a) **3-5kg/kg DM**
b) 8-10kg/kg DM
c) 1-1.5kg/kg DM
d) 0.5-1.2kg/kg DM

Q 217 Water requirement for zebu cattle is __________

a) 3-5kg/100kg B.wt.
b) 8-10kg/100kg B.wt.
c) **2-2.5kg/100kg B.wt.**
d) 3.5-4.2kg/100kg B.wt.

Q 218 Tannin rich grain is __________

a) **Jawar**
b) Wheat
c) Rice
d) Cu

Q 219 Groundnut cake is poor source of __________

a) Methionine
b) Methionine and Lysine
c) **Methionine, Lysine and Cysteine**
d) Lysine and Cysteine

Q 220 The cake has maximum calcium __________

a) GNC
b) **TOC**
c) CSC
d) None

Q 221 The cake has maximum calcium and phosphorus content __________

a) GNC
b) TOC
c) CSC
d) **Mustard cake**

Q 222 The cake that can absorb more molasses __________

a) **Coconut cake**
b) TOC
c) CSC
d) GNC

Q 223 For one litre of milk production, requirement of mineral is __________

a) 0.35%
b) **0.7%**
c) 1.05%
d) 1.4%

Q 224 Level of mineral mixture in cattle feeding is __________

a) 1% of roughage
b) 2% of roughage
c) 1% of concentrate
d) **2% of concentrate**

Q 225 Amount of succulent in cattle feed is __________

a) **2/3 of roughage**
b) 1/3 of roughage
c) 2/3 of concentrate
d) 1/3 of concentrate

Q 226 Requirement of DCP at 5 month of pregnancy is __________

a) 500 g
b) **140 g**
c) 830g
d) 1.2 kg

Q 227 Production ration have concentrate in zebu is __________

a) **1kg/3 kg milk**
b) 1kg/2 kg milk
c) 1kg/1 kg milk
d) 2kg/1 kg milk

Q 228 Production ration have concentrate in crossbreed cattle is __________

a) 1kg/3 kg milk
b) **1kg/2 kg milk**
c) 1kg/1 kg milk
d) 2kg/1 kg milk

Q 229 The first limiting amino acid in the protein of groundnut cake __________

a) Methionine
b) Methionine and Lysine
c) **Lysine**
d) Lysine and Cysteine

Q 230 As per BIS specifications mineral mixture for dairy cattle should be __________

a) 20% Ca and 12% P
b) 16% Ca and 9% P
c) 18% Ca and 9% P
d) **Both a and b**

Q 231 Molasses can be used in livestock ration __________

a) As a source of energy
b) As a binder of pelleting
c) To improve palatability of feed
d) **All the above**

Q 232 The cake that contains the highest DCP __________

a) **GNC**
b) Neem cake
c) CSC
d) Mustard cake

Q 233 The roughage that contains the highest TDN __________

a) **Lucerne hay**
b) Berseem hay
c) Anjan hay
d) All the above

Q 234 A working animal weighing 500kg will require how many kg of DCP and TDN for heavy work?

a) **1.13 and 9.9**
b) 5.13 and 7.9
c) 0.53 and 0.99
d) 1.13 and 2.79

Q 235 The most important for milk production is __________

a) Protein
b) **Energy**
c) Mineral
d) Calcium

Q 236 The concentrate mixture fed to milch cows should contain a protein percentage of __________

a) 10-12%
b) 12-14%
c) **16-18%**
d) 18-20%

Q 237 Daily requirement of mineral mixture for a dairy animal producing 5-7 litres/d of milk __________

a) **50g**
b) 60g
c) 100g
d) 20-30g

Q 238 Daily requirement of mineral mixture for a dairy animal producing 8-10 litres/d of milk __________

a) 50g b) **60g**

c) 100g d) 20-30g

Q 239 Daily requirement of mineral mixture for a dairy animal producing 11-20 litres/d of milk __________

a) 30-50g b) 100-200g

c) **75-100g** d) 20-30g

Q 240 Daily requirement of mineral mixture for calves __________

a) 50g b) 7.5g

c) 10g d) **20-30g**

Q 241 Daily requirement of mineral mixture for a breeding bull __________

a) 50g b) 75g

c) **100g** d) 150g

Q 242 A cow must not be allowed to eat its placenta because it results in reduced milk production due to __________

a) It causes infection in the digestive tract

b) It contains poisonous substances

c) **It is high in protein and appetite is lost**

d) It is high in fat and disturbs the digestion

❑❑❑

Chapter 20

Nutrient Requirements and Feeding of Sheep and Goats

Q 1 Latest feeding standard available for sheep and goat __________

a) NRC (1992)
b) NRC (1994)
c) NRC (2001)
d) **NRC (2007)**

Q 2 Latest Indian feeding standard available for sheep and goat __________

a) NRC (2007)
b) **ICAR (2013)**
c) BIS (2001)
d) None

Q 3 NE requirement for maintenance of sheep and goat is sum of the NE required for __________

a) Basal metabolism
b) Activity increment
c) Body temperature regulation
d) **All**

Q 4 The ruminant with highest BMR is __________

a) Cow
b) **Goat**
c) Buffalo
d) Sheep

Q 5 Nutrient requirements of goat will ________, if it consume cold water during winter.

a) **Increase**
b) Decrease
c) Remains same
d) Wrong statement

Q 6 The most common limiting factor in small ruminant nutrition __________

a) Protein
b) **Energy**
c) Fat
d) Water

Q 7 Requirements for a growing kid is sum of the requirement for __________

a) Maintenance requirement b) Growth requirement
c) **Both a and b** d) None

Q 8 Requirements for a suckling doe that is still growing is sum of the requirement for __________

a) Maintenance requirement
b) Growth requirement
c) Requirement of milk production
d) **All**

Q 9 Goats require more nutrients as compared to sheep and cattle because of __________

a) High metabolic rate
b) More thyroxine production
c) **Both a and b**
d) None

Q 10 Metabolic faecal nitrogen consists of __________

a) Residual bile b) Digestive enzymes
c) Epithelial cell d) **All the above**

Q 11 The conditions of animals which are not essential for measuring metabolic rate are __________

a) Good nutritive condition
b) Environmental temperature
c) Rest
d) **Productive status**

Q 12 The rate of growth in sheep is chiefly measured as __________

a) **Average daily weight gain** b) Age
c) Size d) Height

Q 13 The energy requirement for basal metabolism and activity factor is called as __________

a) Growth requirement
b) **Maintenance requiremen**t
c) Basal requirement
d) Production require

Q 14 For nitrogen balance studies, the plane of nutrition of the animal at the start of the experiment should be in __________

a) High b) Very high

c) Low d) **Adequate**

Q 15 During growth period the critical nutrient in small ruminants is __________

a) Fats b) Carbohydrates

c) **Protein** d) Vitamins

Q 16 True growth involves an increase in structured constituents and not __________

a) **Fats** b) Tissue

c) Bone d) Organs

Q 17 As the animal grows older, the protein requirement is proportionately __________

a) Increases b) **Lower**

c) Double d) Same

Q 18 The accurate method of estimating the protein requirement is by __________

a) **Nitrogen balance study** b) Chemical test

c) Weight gain d) Digestion trial

Q 19 Energy requirement of goats on hilly or semiarid range land need ________% more energy above basic maintenance requirement.

a) 25% b) **50%**

c) 75% d) All

Q 20 Energy requirement of goats on light activity need ________% more energy above basic maintenance requirement.

a) **25%** b) 50%

c) 75% d) All

Q 21 When vegetation is sparse and goats have to travel long distances to graze, their energy requirement is ________% above basic maintenance requirement.

a) 25% b) 50%

c) **75%** d) All

Q 22 Energy requirement of goats are related to ________

a) Age b) Body size

c) Pregnancy and lactation d) **All**

Q 23 Pashmina goats require ________ energy after shearing.

a) **More** b) Less

c) Remains same d) Wrong statement

Q 24 The protein requirement is higher during.

a) Growth (Kid) b) Lactation

c) Mohair growth d) **All**

Q 25 Mineral deficiency rarely occurs in goats since consumption of the following by goats minimizes the deficiency ________

a) Stubbles b) **Tree leaves**

c) Dry fodder d) Grazing

Q 26 Vitamin E and K are obtained from browsing ________

a) Stubbles b) **Tree leaves**

c) Rye grass d) Concentrate mixture

Q 27 Salt should be included in the concentrate mixture of small ruminants ________

a) 2-3% b) 2.5%

c) **0.5-1%** d) 3.5%

Q 28 The grower period in goats is upto ________

a) **12 months** b) 9 months

c) 6 months d) 18 months

Q 29 Concentrate supplementation in grazing goats is important during ________

a) Breeding season b) Throughout the year

c) **Lean season** d) None of the above

Q 30 For lactating goats, the level of concentrate mixture supplying the DM requirement should be ________

a) 10% b) 20%

c) **30%** d) 40%

Q 31 Twining in goats is __________

a) Age specific
b) **Breed specific**
c) Parity specific
d) Level of feeding specific

Q 32 Male and female kids selected for breeding purpose are called as __________

a) **Replacement stock**
b) Culls
c) Finishers
d) Growers

Q 33 Goats have the ability to conserve water by reducing loss through __________

a) Skin
b) Respiration
c) **Urine and faeces**
d) Metabolic water production

Q 34 The quantity of water consumed by an adult goat per day is __________

a) 3000ml
b) 1800ml
c) 300-400ml
d) **400-700ml**

Q 35 The TDN content in lactating goat's concentrate feed should be __________

a) 30-40%
b) **55-60%**
c) 65-70%
d) 72%

Q 36 Feeding hard water continuously for goats causes deficiency of __________

a) Calcium
b) Phosphorus
c) **Both a and b**
d) None of the above

Q 37 Nutrients requirements of calcium (g/kgDM) for growth of kids (ICAR, 2013) __________

a) **1.7-3.8**
b) 3.0-3.9
c) 2.7-3.0
d) 1.0-1.6

Q 38 Nutrients requirements of phosphorus (g/kgDM) for growth of kids (ICAR, 2013) __________

a) 1.7-3.8
b) **3.0-3.9**
c) 2.7-3.0
d) 1.0-1.6s

Q 39 Nutrients requirements of calcium (g/kgDM) for pregnant goat with one kid (ICAR, 2013) __________

a) **2.0-2.9** b) 3.0-3.9
c) 2.7-3.0 d) 1.0-1.6

Q 40 Nutrients requirements of phosphorus (g/kgDM) for pregnant goat with one kid (ICAR, 2013) __________

a) 1.7-3.8 b) 3.0-3.9
c) 2.7-3.0 d) **1.0-1.6**

Q 41 Nutrients requirements of phosphorus (g/kgDM) for lactating goat (ICAR, 2013) __________

a) 1.7-3.8 b) 3.0-3.9
c) **2.7-3.0** d) 1.0-1.6

Q 42 Nutrients requirements of metabolizable protein (g/g daily gain) for growing dairy goats (NRC, 2007) __________

a) **0.29** b) 0.404
c) 0.10 d) 0.281

Q 43 Nutrients requirements of metabolizable protein (g/g daily gain) for growing meat goats (NRC, 2007) __________

a) 0.29 b) **0.404**
c) 0.10 d) 0.281

Q 44 Nutrients requirements of metabolizable protein (g/g daily gain) for growing Angora goats (NRC, 2007) __________

a) 0.29 b) 0.404
c) 0.10 d) **0.281**

Q 45 Requirements of metabolizable protein (g/g) for clean mohair fibre (NRC, 2007)

a) **1.65** b) 1.04
c) 2.70 d) 2.81

Q 46 Meat goats consume dry matter _______ % of their body weight.

a) **3-4%** b) 5-7%
c) 4-5% d) 1-2%

Q 47 Dairy goats consume dry matter ______% of their body weight.

a) 3-4% b) **5-7%**

c) 4-5% d) 1-2%

Q 48 Dry matter requirements for growing kids ranges between __________

a) 40-59 g/$W^{0.75}$ b) **35-50 g/$W^{0.75}$**

c) 50-60 g/$W^{0.75}$ d) None

Q 49 Dry matter requirements for kids with 30 kg body and growing at the rate of 50g/day as per ICAR (1994) is __________

a) 425g/d b) 600 g/d

c) 700 g/d d) **950 g/d**

Q 50 Dry matter requirements for kids with 10 kg body and growing at the rate of 50g/day as per ICAR (1994) is __________

a) **425 g/d** b) 600 g/d

c) 700 g/d d) 950 g/d

Q 51 One kg of kid gain requires _______ kg of milk.

a) **4-5** b) 3-3.5

c) 6-7 d) None

Q 52 Average energy requirement for maintenance in goat ______

a) **101 Kcal ME/$W^{0.75}$ Kg/d** b) 98 Kcal ME/$W^{0.75}$ Kg/d

c) 106 Kcal ME/$W^{0.75}$ Kg/d d) 180 Kcal ME/$W^{0.75}$ Kg/d

Q 53 Average energy requirement for pregnant goat __________

a) 101 Kcal ME/$W^{0.75}$ Kg/d b) 98 Kcal ME/$W^{0.75}$ Kg/d

c) 106 Kcal ME/$W^{0.75}$ Kg/d d) **180 Kcal ME/$W^{0.75}$ Kg/d**

Q 54 Starter/creep ration should contain __________

a) 14-16% DCP and 72% TDN

b) **18-20% DCP and 72% TDN**

c) 20-22% DCP and 72% TDN

d) 22-24% DCP and 72% TDN

Q 55 Growing kid ration should contain __________

a) 12-14% DCP and 60-65% TDN

b) 16-18% DCP and 60-65% TDN

c) 10-12% DCP and 72% TDN

d) **12-14% DCP and 60-65% TDNs**

Q 56 Finisher goat ration should contain __________

a) **6-8% DCP and 60-65% TDN**

b) 12-14% DCP and 60-65% TDN

c) 6-8% DCP and 72% TDN

d) 12-14% DCP and 72% TDN

Q 57 Breeding buck ration should contain __________

a) 6-8% DCP and 60% TDN b) **4-6% DCP and 60% TDN**

c) 6-8% DCP and 72% TDN d) 4-6% DCP and 72% TDN

Q 58 Pregnant doe ration should contain __________

a) 10.5% DCP and 60-65% TDN

b) 8.5% DCP and 60-65% TDN

c) **12.5% DCP and 55-60% TDN**

d) 18.5% DCP and 72% TDN

Q 59 Lactating goat ration should contain __________

a) **9-10% DCP and 60-65% TDN**

b) 4-6% DCP and 60-65% TDN

c) 6-8% DCP and 72% TDN

d) 4-6% DCP and 72% TDN

Q 60 Feeding of extra allowance 2-3 weeks before breeding season to sheep/goats __________

a) **Flushing** b) Breeding diet

c) Heatup diet d) Steaming up

Q 61 The proper ratio of calcium to phosphorus is __________

a) **2.5 to 1.0** b) 1.5-2.0

c) 2.5-3.0 d) None

Q 62 The water requirement of sheep per kg of dry matter consumed is __________

a) 1-2 kg b) **2-3 kg**

c) 3-4 kg d) 12.0 kg

Q 63 Water requirement of sheep is not related to __________

a) Feed intake and its composition

b) Environmental temperature

c) Wool covering

d) **None**

Q 64 For efficient utilization of NPN compounds in rumen of sheep, the nitrogen-sulfur ratio in diet should be __________

a) **10:1** b) 3:1

c) 2:1 d) 5:1

Q 65 In lambs, selenium deficiency may lead to __________

a) **White muscle disease** b) Selenosis

c) Both A and B d) None of above

Q 66 The mineral which is important for wool growth __________

a) Zinc b) **Sulfur**

c) Selenium d) Cobalt

Q 67 Urinary calculi in goats is due to __________

a) Feeding of P and Mg rich concentrates

b) Imbalance Ca and P intake

c) Eating of oxalate/silicate rich forages

d) **All**

Q 68 Incidence of calculi is more in goat __________

a) **Males** b) Females

c) Same d) None

Q 69 Nutritional prevention of urinary calculi in goats includes use of __________

a) Sodium bicarbonate b) **Ammonium chloride**

c) Both A and B d) None

Q 70 Ammonium chloride can be used to prevent urinary calculi in concentrate mixture of goats @__________/100kg feed.

a) 100g b) 10g

c) **0.5%** d) None

Q 71 The first limiting amino acid in the diet of sheep is ________

a) Leucine b) **Methionine**

c) Lysine d) Threonine

Q 72 The amino acid which can replace methionine for wool growth ________

a) Leucine b) Lysine

c) **Cystine** d) Threonine

Q 73 The maximum dry matter requirement per 100kg body weight is of ________

a) Cow b) **Goat**

c) Buffalo d) Sheep

Q 74 Sheep consume dry matter ________% of their body weight to fulfill maintenance requirements.

a) 3.27-4.81% b) 5-7%

c) **2.15-3.5%** d) 2.0-2.3%

Q 75 Lactating sheep consume dry matter ________% of their body weight.

a) **3.27-4.81%** b) 5-7%

c) 2.15-3.5% d) 2.0-2.3%

Q 76 After kidding/lambing, DMI rises and reaches a maximum between ________

a) 4 to 5 weeks b) **6 to 10 weeks**

c) 10 to 15 weeks d) 15 to 18 weeks

Q 77 Dry matter requirement of sheep ________% of their body weight (Ranjan, 1998).

a) **2.2-2.8%** b) 5-7%

c) 4-5% d) 1-2%

Q 78 Sheep may consume ________% more dry matter on pasture than when fed in the stall with same.

a) 20% b) 5%

c) **15%** d) 10%

Q 79 Total digestible nutrient requirement of sheep (ICAR, 2013) __________

a) $76g/W^{0.75}$ b) **$30g/W^{0.75}$**
c) $45g/W^{0.75}$ d) $2.5g/W^{0.75}$

Q 80 Digestible crude protein requirement of sheep (ICAR, 2013) __________

a) $76g/W^{0.75}$ b) $30g/W^{0.75}$
c) $2.97g/W^{0.75}$ d) **$2.5g/W^{0.75}$**

Q 81 Digestible crude protein requirement of sheep (Ranjan, 1998) __________

a) $76g/W^{0.75}$ b) $30g/W^{0.75}$
c) **$2.97g/W^{0.75}$** d) $2.5g/W^{0.75}$

Q 82 Energy requirement of sheep (Ranjan, 1998) __________

a) 27.3g TDN/$W^{0.75}$ Kg b) 98 Kcal ME/$W^{0.75}$ Kg
c) **Both a and b** d) None

Q 83 Efficiency of conversion of metabolizable energy for wool production in sheep __________

a) 65% b) **18%**
c) 96% d) 82%

Q 84 Poorly packed silage may contain harmful molds, which causes a disease in sheep/goat __________

a) **Listeriosis** b) Mycotoxicosis
c) Aflatoxicosis d) Toxemia

Q 85 Feeding of extra feeds to meet heavy demand of the unborn lamb is called __________

a) Flushing b) Breeding diet
c) Heat up d) **Steaming up**

Q 86 Sheep can nibble tiny blades of vegetation because of small muzzle and split __________

a) Lower lips b) Lower jaws
c) **Upper lips** d) Both A and C

Q 87 Flushing increases the ovulation rate by __________

a) **10-20%** b) 5%
c) 15-30% d) 40%

Q 88 Sheep have less faecal water loss than cattle __________

a) **13-24% vs 30-32% for cattle**

b) 3-4% vs 13-24% for cattle %

c) Wrong statement

d) None

Q 89 The energy requirement of ewes is greatest during the _______ of lactation.

a) Last 8-10 weeks
b) **First 8-10 weeks**
c) Both A and B
d) None

Q 90 The mineral deficiency occurs in lamb that impaired testicular growth and complete cessation of spermatogenesis.

a) Cu
b) Mn
c) Fe
d) **Zn**

Q 91 The deficiency of mineral will leads to poor quality wool production.

a) **Sulphur**
b) Zinc
c) Methionine
d) None

Q 92 The deficiency of mineral will lead to stringy wool production __________

a) Sulphur
b) **Copper**
c) Zinc
d) None

Q 93 A technique by which one can measure the amount of muscle and fat a sheep is carrying at a certain time is known as __________

a) **Condition scoring**
b) Back fat thickness
c) Growth index
d) None

Q 94 Generally, considered ideal nutrient level for lamb starter is __________

a) **CP: 18-20% & TDN:75%**
b) CP: 16% & TDN:75%
c) CP: 16% & TDN:80%
d) None

Q 95 Flushing provide ________ percent more nutrients above the maintenance needs.

a) 30%
b) **25%**
c) 20%
d) 15%

Q 96 Special feeding care of ewes during the last six weeks of pregnancy will increase the __________

a) Number of viable lambs
b) Ewes milk yield
c) Growth rate of lambs
d) **All**

Q 97 The Nutritive ratio for lambs of body weight 50 kg or more should be __________

a) **1:7 or 1:8**
b) 1:5 or 1:6
c) 1:6.5
d) None

Q 98 The Nutritive ratio in ewes and nursing lamb should be __________

a) 1:7 or 1:8
b) 1:5 or 1:6
c) **1:6.5**
d) None

Q 99 Nutrients requirements of calcium (g/kg DM) for growth of lambs (ICAR, 2013) __________

a) 1.4-1.6
b) 4.3
c) **4.0**
d) 2.0-2.6

Q 100 Nutrients requirements of calcium (g/kg DM) for lactating sheep (ICAR, 2013) __________

a) 1.4-1.6
b) **4.3**
c) 4.0
d) 2.0-2.6

Q 101 Nutrients requirements of calcium (g/kg DM) for pregnant sheep with one lamb (ICAR, 2013) __________

a) **1.4-1.6**
b) 4.3
c) 4.0
d) 2.0-2.6

Q 102 Nutrients requirements of phosphorus (g/kg DM) for growth of lambs (ICAR, 2013) __________

a) 1.7-3.8
b) **3.9**
c) 3.0
d) 1.0-1.6

Q 103 Nutrients requirements of phosphorus (g/kg DM) for pregnant sheep with one lamb (ICAR, 2013) __________

a) 1.7-3.8
b) 3.0-3.9
c) 2.7-3.0
d) **1.0-1.6**

Q 104 Nutrients requirements of phosphorus (g/kg DM) for lactating sheep (ICAR, 2013) __________

a) 1.7-4.0 b) 3.9
c) **3.0** d) 1.0-1.6

Q 105 Nutrients requirements of sulfur (g/kg DM) for growth of lambs (ICAR, 2013) __________

a) 1.7-3.8 b) **2.2**
c) 3.0 d) 1.0-1.6

Q 106 Ideal body condition score of sheep on maintenance ration __________

a) **2.5** b) 3.5
c) 4.0-5.0 d) None

Q 107 For effectiveness of flushing the body condition score of sheep should be __________

a) 2.5 b) **3.5**
c) 4.0-5.0 d) None

Q 108 Stiff lamb disease can be prevented by supplementation of __________

a) **Vitamin E** b) Keratine
c) Copper d) Methionine

Q 109 Which ruminant is most prone to both cobalt deficiency and copper toxicity?

a) Cow b) Goat
c) Buffalo d) **Sheep**

Q 110 Pregnancy toxemia is seen in __________

a) Sheep and Goat b) Sheep and Rat
c) **Sheep and Guinea pig** d) Sheep and Rabbit

Q 111 The minimum percentage of fat to be maintained in sheep ration is __________

a) 2% b) 1%
c) **3%** d) 5%

Q 112 The requirement of TDN during first 10 weeks of lactation will be more by ________

a) 10% b) **100%**

c) 50% d) 20%

Q 113 Copper deficiency in sheep results in ________

a) **Stringy wool** b) Short wool

c) Brittle wool d) Crispy wool

Q 114 Vitamin E deficiency in sheep causes ________

a) Blindness b) Stunted growth

c) Scours d) **Stiff lamb disease**

Q 115 Lambs can be allowed to suckle upto ________

a) 4 weeks b) 8 weeks

c) **12 weeks** d) 16 weeks

Q 116 High concentrate feeding leads to swollen udder in sheep ________

a) **True** b) False

c) Wrong statement d) Can't say

Q 117 Alternative to concentrate feeding in sheep ________

a) Maize straw b) Green grass

c) Rice straw d) **Legumes**

Q 118 Concentrate mixture can be started (lambs) at the age of ________

a) 2 months b) 8 weeks

c) **2 weeks** d) 16 weeks

Q 119 The common supplement in creep mixture is ________

a) Oils b) **Vitamin mixture**

c) Antifungal compounds d) Prebiotics

Q 120 Fatty breeding ram in the flock causes ________

a) Abortion b) Weak lambs

c) High fertility d) **Poor fertility**

Q 121 The result of flushing is more prominent in ________

a) Well maintained ewes b) Fatty ewes

c) Young ewes d) **Underfed ewes**

Q 122 The daily dry matter intake in fattening rams upto ________

a) 2% b) 2.5%

c) 3% d) **4-5%**

Q 123 Flushing in small ruminants improves ________

a) **Conception rate** b) Lamb survival

c) Immunity d) No effect

Q 124 Flushing is practiced ________

a) Throughout the year

b) One week before breeding season

c) 3 weeks before breeding season

d) 8 weeks before breeding season

Q 125 When sufficient pasture land is not available, adult sheep should be fed with straw plus ________ g of concentrate mixture.

a) **300-400g** b) 100-200g

c) 400-500g d) 150-200g

Q 126 The adult sheep should be allowed to graze free of choice on pasture and supplemented with ________ g of concentrates mixture.

a) 300g b) **100g**

c) 400g d) 150-200g

Q 127 For lactating sheep, legumes can be fed upto ________

a) 300g b) 400g

c) **800g** d) 150-200g

Q 128 The quantity of calcium to supplemented for every kg of milk produced is ________

a) 20g b) 5g

c) 10g d) **1.3g**

Q 129 Biological value of protein for sheep is __________

a) 50% b) **65%**

c) 70% d) 100%

Q 130 In Copper deficiency in wool losses its __________

a) Colour b) Appearance

c) Weight d) **Crimp**

Q 131 The chief amino acid present in keratin is __________

a) **Cystine** b) Methionine

c) Leucine d) Arginine

Q 132 The wool fibre contains __________

a) Fats b) Carbohydrates

c) **Protein** d) NFE

Q 133 Feeder lamb refers to __________

a) **Under one years age used for slaughter**

b) Castrated lambs

c) Under two years age used for slaughter

d) Lambs ready for mating

Q 134 Feeder sheep refers to __________

a) **Over two years old fattened sheep for marketing purpose**

b) Under one years old fattened sheep

c) Under two years old fattened sheep for marketing purpose

d) None of above

Q 135 The amount of creep feed consumed is inversely proportional to __________

a) Weight gain of lambs b) Body weight of lambs

c) **Ewe's milk production** d) Heart girth of lambs

Q 136 Colostrum should be preserved with __________

a) 200ml b) 50ml

c) 150ml d) **100ml**

Q 137 Colostrum should be given to kids at the rate of ________ per kg live weight.

a) 1-1.5% propionic acid
b) 0.1% formaldehyde
c) **Both a and b**
d) None

Q 138 Propionic acid is preferred to preserve colostrums because ____

a) **It keeps pH value low**
b) Excellent source of energy
c) Not react with immunoglobulins
d) All the above

Q 139 The milking doe should be provided concentrate mixture @ ________ g for each liter of milk production.

a) **350g**
b) 250g
c) 500g
d) 100g

Q 140 Pregnant doe having free access to good pasture must be given concentrate __________

a) 0.1-0.2kg
b) 0.2-0.36kg
c) **0.2-0.5kg**
d) 1.0-2.0kg

Q 141 During lean period, yearling doe must feed __________ kg concentrate mixture.

a) 0.1-0.2kg
b) 0.2-0.36kg
c) **0.2-0.5kg**
d) 1.0-2.0kg

Q 142 During breeding season, a ram must be given ________ g concentrate mixture.

a) 100-200g
b) **250-500g**
c) 1000-1500g
d) 450-700g

Q 143 The ingredient used to make the ration bulky for starter kids __________

a) Maize
b) Wheat
c) Groundnut cake
d) **Rice bran**

Q 144 Which of following may not cause the deficiency of energy to sheep?

a) Over matured pasture
b) **Inadequate DM content of pasture**
c) Lack of available feeds due to draught
d) Lack of available feeds due to snow

❑❑❑

Chapter 21

Nutrients Requirements and Feeding of Pigs

Q 1 Estimation of protein requirements for maintenance and growth in pig by __________

a) Factorial method
b) Nitrogen balance method
c) Feeding trial method
d) **All**

Q 2 For pig, the protein requirements are usually stated together for maintenance and __________

a) Growth
b) Reproduction
c) **Both a and b**
d) Production

Q 3 NE requirement for growth of pig is sum of the NE required for __________

a) Basal metabolism
b) Activity increment
c) Tissue growth
d) **All**

Q 4 Feeding standards available for pigs are __________

a) **NRC, ARC, BIS and ICAR**
b) NRC, BIS and ICAR
c) NRC, ARC, BIS, ICAR and CARI
d) NRC, BIS and ARC

Q 5 Latest feeding standard available for pigs __________

a) NRC (1992)
b) NRC (1994)
c) NRC (2001)
d) **NRC (1998)**

Q 6 Latest Indian feeding standard available for pigs __________

a) NRC
b) **ICAR**
c) BIS
d) None

Q 7 Latest Indian feeding standard available for pigs (year) ______

a) **2013** b) 2009

c) 2007 d) 1998

Q 8 In pigs, the ME for maintenance is (kcal/day) _________

a) **106 × BW$^{0.75}$** b) 83 × BW$^{0.75}$

c) 110 × BW$^{0.75}$ d) None

Q 9 In pigs, the DE for maintenance is (kcal/day) _________

a) 106 × BW$^{0.75}$ b) 83 × BW$^{0.75}$

c) **110 × BW$^{0.75}$** d) None

Q 10 The daily maintenance requirement of the lactating sow is_______ of ME/kg BW$^{0.75}$.

a) **0.44. MJ** b) 0.46. MJ

c) 0.40. MJ d) None

Q 11 The NE requirements are approximately _______ of the ME requirements.

a) 96% b) 83%

c) 75% d) **82%**

Q 12 The requirement for ME is the requirement for DE × _________

a) **0.96** b) 0.82

c) 0.75 d) None

Q 13 Digestible lysine requirement (g/day) for maintenance in swine (NRC, 1998) is _________

a) **0.036 × BW$^{0.75}$** b) 0. 36 × BW$^{0.75}$

c) 36 × BW$^{0.75}$ d) None

Q 14 Energy cost of protein accretion in growing pigs is _________

a) **10.6 kcal ME/g** b) 12.5 kcal ME/g

c) 106 kcal ME/g d) 110 kcal ME/g

Q 15 Energy cost of fat accretion in growing pigs is _________

a) 10.6 kcal ME/g b) **12.5 kcal ME**

c) 106 kcal ME/g d) 110kcal ME/g

Q 16 Lean muscle tissue contains protein __________

a) 16-18%
b) 80-95%
c) **20-23%**
d) Variable

Q 17 Adipose tissue contains fat __________

a) 16-18%
b) **80-95%**
c) 20-23%
d) Variable

Q 18 The energy requirement for milk production can be estimated from the __________

a) Litter gain
b) Number of piglets
c) **Both**
d) None

Q 19 Estimation of nutrient requirements for lactating sows is complicated because __________

a) **Sow contribute nutrients from her own body**
b) Suckling piglets
c) Both
d) None

Q 20 The energy cost for muscle tissue production is _______ as compared to that for fat tissue deposition.

a) Same
b) **Less**
c) More
d) None

Q 21 The daily energy requirement for growth of the products of conception is _______ kcal of ME/pig.

a) **35.8**
b) 12.5
c) 10.6
d) None

Q 22 Marginal efficiency of use of ME for milk production in sow is __________

a) **72%**
b) 82%
c) 61%
d) 100%

Q 23 For growing-finishing pigs, the daily lysine requirement is the sum of the requirements for __________

a) Maintenance
b) Protein accretion
c) **Both a and b**
d) Variable

Q 24 Average daily nitrogen retention in pregnant sow is the sum of maternal nitrogen retention and nitrogen in ________

a) Tissue
b) Placenta
c) Both a and b
d) **Products of conceptus**

Q 25 N retention (g/day) in the products of conception is given by number of pigs×________ g/day.

a) 0.036
b) **0.34**
c) 0.23
d) None

Q 26 Feed conversion efficiency of pigs ________

a) 2.5:1
b) **3:1**
c) 3.5:1
d) 1.9:1

Q 27 BIS (1986, reaffirmed in 2001) nutrients requirements for pig creep feed are ________

a) **CP 20%; ME 3360 Kcal/d**
b) CP 20%; ME 3170 Kcal/d
c) CP 18%; ME 3360 Kcal/d
d) CP 18%; ME 3170 Kcal/d

Q 28 BIS (1986, reaffirmed in 2001) nutrients requirements for pig grower feed are ________

a) CP 20%; ME 3360 Kcal/d
b) CP 20%; ME 3170 Kcal/d
c) **CP 18%; ME 3170 Kcal/d**
d) CP 16%; ME 3170 Kcal/d

Q 29 BIS (1986, reaffirmed in 2001) nutrients requirements for pig finisher/breeding meal are ________

a) CP 20%; ME 3360 Kcal/d
b) CP 20%; ME 3170 Kcal/d
c) CP 18%; ME 3170 Kcal/d
d) **CP 16%; ME 3170 Kcal/d**

Q 30 Energy requirements (ME Kcal/d) for pigs from 1-5kg, 5-10kg, 10-20kg, 20-50kg and 50-80kg body weights (NRC, 1998) are ________

a) 3360, 3360, 3200, 3170 and 3170
b) 3265, 3265, 3200, 3170 and 3100
c) **3265**
d) None of above

Q 31 Protein requirements (%) pigs from 1-5kg, 5-10kg and 10-20kg body weights (NRC, 1998) are ________

a) 20.0, 17.7 and 15.9
b) **18.0, 15.5 and 13.2**
c) 20.0, 18.0 and 16.0
d) 18.0, 16.0 and 15.0

Q 32 Protein requirements (%) pigs from 20-50 kg, 50-80kg and 80-120kg body weights (NRC, 1998) are __________

a) **26.0, 23.7 and 20.9** b) 23.0, 20.0 and 18.9

c) 25.0, 23.7 and 21.9 d) 23.7, 20.0 and 18.9

Q 33 NRC (1998) nutrients requirements (per kg feed) for lactating sow is __________

a) CP 20%; ME 3265 Kcal b) CP 16%; ME 3170 Kcal

c) CP 16%; ME 3265 Kcal d) **CP 18.4%; ME 3265 Kcal**

Q 34 NRC (1998) nutrients requirements(per kg feed) for pregnant sow is __________

a) CP 13%; ME 3265 Kcal b) CP 16%; ME 3170 Kcal

c) **CP 12.4%; ME 3265 Kcal** d) CP 18.4%; ME 3265 Kcal

Q 35 NRC (1998) nutrients requirements (per kg feed) for boar is __________

a) **CP 13%; ME 3265 Kcal** b) CP 16%; ME 3170 Kcal

c) CP 12.4%; ME 3265 Kcal d) CP 18.4%; ME 3265 Kcal

Q 36 Lysine requirements for pig in starter phase (NRC, 1998) is __________

a) **Above 1%** b) 0.5%

c) Between 0.5 to 1.0% d) None

Q 37 Nutrients requirements of calcium (%) for pregnant/lactating sow (NRC, 1998) __________

a) 0.55 b) 1.00

c) **0.75** d) 0.90

Q 38 The NRC (1998) estimates requirements of calcium and phosphorus for growing pigs of 10-20 kg body weight are __________

a) 0.6 and 0.5% b) 0.5 and 0.6%

c) 0.6 and 0.7% d) **0.7 and 0.6%**

Q 39 Iron requirements (mg/kg feed) for pig in starter phase (NRC, 1998) are __________

a) 50 b) **100**

c) 80 d) 150

Q 40 Iron requirements (mg/kg feed) for lactating sow (NRC, 1998) are __________

a) 50 b) 100

c) **80** d) 150

Q 41 Nutrients requirements of Vitamin A (IU/kg of diet) for pregnant and lactating sow (NRC, 1998) are __________

a) **2000 and 4000** b) 4000 and 4000

c) 4000and 2000 d) 2200and 1300

Q 42 Energy requirements (ME Kcal/kg diet) for crossbreed pigs with medium to higher growth potential from 8-16 weeks, 17-24 weeks and 25-32 weeks of age (ICAR, 2013) are __________

a) 3360, 3170 and 3050 b) 3300, 3265 and 3100

c) **3400, 2670 and 2270** d) None of above

Q 43 Protein requirements (%) for crossbred pigs with medium to higher growth potential from 8-16 weeks, 17-24 weeks and 25-32 weeks of age (ICAR, 2013) are __________

a) 20.0, 17.7 and 15.9 b) **22.7, 15.2 and 14.0**

c) 20.0, 18.0 and 16.0 d) 18.0, 16.0 and 14.0

Q 44 Energy requirements (ME Kcal/kg diet) for exotic pigs under Indian agro-climatic conditions from 8-16 weeks, 17-24 weeks and 25-32 weeks of age (ICAR, 2013) are __________

a) **2886, 3054 and 2497** b) 3040, 3060 and 2470

c) 3400, 2670 and 2270 d) None of above

Q 45 Protein requirements (%) for exotic pigs under Indian agro-climatic conditions from 8-16 weeks, 17-24 weeks and 25-32 weeks of age (ICAR, 2013) are __________

a) 20.0, 17.7 and 15.9 b) 22.7, 15.2 and 14.0

c) 20.0, 18.7 and 15.3 d) **18.4, 16.7 and 15.0**

Q 46 Energy requirements (ME Kcal/kg diet) for indigenous pigs from 8-20 weeks, 21-28 weeks and 29-32 weeks of age (ICAR, 2013) are __________

a) 2886, 3054 and 2497 b) **3040, 3060 and 2470**

c) 3400, 2670 and 2270 d) None of above

Q 47 Protein requirements (%) for exotic pigs under Indian agro-climatic conditions from 8-20 weeks, 21-28 weeks and 29-32 weeks of age (ICAR, 2013) are __________

a) 20.0, 17.7 and 15.9 b) 22.7, 15.2 and 14.0

c) **20.0, 18.7 and 15.3** d) 18.4, 16.7 and 15.0

Q 48 Lysine requirements (%) for crossbred pigs with medium to higher growth potential from 8-16 weeks, 17-24 weeks and 25-32 weeks of age (ICAR, 2013) are __________

a) 0.70, 0.65 and 0.60 b) **0.91, 0.75 and 0.81**

c) 0.83, 0.99 and 0.79 d) 0.3, 0.45 and 0.55

Q 49 Lysine requirements (%) for exotic pigs under Indian agro-climatic conditions from 8-16 weeks, 17-24 weeks and 25-32 weeks of age (ICAR, 2013) are __________

a) **0.70, 0.65 and 0.60** b) 0.91, 0.75 and 0.81

c) 0.83, 0.99 and 0.79 d) 0.70, for all

Q 50 Lysine requirements (%) for indigenous pigs from 8-20 weeks, 21-28 weeks and 29-32 weeks of age (ICAR, 2013) are __________

a) 0.70, 0.65 and 0.60 b) 0.91, 0.75 and 0.81

c) **0.83, 0.99 and 0.79** d) None

Q 51 Moisture (%, Max) as per BIS (1986, reaffirmed in 2001) nutrient requirements for pig feed is __________

a) 6% b) 8%

c) **11%** d) 12%

Q 52 Crude fibre (%) content of creep feed (BIS (1986, reaffirmed in 2001)) are __________

a) **5%** b) 6%

c) 8% d) 4%

Q 53 Crude fibre (%) content of grower feed (BIS (1986, reaffirmed in 2001)) are __________

a) 5% b) **6%**

c) 8% d) 4%

Q 54 Crude fibre (%) content of finisher/breeding meal (BIS (1986, reaffirmed in 2001)) are __________

a) 5% b) 6%

c) **8%** d) 10%

Q 55 The first limiting amino acid in the diet of swine is __________

a) Leucine b) Methionine

c) **Lysine** d) Threonine

Q 56 The problems in feeding of poultry manure to pigs are __________

a) High uric acid content
b) Presence of pathogens
c) **Both**
d) None

Q 57 The free fatty acids in fat sources used for pig feeding should not exceed __________

a) **15%**
b) 18%
c) 1%
d) None

Q 58 The maximum level of inclusion of Brewer's grain in pig diet is __________

a) 20%
b) **15%**
c) 10%
d) 5%

Q 59 The available amino acids asthe proportions of dietary amino acids which are digested, absorbed and utilized to sustain life and/or the growth of new tissue __________

a) Limiting amino acid
b) Essential amino acid
c) **Ideal protein**
d) None

Q 60 Water requirement of pigs are related to __________

a) Feed intake and it composition
b) Environmental temperature
c) Physiological status
d) **All**

Q 61 Usually pigs consume water ________ the quantity of feed they consume.

a) **Double**
b) 1.5 times
c) Same
d) No relation between these two

Q 62 The water requirement of growing pigs (20-90kg) per kilogram of feed consumed under normal, adlib and restricted feeding is __________

a) **2.0, 2.5 and 3.7 kg**
b) 3.0, 3.5 and 4.7 kg
c) 3.0, 3.5 and 3.7 kg
d) None

Q 63 The water requirement of non-pregnant gilt, pregnant gilt and lactating sow per day is ________

a) 15.0, 20.0 and 18.0 kg b) 8.5, 10.0 and 11.0 kg

c) **11.5, 20.0 and 18.0 kg** d) 7.5, 8.0 and 10.0 kg

Q 64 The biological value of an ideal protein should be ________

a) 0.7 b) **1.0**

c) 0.8 d) 0.6

Q 65 If the pig diet is formulated on a ________ basis, the requirements of other amino acids should be met.

a) **Lysine** b) Tryptophan

c) Leucine d) Methionine

Q 66 Due to antagonism excessive dietary lysine in pig ration increases the requirements for ________

a) Cystiene b) Methionine

c) Leucine d) **Arginine**

Q 67 In pigs, deficiency of fatty acids causes ________

a) Sclerosis b) Posterior paralysis

c) **Dermatitis** d) Arginine

Q 68 The ratio of total Ca: total P should be kept between ________ for maximal utilization of both minerals in pigs.

a) 1:1.25 and 1:1 b) **1.25:1 and 1:1**

c) 1.25:1 and 2:1 d) None

Q 69 In sow, calcium-phosphorus deficiency is often associated with ________

a) Atopy dermatitis b) **Posterior paralysis**

c) Dermatitis d) Arginine

Q 70 The mineral which is poorly transferred in the milk of swine ________

a) Phosphorus b) Calcium

c) Both a and b d) **Iron**

Q 71 The iron requirement is very high in baby pigs because of its __________

a) Rapid growth rate
b) High rate of haemoglobin synthesis
c) Low iron content of milk
d) **All the above**

Q 72 Cotton seed meals with are generally not recommended for pigs because of __________

a) **Gossypol** b) High fibre
c) Growth inhibitors d) Both a and b

Q 73 Maximum level of inclusion of Brewer's grain in pig ration __________

a) Upto 5% b) 10%
c) **Upto 15%** d) 2%

Q 74 Maximum level of inclusion of Poultry droppings in pig ration __________

a) 5% b) Upto 7%
c) 6% d) **Upto 3%**

Q 75 Maximum level of inclusion of fat in pig ration __________

a) **5-7%** b) 8-10%
c) 1.5% d) 2-3%

Q 76 Maximum level of inclusion of Milk whey in pig ration __________

a) Upto 5% b) **Upto 10%**
c) Upto 15% d) Upto 2%

Q 77 After birth, piglets can sustain exclusively on sow's milk for __________

a) 1-3 days b) 10-14 days
c) 7-10 days d) **Both a and c**

Q 78 Piglets need to consume ________ of colostrums or milk to remain in energy balance during first week of their age.

a) **250-300 ml** b) 500 ml
c) 150-200 ml d) None

Q 79 Piglet lacks intestinal sucrase activity, hence dietary sucrose may cause digestive disturbances, if it exceeds ________ of diet.

a) 0.5% b) 2%
c) 0.3% d) **1%**

Q 80 The purpose of creep feeding programme in pigs ________

a) Improve growth

b) Reduces demand on sow's milk

c) **Both a and b**

d) None

Q 81 Pre-starter ration given to piglets upto body weight (NRC, 1998) ________

a) 2-3 kg
b) 1-1.5 kg
c) **1-5 kg**
d) None

Q 82 Starter rations are usually given, when piglets attain the weight of (NRC, 1998).

a) 2 kg
b) **5 kg**
c) 3 kg
d) None

Q 83 Benefits of phase feeding as recommended by NRC (1998) ________

a) Progressive reduction in diet cost

b) Improvement in feed efficiency

c) Less nutrients excretion

d) **All**

Q 84 Young piglets may suffer from piglet anaemia as sow's milk is poor source ________

a) Iron
b) Copper
c) **Both**
d) None

Q 85 Which of following is helpful in prevention of piglet anaemia?

a) intramuscular injection of 200 mg of iron dextran given at 1 to 3 days of age

b) Supplementation of iron and copper in pig's diet @ 25 mg iron and 5 mg of copper/day/pig

c) Daily paint the udder of sow with 5% iron and copper sulphate solution

d) **All**

Q 86 Grower phase of pigs (NRC, 1998) ________

a) **20-50 kg**
b) 20-30 kg
c) 10-20 kg
d) 30-50 kg

Q 87 Finisher phase of pigs (NRC, 1998) __________

a) 20-50 kg
b) 30-80 kg
c) **50-120 kg**
d) 40-70 kg

Q 88 Average feed consumption during grower phase of pigs (NRC, 1998) __________

a) 1.5 kg
b) **2 kg**
c) 3.1 kg
d) 4 kg

Q 89 Average feed consumption during finisher phase of pigs (NRC, 1998) __________

a) 1.5 kg
b) 2 kg
c) **3.1 kg**
d) 4 kg

Q 90 Average feed consumption during prestarter (1-5kg), Starter-I (5-10kg) and Starter-II (10-20kg) phase of pigs (NRC, 1998) __________

a) 150, 360 and 650g
b) 150, 260 and 550g
c) 150, 260 and 450g
d) **250, 460 and 950g**

Q 91 BIS (1986, reaffirmed in 2001) recommended following phases for pig feeding __________

a) **Starter, Grower and Finisher**
b) Pre-starter, Starter, Grower and Finisher
c) Starter-I, Starter-II, Grower and Finisher
d) None

Q 92 The feeding programme recommended for pregnant sows __________

a) Normal Feeding
b) **Restricted feeding**
c) Adlib feeding
d) None

Q 93 Excessive energy intake by sows results in __________

a) Reduced reproductive efficiency
b) High embryonic mortality
c) Smaller litter size
d) **All**

Q 94 Feeding extra allowance of grains by about 0.5-0.7 kg before breeding season __________

a) **Flushing**
b) Breeding diet
c) Heatup diet
d) All

Q 95 Fattening ration for pigs is __________

a) Growing ration
b) **Finisher ration**
c) Flushing
d) Both A and B

Q 96 With the floor feeding cost of feeding equipments and the cleanliness factor get __________

a) Increased
b) Remains same
c) **Reduced**
d) None

Q 97 Backyard pig producers prefer to feed pigs with __________

a) Crumbled feed
b) Dry feed
c) Ground feed
d) **Wet feed**

Q 98 Fine grinding of feeds for pig is not recommended because such feed sticks to the feeder and there is increased incidence of __________

a) **Gastric ulcers**
b) Porcine proliferative enteritis
c) Stomatitis
d) Ileitis

❑❑❑

Chapter 22

Nutrients Requirements and Feeding of Poultry

Q 1 The amount of food energy required to keep the animal at a constant body weight and composition is called __________

a) **Maintenance energy** b) Net energy
c) Gross energy d) Heat Increment

Q 2 The methods adopted to arrive at energy requirements for maintenance as well as growth is __________

a) Fasting metabolism b) Feeding trial method
c) Comparative slaughter d) **All**

Q 3 The heat production at specified times after the last feeding __________

a) **Fasting metabolism** b) Fasting catabolism
c) Basal metabolism d) All

Q 4 Fasting metabolism is preferred to basal metabolism because __________

a) Easy to calculate
b) Simple method
c) **Strict basal conditions are unlikely to observe**
d) Both a and b

Q 5 Estimates of maintenance energy requirements include the __________

a) Effects of food consumption
b) Effects of digestion
c) Environment effects
d) **All**

Q 6 In comparative slaughter, the amount of energy retained in the body is calculated from __________

a) Live weight gain

b) Change in body composition

c) **Both a and b**

d) Growth rate

Q 7 Nutrients requirements of animals are related with __________

a) Body weight b) Stage of maturity

c) **Both** d) None

Q 8 Estimation of protein requirements for maintenance and growth in poultry by __________

a) Factorial method b) Nitrogen balance method

c) Feeding trial method d) **All**

Q 9 For poultry, the protein requirements are usually stated together for maintenance and __________

a) Growth b) Reproduction

c) **Both a and b** d) Production

Q 10 NE requirement for growth of poultry is sum of the NE required for __________

a) Basal metabolism b) Activity increment

c) Tissue growth d) **All**

Q 11 The amount of energy required for moderate activity is referred as __________

a) **Activity increment** b) Heat increment

c) Basal energy d) None

Q 12 Prior to sexual maturity nutrients requirements of males are __________ than that of females.

a) **Same** b) Greater

c) Lesser d) None

Q 13 Metabolic body weight is defined as body weight raised to the power __________

a) 0.78 b) **0.75**

c) 0.72 d) 0.68

Q 14 Latest feeding standard available for poultry birds __________

a) NRC (1992) b) **NRC (1994)**

c) NRC (2001) d) NRC (1998)

Q 15 ARC stands for __________

a) Animal Research Council

b) American Research Council

c) **Agriculture Research Council**

d) None

Q 16 Feeding standards available for poultry are __________

a) NRC, ARC and CARI

b) NRC, ARC and BIS

c) **NRC, ARC, BIS, ICAR and CARI**

d) NRC, BIS and CARI

Q 17 Feeding standards which is almost outdated for poultry __________

a) NRC b) BIS

c) CARI d) **ARC**

Q 18 CARI stands for __________

a) **Central Avian Research Institute**

b) Central Agricultural Research Institute

c) Council of Avian Research and Innovations

d) None

Q 19 The amount of energy required for moderate activity is referred as __________

a) **Activity increment** b) Heat increment

c) Basal energy d) None

Q 20 NRC (1994) specifications of nutrients for poultry as percentages or units per kilogram of diet on the basis of __________

a) **90% DM** b) 100% DM
c) Both d) None

Q 21 In poultry, the net energy for maintenance is (kcal/day) __________

a) $106 \times BW^{0.75}$ b) **$83 \times BW^{0.75}$**
c) $110 \times BW^{0.75}$ d) None

Q 22 The efficiency of protein utilization for maintenance and egg production __________

a) 70% b) 61%
c) **55%** d) None

Q 23 Efficiency of utilization of protein in growing chicken __________

a) 72% b) 82%
c) **61%** d) 65%

Q 24 The activity increment for birds kept in cages is __________

a) **37%** b) 50%
c) 25% d) None

Q 25 The activity increment for birds kept in deep litter system is __________

a) 37% b) **50%**
c) 25% d) None

Q 26 NE_m requirement for 2 kg hen is __________

a) **139.5 kcal/d** b) 2 kcal/d
c) 149.5 kcal/d d) None

Q 27 Energy content of medium-sized egg __________

a) 86 kcal b) **84 kcal**
c) 82 kcal d) None

Q 28 In growing chicks, the maintenance requirements for protein (per kg B wt/d) is __________

a) 0.16g b) **1.6g**
c) 16g d) None

Q 29 NRC (1994) nutrients requirements for broiler finisher are __________

a) **CP 18%; ME 3200 Kcal/d**

b) CP 20%; ME 2800 Kcal/d

c) CP 17%; ME 2700 Kcal/d

d) None of the above

Q 30 NRC (1994) nutrients requirements for broiler starter are __________

a) CP 23%; ME 2900 Kcal/d

b) **CP 23%; ME 3200 Kcal/d**

c) CP 20%; ME 3200 Kcal/d

d) None of the above

Q 31 NRC (1994) nutrients requirements for layer starter are __________

a) CP 18%; ME 2900 Kcal/d

b) **CP 18%; ME 2850 Kcal/d**

c) CP 23%; ME 2850 Kcal/d

d) None of the above

Q 32 NRC (1994) nutrients requirements for layer are __________

a) CP 18%; ME 2900 Kcal/d

b) CP 17%; ME 2800 Kcal/d

c) **CP 15%; ME 2900 Kcal/d**

d) None of the above

Q 33 BIS (1992) nutrients requirements for breeder are __________

a) **CP 18%; ME 2800 Kcal/d**

b) CP 22%; ME 2800 Kcal/d

c) CP 18%; ME 2900 Kcal/d

d) None of the above

Q 34 BIS (1992) nutrients requirements for broiler starter are __________

a) CP 17%; ME 3000 Kcal/d

b) CP 22%; ME 2700 Kcal/d

c) **CP 22%; ME 2900 Kcal/d**

d) CP 16%; ME 2700 Kcal/d

Q 35 BIS (1992) nutrients requirements for broiler finisher are __________

a) **CP 17%; ME 3000 Kcal/d**
b) CP 22%; ME 2700 Kcal/d
c) CP 22%; ME 2900 Kcal/d
d) CP 16%; ME 2700 Kcal/d

Q 36 BIS (1992) nutrients requirements for egg type chick starter are __________

a) CP 17%; ME 3000 Kcal/d
b) **CP 22%; ME 2700 Kcal/d**
c) CP 22%; ME 2900 Kcal/d
d) CP 16%; ME 2700 Kcal/d

Q 37 BIS (1992) nutrients requirements for egg type grower are __________

a) CP 17%; ME 3000 Kcal/d
b) CP 22%; ME 2700 Kcal/d
c) CP 22%; ME 2900 Kcal/d
d) **CP 16%; ME 2700 Kcal/d**

Q 38 BIS (1992) nutrients requirements for layer chicks are __________

a) CP 18%; ME 2800 Kcal/d
b) **CP 22%; ME 2700 Kcal/d**
c) CP 22%; ME 2800 Kcal/d
d) None of the above

Q 39 BIS (1992) nutrients requirements of Vitamin A (IU/Kg) for breeder and layers are __________

a) **8000** b) 6000
c) 4000 d) 7000

Q 40 BIS (1992) nutrients requirements of Vitamin A (IU/Kg) for broilers are __________

a) 8000 b) **6000**
c) 4000 d) 7000

Q 41 Moisture (%, Max) as per BIS (1992) nutrients requirements for poultry feed is __________

a) 6% b) 8%
c) **10%** d) 12%

Q 42 BIS (1992) nutrients requirements for breeder are __________

a) **CP 18%; ME 2800 Kcal/d**

b) CP 22%; ME 2800 Kcal/d

c) CP 18%; ME 2900 Kcal/d

d) None of the above

Q 43 BIS (2007) nutrients requirements for broiler starter are ______

a) CP 17%; ME 3000 Kcal/d

b) CP 22%; ME 3200 Kcal/d

c) **CP 22%; ME 3100 Kcal/d**

d) CP 16%; ME 3000 Kcal/d

Q 44 BIS (2007) nutrients requirements for broiler finisher are _____

a) **CP 20%; ME 3200 Kcal/d**

b) CP 22%; ME 3200 Kcal/d

c) CP 22%; ME 3100 Kcal/d

d) CP 20%; ME 3000 Kcal/d

Q 45 BIS (2007) nutrients requirements for egg type chick starter are __________

a) CP 22%; ME 2800 Kcal/d

b) **CP 20%; ME 2800 Kcal/d**

c) CP 18%; ME 2600 Kcal/d

d) CP 16%; ME 2500 Kcal/d

Q 46 BIS (2007) nutrients requirements for egg type grower are _____

a) CP 17%; ME 2500 Kcal/d

b) CP 20%; ME 2800 Kcal/d

c) CP 18%; ME 2600 Kcal/d

d) **CP 16%; ME 2500 Kcal/d**

Q 47 BIS (2007) nutrients requirements for layer chicks (21-45 weeks) are __________

a) CP 16%; ME 2500 Kcal/d

b) **CP 18%; ME 2600 Kcal/d**

c) CP 20%; ME 2600 Kcal/d

d) None of the above

Q 48 BIS (2007) nutrients requirements of Vitamin A (IU/Kg) for grower and layers are ________

a) **8000** b) 6000

c) 4000 d) 7000

Q 49 BIS (2007) nutrients requirements of Vitamin A (IU/Kg) for broilers finisher are ________

a) 8000 b) **10000**

c) 9000 d) 11000

Q 50 Moisture (%, Max) as per BIS (2007) nutrients requirements for poultry feed is ________

a) 6% b) 10%

c) **11%** d) 12%

Q 51 ICAR (2013) nutrients requirements for broiler starter are ____

a) CP 21.5%; ME 3050 Kcal/d

b) CP 19.5%; ME 3100 Kcal/d

c) **CP 22%; ME 3000 Kcal/d**

d) CP 21.5%; ME 3000 Kcal/d

Q 52 ICAR (2013) nutrients requirements for broiler grower are ________

a) **CP 21.5%; ME 3050 Kcal/d**

b) CP 19.5%; ME 3100 Kcal/d

c) CP 22%; ME 3000 Kcal/d

d) None of the above

Q 53 ICAR (2013) nutrients requirements for broiler finisher are ________

a) CP 21.5%; ME 3050 Kcal/d

b) **CP 19.5%; ME 3100 Kcal/d**

c) CP 22%; ME 3000 Kcal/d

d) CP 20%; ME 3100 Kcal/d

Q 54 ICAR (2013) nutrients requirements for egg type chick starter are ________

a) CP 18.5%; ME 2800 Kcal/d

b) **CP 18.5%; ME 2600 Kcal/d**

c) CP 15.5%; ME 2800 Kcal/d

d) CP 15.5%; ME 2600 Kcal/d

Q 55 ICAR (2013) nutrients requirements for egg type grower are __________

a) CP 18.5%; ME 2800 Kcal/d

b) CP 20%; ME 2800 Kcal/d

c) CP 15.5%; ME 2800 Kcal/d

d) **CP 15.5%; ME 2600 Kcal/d**

Q 56 ICAR (2013) nutrients requirements for layer chicks above 30 weeks of age (for live wt 1400g, egg mass 45g and feed intake 100g/day) are __________

a) CP 16%; ME 2600 Kcal/d

b) **CP 16.5%; ME 2600 Kcal/d**

c) CP 15.5%; ME 2800 Kcal/d

d) None of the above

Q 57 ICAR (2013) nutrients requirements of Vitamin A (IU/Kg) for grower are __________

a) **2500**
b) 3500
c) 4500
d) 5000

Q 58 ICAR (2013) nutrients requirements of Vitamin A (IU/Kg) for layers (for live wt 1400g, egg mass 45g and feed intake 100g/day) are __________

a) 2500
b) 3500
c) **4500**
d) 5000

Q 59 ICAR (2013) nutrients requirements of Vitamin A (IU/Kg) for broilers are __________

a) 8000
b) **5000**
c) 9000
d) 6000

Q 60 ARC nutrients requirements for chick starter are __________

a) **CP 16%; DE 2700 Kcal/d**

b) CP 16%; ME 2900 Kcal/d

c) CP 15%; ME 2700 Kcal/d

d) None of the above

Q 61 The amino acids which can be synthesized from other amino acids in animal body are called dietary __________

a) Essential amino acids

b) **Non-essential amino acids**

c) Ideal amino acids

d) Semi-indispensible amino acids

Q 62 The amino acids either not synthesized at all or are synthesized too slowly to meet the metabolic requirements of poultry are called dietary __________

a) **Essential amino acids**

b) Non-essential amino acids

c) Ideal amino acids

d) Semi-indispensible amino acids

Q 63 Number of amino acids required for the synthesis of various proteins in the body of birds __________

a) 20 b) **22**

c) 10 d) 12

Q 64 Number of essential amino acids required by poultry birds _____

a) 20 b) 22

c) **10** d) 12

Q 65 The amino acid which is not essential in the diet of poultry ___

a) Histidine b) Leucine

c) Threonine d) **Glutamine**

Q 66 The amino acid which is essential in the diet of poultry _______

a) Alanine b) Asparagine

c) **Arginine** d) Glutamine

Q 67 The amino acid which is essential in the diet of poultry _______

a) Alanine b) Asparagine

c) Proline d) **Valine**

Q 68 Semi-essential amino acids in the diet of poultry are _______

a) **Cysteine & tyrosine**

b) Lysine & leucine

c) Methionine & phenylalanine

d) Arginine and valine

Q 69 The first limiting amino acid in maize-soya based diets for poultry is ________

a) Arginine b) Lysine

c) **Methionine** d) None

Q 70 Cysteine can be synthesized in poultry birds from ________

a) Arginine b) Glycine

c) **Methionine** d) Phenylalanine

Q 71 Tyrosine can be synthesized in poultry birds from ________

a) Arginine b) Glycine

c) Methionine d) **Phenylalanine**

Q 72 Amino acid required by young birds for biosynthesis of uric acid is ________

a) Arginine b) **Glycine**

c) Methionine d) Phenylalanine

Q 73 To develop ideal amino acid ratio for poultry diets, which amino acid used as reference?

a) **Lysine** b) Methionine

c) Threonine d) None

Q 74 BIS (1992) nutrients requirements of lysine (%) for layers and broilers are ________

a) 0.7 and 0.9 b) 0.7 and 0.9

c) **0.5 and 0.9** d) 0.5 and 0.7

Q 75 BIS (2007) nutrients requirements of methionine (%) for layers are ________

a) 0.4 b) 0.2

c) 0.5 d) **0.3**

Q 76 BIS (2007) nutrients requirements of lysine (%) for layers are ________

a) 0.70-0.75 b) 1.0-2.0

c) **0.65-0.70** d) 0.55-0.65

Q 77 BIS (2007) nutrients requirements of lysine (%) for broilers are ________

a) 1.0-2.0 b) 1.3-1.4

c) 0.7-1.0 d) **1.0-1.3**

Q 78 ICAR (2013) nutrients requirements of lysine (%) for layers are __________

a) 0.70-0.75 b) 0.65-0.70

c) **0.76-0.82** d) 0.55-0.65

Q 79 ICAR (2013) nutrients requirements of lysine (%) for broilers are __________

a) 1.0-2.0 b) 0.80-0.85

c) **0.94-1.20** d) None of above

Q 80 ICAR (2013) nutrients requirements of methionine (%) for layers are __________

a) 0.4-0.5 b) 0.24-0.32

c) 0.5-0.6 d) **0.34-0.36**

Q 81 After hatching, body weights of commercial broilers will increase in 6 weeks by __________

a) 20 to 25 fold b) 100 fold

c) **50 to 55 fold** d) 10-20 fold

Q 82 High levels of lean meat deposition require relatively high levels of __________

a) Methionine b) **Lysine**

c) Threonine d) All

Q 83 High levels of egg output require relatively high levels of ______

a) **Methionine** b) Lysine

c) Threonine d) All

Q 84 High levels of feather growth require relatively high levels of __________

a) **Methionine** b) Lysine

c) Threonine d) All

Q 85 In practical feed formulation, methionine can spare ________ as a methyl donor.

a) Glycine b) Leucine

c) Threonine d) **Choline**

Q 86 Essential fatty acid in the diets of poultry is __________

a) Butyric acid b) Lysine

c) **Linoleic acid** d) Ecosanoic acid

Q 87 Linoleic acid (%) recommendations for layer (BIS,1992, 2007); NRC,1994); ICAR (2013) is ________

a) **1%** b) 1.5%

c) 2% d) 0.5%

Q 88 Energy required for poultry birds to gain 1 g body weight is __

a) 1-2 kcal b) **2-3 kcal**

c) 3-4 kcal d) None

Q 89 The ME requirements are higher than the NE requirements ________

a) 10% b) 9%

c) **18%** d) 10%

Q 90 The nutrients requirements of growing chicks are ________ than that of pullets.

a) **Higher** b) Lower

c) Same d) Variable

Q 91 The limiting factor for growth of egg-strain birds reared under most environmental conditions ________

a) Protein b) **Energy**

c) Both d) None

Q 92 The environmental temperature and energy intake (feed intake) are related ________

a) Directly b) **Inversely**

c) Variable d) None

Q 93 In general egg contains ________ protein by weight.

a) 4-5 g b) 8-9 g

c) **6-7 g** d) None

Q 94 The estimated nutrient requirements (NRC, 1994) of brown-egg layers are greater than those of the white-egg-laying layers ________

a) 2% b) **10%**

c) 8% d) Same

Q 95 Crude fibre (%) content of broiler finisher diet (BIS, 1992 and BIS, 2007) are ________

a) **6% and 5%** b) 7% and 8%

c) 4% and 5% d) 6% and 4%

Q 96 Crude fibre (%) content of layer diet from 21-45 weeks (BIS, 1992 and BIS, 2007) are ________

a) 6% and 5% b) **8% and 9%**

c) 9% and 10% d) None of above

Q 97 Common salt (%) required for poultry birds (BIS, 1992 and BIS, 2007) are ________

A) 1% and 0.6% B) 0.6% and 0.6%

C) 0.6% and 0.5% D) None of the above

Q 98 Calcium (%) required for layers (BIS, 1992 and BIS, 2007) are ________

a) 2.75% b) **2.75% and 3.5%**

c) 0.6% d) None of the above

Q 99 Calcium (%) required for layers (ICAR, 2013) is ________

a) 2.75% b) 3.18

c) **3.61%** d) None of the above

Q 100 The vitamin which can be synthesized by the poultry birds ________

a) Vitamin B b) **Vitamin C**

c) Vitamin E d) Vitamin A

Q 101 Macro-minerals are elements required in the diet at concentrations of more than ________

a) 50 mg/kg b) 75mg/kg

c) **100 mg / kg** d) 1g /kg

Q 102 The recommended ratio calcium and non-phytate phosphorus in growing birds' diets is ________

a) **2:1** b) 1:1

c) 12:1 d) 6:1

Q 103 The recommended ratio of calcium and non-phytate phosphorus in laying birds' diets is ________

a) 2:1 b) 1:1

c) **12:1** d) 6:1

Q 104 Metabolizable energy (kcal) per kilogram divided by the percentage of crude protein in the ration is __________

a) Ideal protein ratio b) **Calorie-protein ratio**
c) Ration density d) ME ratio

Q 105 Calorie-protein ratio (BIS, 1992) for layer ration is __________

a) 122 b) 130
c) 145 d) **144**

Q 106 Calorie-protein ratio (BIS, 1992) for broiler starter ration is __________

a) **122** b) 130
c) 145 d) 144

Q 107 Calorie-protein ratio (BIS, 1992) for broiler finisher ration is __________

a) 122 b) 130
c) **145** d) 144

Q 108 Calorie-protein ratio (BIS, 1992) for chick starter ration is __________

a) 156 b) **130**
c) 145 d) 144

Q 109 Calorie-protein ratio (BIS, 1992) for chick grower ration is __________

a) **156** b) 130
c) 145 d) 144

Q 110 The electrolyte balance of diet considered satisfactory for optimum growth of poultry is __________

a) 25 mEq / kg b) 2.5 mEq / kg
c) **250 mEq / kg** d) None

Q 111 Dietary proportions of elements largely determine the acid-base balance in the body __________

a) Na, Cl and Mg b) Na, Cl and Ca
c) **Na, Cl and K** d) Na, Cl and P

Q 112 Maximum level of inclusion of fish meal in poultry ration _____

a) 5% b) **10%**
c) 15% d) 2%

Q 113 Maximum level of inclusion of wheat bran in grower ration __________

a) 5% b) **10%**
c) 15% d) 2%

Q 114 Maximum level of inclusion of soybean meal in chick ration __________

a) 5% b) 10%
c) **35%** d) 2%

Q 115 Maximum level of inclusion of fat in poultry ration __________

a) **5%** b) 10%
c) 15% d) 2%

Q 116 Feed represents total cost of broiler production is about __________

a) 70% b) **55%**
c) 80% d) None

Q 117 Poultry birds are __________

a) Herbivores b) **Omnivores**
c) Carnivores d) None

Q 118 Poultry birds have __________

a) **Simple stomach** b) Compound stomach
c) 3-compartment stomach d) None

Q 119 Poultry birds require more concentrated ration because of v

a) Simple stomach b) No teeth
c) No lips d) **All**

Q 120 Organ act as storage pouch of feed in poultry birds __________

a) Gizzard b) Proventriculus
c) **Crop** d) Duodenum loops

Q 121 Organ helps in grinding of feed in poultry birds __________

a) **Gizzard** b) Proventriculus
c) Crop d) Duodenum loops

Q 122 Organ positioned in center of body to facilitate flight in poultry birds __________

a) **Gizzard** b) Proventriculus

c) Crop d) Oesophagus

Q 123 In poultry birds, digestion mainly takes place in __________

a) Gizzard b) Proventriculus

c) Crop d) **Small intestine**

Q 124 In poultry birds, saliva and secretions soften the feed in ______

a) Gizzard b) Proventriculus

c) **Crop** d) Small intestine

Q 125 In poultry birds, the site where undigested food and urine meet __________

a) Vent b) **Cloaca**

c) Ceca d) Gullet

Q 126 Poultry birds eats to satisfy their __________

a) **Energy needs** b) Protein needs

c) Productive needs d) Maintenance needs

Q 127 Chick starter ration (BIS, 1992 and BIS, 2007) are __________

a) 0-8 weeks and 0-6 weeks b) 0-6 weeksand 0-8 weeks

c) 0-5 weeks and 0-8 weeks d) **0-8 weeks**

Q 128 Chick grower ration (BIS, 1992 and BIS, 2007) __________

a) **9-20 weeks** b) Above 20 weeks

c) 5-15 weeks d) 0-8 weeks

Q 129 Chick layer ration (BIS, 1992 and BIS, 2007) __________

a) 8-20 weeks b) **Above 20 weeks**

c) 5-15 weeks d) 0-8 weeks

Q 130 Broiler pre-starter ration (BIS, 2007) __________

a) 0-14 days b) 0-3 days

c) 0-10 days d) **1-7 days**

Q 131 Broiler starter ration (BIS, 1992 and BIS, 2007) are ________

a) 0-14 days and 8-21 days b) 0-28 days and 0-21 days

c) **0-28 days and 8-21 days** d) 8-28 days and 0-21 days

Q 132 Broiler finisher ration (BIS, 1992 and BIS, 2007) are ________

a) 3-6 weeks and above 4 weeks

b) **4-6 weeks and above 3 weeks**

c) 2-6 weeks and above 3 weeks

d) None of above

Q 133 Chick starter ration (ICAR, 2013) for layer ________

a) 0-6 weeks b) 0-7 weeks

c) **0-8 weeks** d) 0-50 days

Q 134 Chick grower ration (ICAR, 2013) ________

a) **9-20 weeks** b) 8-19 weeks

c) 8-16 weeks d) None of above

Q 135 Chick layer ration starts from (ICAR, 2013) ________

a) 20 weeks b) **18 weeks**

c) 16 weeks d) 14 weeks

Q 136 Chick pre-layer ration (ICAR, 2013) ________

a) 18-20 weeks b) 14-16 weeks

c) **16-18 weeks** d) 16-20 weeks

Q 137 Broiler starter, grower and finisher ration (ICAR, 2013) ________

a) **0-14, 14-21 and 21-42 days**

b) 0-14, 14-28 and 28-42 days

c) 0-10, 10-18 and 18-35 days

d) None of above

Q 138 Water is required for poultry birds for ________

a) Digestion and absorption

b) Excretion of waste products

c) Regulation of body temperature

d) **All**

Q 139 Usually birds drink water ________ the quantity of feed they consume.

a) **Double**

b) 1.5 times

c) Same

d) No relation between these two

Q 140 Water intake increase if birds consume more ________

a) Dietary salt b) Crude protein

c) Starch d) **Both a and b**

Q 141 For each 1°C rise in environment temperature above 21°C, water consumption increases about ________

a) **5%** b) 2%

c) 7% d) Remains same

Q 142 Representative poultry diet contains energy around ________

a) **2.8 M cal ME/kg feed** b) 2.0 M cal ME/kg feed

c) 2.4 M cal ME/kg feed d) None

Q 143 Daily energy consumption of poultry will vary with ________

a) Age b) Production status

c) Environmental temperature d) **All**

Q 144 Few weeks before the onset of egg production, switch pullets from growing diet to ________

a) High-protein laying diet b) **High-calcium laying diet**

c) High-energy laying diet d) None

Q 145 Adequate dietary vitamin B_{12} helps pullets develop the ability to biosynthesize ________

a) **Choline** b) Biotin

c) Betaine d) Pyridoxine

Q 146 The vegetable proteins are generally deficient in ________

a) Methionine b) Lysine

c) Tryptophan d) **All**

Q 147 What limit the use of cotton seed meal in layer diets?

a) Gossypol b) High fibre

c) **Both** d) None

Q 148 What limit the use of blood meal in poultry diets?

a) Deficient isoleucine
b) Poor palatability
c) **Both**
d) None

Q 149 Pelleting of feed is done to __________

a) Increase feed density
b) Facilitate handling
c) Reduce feed wastage
d) **All**

Q 150 Feed more prone to mould formation and rancidity __________

a) **Dry mash**
b) Pellet feed
c) Crumble feed
d) Both B and C

Q 151 Various methods of feed restriction in poultry __________

a) Quantitative feed restriction
b) Feeding of low energy diets
c) Restriction of dietary protein levels
d) **All**

Q 152 The feeding programs based on the assumption that the amount of nutrient needed each day is different at different stages of the production cycle __________

a) Force feeding
b) **Phase feeding**
c) Restricted feeding
d) None

Q 153 First phase of production cycle of layer is __________

a) **Onset of egg production to 36 weeks**
b) 36 weeks to 52 weeks
c) 52 weeks to end of the production cycle
d) 30 weeks to 40 weeks

Q 154 Second phase of production cycle of layer is __________

a) Onset of egg production to 36 weeks
b) **36 weeks to 52 weeks**
c) 52 weeks to end of the production cycle
d) 30 weeks to 40 weeks

Q 155 Third phase of production cycle of layer is __________

a) Onset of egg production to 36 weeks
b) 36 weeks to 52 weeks
c) **52 weeks to end of the production cycle**
d) 30 weeks to 40 weeks

Q 156 The phase critical to provide mature hens with vigour and tissue reserve needed for maximum production throughout her productive life ________

a) **Phase I** b) Phase II
c) Phase III d) None

Q 157 In winter months, the calorie (ME)/protein ratio during laying phase-I should range from ________

a) 193-195 b) **166-170**
c) 196-200 d) None

Q 158 In winter months, the calorie (ME)/protein ratio during laying phase-II should range from ________

a) **193-195** b) 166-170
c) 196-200 d) None

Q 159 In winter months, the calorie (ME)/protein ratio during laying phase-III should range from ________

a) 193-195 b) 166-170
c) **196-200** d) None

Q 160 The inorganic phosphates sources used in poultry diets are ________

a) Dicalcium phosphate b) Rock phosphate
c) Defluorinated phosphate d) **All**

Q 161 Limestone powder contains calcium phosphorus ________

a) 22% and 18% b) 29% and 12%
c) **38% and 0%** d) 32% and 18%

Q 162 Calcium carbonate contains calcium phosphorus ________

a) 22% and 18% b) 29% and 12%
c) **38% and 0%** d) 32% and 18%

Q 163 Dicalcium phosphate (DCP) contains calcium phosphorus ________

a) **22% and 18%** b) 29% and 12%
c) 38% and 0% d) 32% and 18%

Q 164 Bone meal contains calcium phosphorus ________

a) 22% and 18% b) **29% and 12%**

c) 38% and 0% d) 32% and 18%

Q 165 Rock phosphate (defluorinated) contains calcium phosphorus ________

a) 22% and 18% b) 29% and 12%

c) 38% and 0% d) **32% and 18%**

Q 166 Excess dietary phosphorus may ________ eggshell strength in layers.

a) **Decrease** b) Increase

c) No effect d) All

Q 167 Excessive salt in poultry diet lead to ________

a) Increase in water consumption

b) Wet excreta

c) **Both a and b**

d) None

Q 168 The pigments used to improve egg yolk colour/skin colour ________

a) Zeaxanthin b) Canthaxanthin

c) **Both a and b** d) None

Q 169 Anti-microbial proteins/peptides used to prevent the growth of harmful bacteria in poultry diets ________

a) Lysozyme b) Lactacin F

c) α-lactalbumin d) **All**

Q 170 Anti-nutritional factor present in barley is ________

a) **β-glucans** b) Phytate

c) Arabinoxylans d) All

Q 171 Example of an anti-oxidant ________

a) Tylosin b) **Ethoxyquine**

c) Roxarsone d) None

Q 172 Which drug is not used as coccidiostat in poultry diet?

a) Monensin b) Amprolium

c) Narasin d) **Avoparcin**

Q 173 High levels of limestone and calcium phosphates in diet make it __________

a) Unpalatable

b) Dilute other dietary components

c) **Both a and b**

d) None

Q 174 Dietary requirement for vitamin E depends on the concentration /presence of __________ in diet.

a) Selenium b) Antioxidants

c) Pro-oxidants d) **All**

Q 175 In the poultry diet, the energy feeds forms __________

a) **70-75%** b) 40-45%

c) 25-30% d) None

Q 176 In the poultry diet, the protein feeds forms __________

a) 70-75% b) 40-45%

c) **25-30%** d) None

Q 177 Most commonly used high energy cereal grain in poultry ration is __________

a) Sorghum b) **Maize**

c) Fat d) Wheat

Q 178 The most commonly used vegetable protein feed in poultry ration is __________

a) Fish meal b) Maize

c) Groundnut meal d) **Soyabean meal**

Q 179 In hot climates, use 0.2 to 0.3% ________ in poultry ration.

a) **Sodium bicarbonate** b) Calcium carbonate

c) Calcium sulphate d) Shell grit

Q 180 If diet contains 5% fish meal, there is no need to supplement __________

a) Sodium bicarbonate b) **Sodium chloride**

c) Soyabean meal d) Both a and b

Q 181 Wet litter problem in poultry may result from feeding of __________

a) **Molasses** b) Bentonite

c) Rubber seed meal d) Sesame meal

Q 182 Cheapest method of feeding compounded rations __________

a) **Dry mash** b) Pellet form

c) Crumble form d) Both a and c

Q 183 The method of feeding not practiced in poultry birds _______

a) Ad-libitum feeding b) Force feeding

c) Restricted feeding d) **None**

Q 184 Force feeding recommended during __________

a) Breeding phase b) **During first week of age**

c) Molting phase d) After 80 weeks of age

Q 185 To prevent feed wastage and to keep the litter out of the feeder, put the feeders as high as __________

a) Chicken hackles b) Chicken beak

c) **Chicken back** d) Chicken comb

Q 186 Which is not essential for egg shell formation?

a) Calcium b) Manganese

c) Zinc d) **None**

Q 187 The vitamin that can influence the thickness of egg shell __________

a) Vitamin A b) **Vitamin D**

c) Vitamin E d) None

Q 188 The feed ingredient that do not improve yolk colour __________

a) Yellow maize b) Lucerne meal

c) **Mustard meal** d) Maize gluten meal

Q 189 Lutin an example of carotenoid pigments present in __________

a) Lupin meal b) Maize

c) **Alfalfa meal** d) None

Q 190 Choline is required by birds as an integral part/source of ________

a) Body phospholipids
b) Acetylcholine
c) Methyl groups
d) **All**

Q 191 If the recommended concentration of a medication in the feed is 12 parts per million (ppm), what percentage does it mean?

a) 0.12 %
b) 0.012%
c) **0.0012%**
d) 0.00012%

Q 192 Loss of pigmentation of egg shell and increase in mottled yolk are features of toxicity with which of the following anti-coccidials?

a) Amprolium
b) Roxarsone
c) **Nicarbazine**
d) Halofuginone

Q 193 The vitamin should not be given in combination with amprolium ________

a) **Vitamin B_1**
b) Folic acid
c) Vitamin K
d) Biotin

Q 194 The anticoccidial increases metabolic rate and makes bird more susceptible to the heat stress ________

a) Narasine
b) Tetracycline
c) **Nicarbazine**
d) Halofuginone

Q 195 From gastrointestinal tract, Ca reduces the absorption of ________

a) Sulfonamides
b) **Tetracycline**
c) Penicillin
d) Lincomycin

Q 196 The antibiotic medication has the longest withdrawal period for chicken ________

a) Erythromycin
b) Tetracycline
c) Penicillin
d) **Sulphaquinoxaline**

Q 197 Anti-coccidial required in the feed of ________

a) Starters
b) Layer
c) Grower
d) **Both a and c**

Q 198 The conditions facilitate mycotoxin production in feed are __________

a) Humidity above 62%, b) Temperature above 80°F
c) Moisture above 14% d) **All**

Q 199 Mycotoxins produced in poultry feed mainly by __________

a) Penicillium b) Fusarium
c) Aspergillus d) **All**

Q 200 Which is not a mycotoxin binder?

a) Activated charcoal b) Extracts of yeast cell wall
c) Aluminosilicates d) **None**

Q 201 Coccidiostat used in ration of broiler @ ________/ton of feed.

a) **50g** b) 100g
c) 75g d) 150g

Q 202 Mycotoxin binders used in poultry feed @ __________

a) **1.0 %** b) 2.0%
c) 3.0 % d) 0.5%

Q 203 The upper limit level of aflatoxins in poultry feed to prevent adverse effects __________

a) **50 parts per billion** b) 50 parts per million
c) 20 parts per billion d) 20 parts per million

Q 204 Ducks do not have __________

a) Gizzard b) Proventriculus
c) **Crop** d) Duodenum loops

Q 205 Organ which is cylindrical in duckd __________

a) Gizzard b) **Proventriculus**
c) Crop d) Duodenum loops

Q 206 Faster rate of passage of ingesta in ducks than in broilers is due __________

a) Faster metabolic rate
b) Faster peristaltic movements
c) **Absence of crop**
d) Statement is wrong

Q 207 Latest feeding standard available for ducks, quail and turkey __________

a) NRC (1992) b) **NRC (1994)**
c) NRC (2001) d) NRC (1998)

Q 208 NRC (1994) energy requirements (ME Kcal/d) for ducks from 0-3 weeks and from 3-7 weeks are __________

a) **2900 and 3000** b) 3000 and 2900
c) 2750 and 2700 d) None of the above

Q 209 NRC (1994) protein requirements (%) for ducks from 0-3 weeks and from 3-7 weeks are __________

a) 22 and 18 b) 20 and 18
c) **22 and 16** d) 18 and 16

Q 210 BIS (1992) energy requirements (ME Kcal/d) for ducks from 0-3 weeks, 3-8 weeks and 9-20 weeks are __________

a) 2750, 2700 and 2700 b) 3000, 2900 and 2700
c) **2750, 2750 and 2700** d) 3000, 2900 and 2750

Q 211 BIS (1992) protein requirements (%) for ducks from 0-3 weeks, 3-8 weeks and 9-20 weeks are __________

a) **20, 18 and 15** b) 18, 16 and 15
c) 20, 16 and 15 d) 20, 18 and 15

Q 212 BIS (1992) nutrients requirements for duck layer are __________

a) CP 18%; ME 2900 Kcal/d b) **CP 18%; ME 2650 Kcal/d**
c) CP 16%; ME 2650 Kcal/d d) CP 16%; ME 2750 Kcal/d

Q 213 BIS (1992) nutrients requirements of lysine (%) for ducks are __________

a) 0.9 and 1.0 b) 0.8 and 0.9
c) 0.35 and 0.45 d) **0.5 and 0.7**

Q 214 BIS (1992) nutrients requirements of methionine (%) for ducks are __________

a) 0.40-0.65 b) **0.27-0.40**
c) 0.18-0.28 d) Not required

Q 215 BIS (1992) nutrient requirements of calcium (%) and phosphorus (%) for ducks are ________

a) **0.60-0.65 and 0.60** b) 0.5-0.55 and 0.50

c) 0.40-0.45 and 0.30 d) None of above

Q 216 BIS (1992) nutrient requirements of vitamin A (IU) for ducks are ________

a) 500-1500 b) 1500-3000

c) 1500-2000 d) **2500-4000**

Q 217 The upper limit level of aflatoxins in duck feed is ________

a) 50 parts per billion b) 50 parts per million

c) **30 parts per billion** d) 30 parts per million

Q 218 On an average ducks consume feed/day ________

a) **170-230g** b) 100-130g

c) 270-330g d) 250-300g

Q 219 Quail eggs as compared to hen eggs ________

a) **4.3% less fat and 5% more protein**

b) 5% less fat and 4.3% more protein

c) 4.3% less fat and same protein content

d) Same nutritive value

Q 220 Quail start to lay egg at age ________

a) 8 weeks b) **6 weeks**

c) 12 weeks d) 21 weeks

Q 221 Energy requirements (ME Kcal/d) for quail from 0-3 weeks and from 3-5 weeks (NRC, 1994; ICAR, 2013) are ________

a) 2900 and 3000 b) **2900 and 2950**

c) 2900 and 2850 d) 2900 and 2700

Q 222 Protein requirements (%) for quail from 0-3 weeks and from 3-5 weeks (NRC, 1994; ICAR, 2013) are ________

a) 25 and 22 b) 22 and 18

c) **25 and 21.5** d) 22 and 21.5

Q 223 Nutrients requirements for egg line quail breeders/layer (NRC, 1994; ICAR, 2013) are __________

a) **CP 18.6%; ME 2850 Kcal/d**

b) CP 18%; ME 2850 Kcal/d

c) CP 18%; ME 2650 Kcal/d

d) CP 18.6%; ME 2750 Kcal/d

Q 224 Nutrients requirements for quail broiler breeders (NRC, 1994; ICAR, 2013) are __________

a) CP 18.6%; ME 2850 Kcal/d

b) CP 18%; ME 2850 Kcal/d

c) CP 18%; ME 2650 Kcal/d

d) **CP 20%; ME 2950 Kcal/d**

Q 225 Nutrients requirements of lysine (%) for growing quails is (NRC, 1994; ICAR, 2013) __________

a) 0.20- 0.45 b) 1.00- 1.10

c) **1.20- 1.45** d) 1.50- 1.65

Q 226 Nutrients requirements of lysine (%) for breeder quails is (NRC, 1994; ICAR, 2013) __________

a) 0.20- 0.45 b) **1.00- 1.10**

c) 1.20- 1.45 d) 1.50- 1.65

Q 227 Nutrients requirements of methionine (%) for quails is (NRC, 1994; ICAR, 2013) __________

a) **0.40-0.55** b) 0.27-0.35

c) 0.18-0.28 d) Not required

Q 228 Nutrients requirements of calcium (%) in growing and laying quail mash is (NRC, 1994; ICAR, 2013) __________

a) 0.85 and 2.0% b) 1.0 and 2.8%

c) **0.85 and 3.0%** d) None of the above

Q 229 Nutrients requirement of Vitamin A, D_3 and E in growing quail feed (NRC, 1994; ICAR, 2013) __________

a) **2500 IU/kg, 400 ICU/kg and 10 IU/kg**

b) 2970 IU/kg, 810 ICU/kg and 22.5 IU/kg

c) 2600 IU/kg, 708 ICU/kg and 12.5 IU/kg

d) None of the above

Q 230 Nutrients requirement of Vitamin A, D_3 and E in laying quail feed (NRC, 1994; ICAR, 2013) __________

a) 2500 IU/kg, 400 ICU/kg and 10 IU/kg
b) **2970 IU/kg, 810 ICU/kg and 22.5 IU/kg**
c) 2500 IU/kg, 400 ICU/kg and 10 IU/kg
d) None of the above

Q 231 On an average quail consume feed/day __________

a) **25g** b) 45g
c) 15g d) 40g

Q 232 NRC (1994) nutrients requirements for geese starter are ______

a) **CP 20%; ME 2900 Kcal/d**
b) CP 15%; ME 3000 Kcal/d
c) CP 15%; ME 2900 Kcal/d
d) CP 18.6%; ME 2750 Kcal/d

Q 233 NRC (1994) nutrients requirements for geese grower are ______

a) CP 20%; ME 2900 Kcal/d
b) **CP 15%; ME 3000 Kcal/d**
c) CP 15%; ME 2900 Kcal/d
d) CP 18.6%; ME 2750 Kcal/d

Q 234 NRC (1994) nutrients requirements for geese breeder are ______

a) CP 20%; ME 2900 Kcal/d
b) CP 15%; ME 3000 Kcal/d
a) **CP 15%; ME 2900 Kcal/d**
d) CP 18.6%; ME 2750 Kcal/d

Q 235 Nutrients requirements of lysine (%) for growing geese is (NRC, 1994) __________

a) **0.85** b) 1.00
c) 0.45 d) 0.60

Q 236 Nutrients requirements of lysine (%) for breeder geese is (NRC, 1994) __________

a) 0.85 b) 1.00
c) 0.45 d) **0.60**

Q 237 Nutrients requirements of calcium (%) for growing geese is (NRC, 1994) __________

A) 0.85 B) 0.80
C) 0.40 D) **0.60**

Q 238 Nutrients requirements of calcium (%) for breeder geese is (NRC, 1994) __________

a) 3.00 b) 1.80
c) **2.25** d) 3.60

Q 239 Nutrients requirement of Vitamin A and D_3 for geese (NRC, 1994) is __________

a) **1500 IU/kg and 200 IU/kg**
b) 1700 IU/kg and 300 IU/kg
c) 1000 IU/kg and 150 IU/kg
d) None of above

Q 240 Green geese is __________

a) **Young geese** b) Adult male
c) Adult female d) None of the above

Q 241 Gander is __________

a) Young geese b) **Adult male**
c) Adult female d) None of the above

Q 242 Goose is __________

a) Young geese b) Adult male
c) **Adult female** d) None of the above

Q 243 Excellent forager is __________

a) **Geese** b) Quail
c) Duck d) None of the above

Q 244 Turkey start to lay egg at age __________

a) 24 weeks b) 21 weeks
c) 18 weeks d) **30 weeks**

Q 245 Eggs are tinted __________

a) Geese b) Quail
c) Duck d) **Turkey**

Q 246 Energy requirements (ME Kcal/d) for turkeys from 0-6 weeks, 6-12 weeks and 12-18 weeks (NRC, 1994; ICAR, 2013) are __________

a) 2800, 2700 and 2650 b) 3000, 2900 and 2700

c) **2800, 2900 and 2650** d) 3000, 2900 and 2750

Q 247 Protein requirements (%) for turkeys from 0-6 weeks, 6-12 weeks and 12-18 weeks (NRC, 1994; ICAR, 2013) are __________

a) **24, 22 and 18** b) 22, 18 and 16

c) 22, 20 and 18 d) 23, 20 and 18

Q 248 Energy requirements (ME Kcal/d) for turkeys during pre lay and laying period (NRC, 1994; ICAR, 2013) are __________

a) **2600 and 2650** b) 2600 and 2700

c) 2800 and 2900 d) 2900 and 2750

Q 249 Protein requirements (%) for turkeys during pre lay and laying period (NRC, 1994; ICAR, 2013) are __________

a) 16 and 15 b) 18 and 16

c) 15 and 16 d) **15 and 15**

Q 250 Lysine requirements (%) for turkeys from 0-6 weeks, 6-12 weeks and 12-18 weeks (NRC, 1994; ICAR, 2013) are __________

a) **1.5, 1.2 and 1.05** b) 1.0, 0.8 and 1.05

c) 1.2, 0.8 and 0.85 d) 0.75, 0.62 and 0.55

Q 251 Methionine requirements (%) for turkeys from 0-6 weeks, 6-12 weeks and 12-18 weeks (NRC, 1994; ICAR, 2013) are __________

a) 0.3, 0.2 and 0.1 b) 0.45, 0.35 and 0.25

c) 0.75, 0.55 and 0.65 d) **0.55, 0.45 and 0.35**

Q 252 Nutrients requirements of calcium (%) for layer turkey (NRC, 1994; ICAR, 2013) __________

a) 3.00 b) 1.80

c) **2.25** d) 3.60

Q 253 Nutrient requirements of Vitamin A and D_3 for turkey (NRC, 1994; ICAR, 2013) are __________

a) **5000 IU/kg and 1100 IU/kg**

b) 4000 IU/kg and 1300 IU/kg

c) 1000 IU/kg and 1500 IU/kg

d) None of the above

❑❑❑

Chapter 23

Nutrients Requirements and Feeding of Equine

Q 1 The organ contains many microbial populations which allow the digestion of fibrous feeds in horse similar to ruminants __________

a) Caecum
b) Colon
c) **Both a and b**
d) Wrong statement

Q 2 Synthesis of the B vitamins and amino acids in horse takes place in __________

a) Caecum
b) Colon
c) Not synthesized
d) **Both a and b**

Q 3 The digestive capacity of lower gut of horse is __________

a) 72%
b) 82%
c) 55%
d) **65%**

Q 4 Lower digestion efficiency in horses than in ruminants is due to __________

a) Faster rate of food passage of digesta
b) Caecum's location toward the end of the digestive tract
c) **Both a and b**
d) None of above

Q 5 Latest NRC feeding standard available for horses __________

a) NRC (2001)
b) NRC (2013)
c) **NRC (2007)**
d) NRC (1998)

Q 6 In feeding standard ICAR (2013), the nutrient requirements of horses are adapted as such from ________

a) BIS (2001) b) **NRC (2007)**

c) Pagan and Hintz, 1986 d) None of the above

Q 7 Highest energy is required for ________

a) Standing b) Trotting

c) **Cantering** d) Walking

Q 8 The nutrient requirements of horses is influenced by ________

a) Roughage concentrate ratio b) Type of feed

c) Feed intake d) **Level of activity**

Q 9 Horses will normally consume from ________ % of the body weight daily in dry matter.

a) **1.5-2.5** b) 1.0-2.0

c) 1.0 d) None

Q 10 The digestible energy requirement for pregnant mare remains same upto ________

a) 7th month of gestation b) 9th month of gestation

c) **8th month of gestation** d) Throughout the gestation

Q 11 For 9 months pregnant mare ________

a) $DE = 1.20 \times DE_m$ b) $DE = 1.13 \times DE_m$

c) **$DE = 1.11 \times DE_m$** d) $DE = 1.50 \times DE_m$

Q 12 For 10 months pregnant mare ________

a) $DE = 1.20 \times DE_m$ b) $DE = 1.13 \times DE_m$

c) **$DE = 1.11 \times DE_m$** d) $DE = 1.50 \times DE_m$

Q 13 For 11 months pregnant mare ________

a) **$DE = 1.20 \times DE_m$** b) $DE = 1.25 \times DE_m$

c) $DE = 1.11 \times DE_m$ d) $DE = 1.50 \times DE_m$

Q 14 In horses, for light work ________

a) $DE = 1.20 \times DE_m$ b) **$DE = 1.25 \times DE_m$**

c) $DE = 2.00 \times DE_m$ d) $DE = 1.50 \times DE_m$

Q 15 In horses, for moderate work __________

a) $DE = 1.20 \times DE_m$
b) $DE = 1.25 \times DE_m$
c) $DE = 2.00 \times DE_m$
d) **$DE = 1.50 \times DE_m$**

Q 16 In horses, for heavy work __________

a) $DE = 1.20 \times DE_m$
b) $DE = 1.25 \times DE_m$
c) **$DE = 2.00 \times DE_m$**
d) $DE = 1.50 \times DE_m$

Q 17 Protein requirements for growth of weanlings is estimated as CP = __________

a) **(50) (Mcal of DE/day)**
b) (45) (Mcal of DE/day)
c) (40) (Mcal of DE/day)
d) (42.5) (Mcal of DE/day)

Q 18 Protein requirements for growth of 2 year old horse is estimated as CP = __________

a) (50) (Mcal of DE/day)
b) (45) (Mcal of DE/day)
c) (40) (Mcal of DE/day)
d) **(42.5) (Mcal of DE/day)**

Q 19 Protein required by horse for work is estimated as CP = ______

a) (50) (Mcal of DE/day)
b) (45) (Mcal of DE/day)
c) **(40) (Mcal of DE/day)**
d) (42.5) (Mcal of DE/day)

Q 20 The efficiency of utilization of digestible protein for milk production in mare is __________

a) 72%
b) 82%
c) 61%
d) **65%**

Q 21 Estimates of the DP requirements for maintenance of horses have ranged from ____ to ___ g of DP/kg of body weight/ day.

a) 0.29 to 0.38
b) **0.49 to 0.68**
c) 0.69 to 0.88
d) None

Q 22 Digestible energy requirement for weanlings, 4 months per kilogram of gain (Mcal/d) __________

a) **9.1**
b) 11.0
c) 15.5
d) 18.4s

Q 23 Digestible energy requirement for weanlings, 6 months per kilogram of gain (Mcal/d) ________

a) 9.1 b) **11.0**

c) 15.5 d) 18.4

Q 24 Digestible energy requirement for yearling per kilogram of gain (Mcal/d) ________

a) 9.1 b) 11.0

c) **15.5** d) 18.4

Q 25 Digestible energy requirement for long yearling per kilogram of gain (Mcal/d) ________

a) 9.1 b) 11.0

c) 15.5 d) **18.4**

Q 26 Digestible energy requirement for 2 year old horse per kilogram of gain (Mcal/d) ________

a) **19.6** b) 11.0

c) 15.5 d) 18.4

Q 27 Mares (light breeds) produce amounts of milk during early and during late lactation equivalent to_____ and _____ percent of their body weight ________

a) 4 and 3 b) 4 and 2

c) **3 and 2** d) 5 and 2

Q 28 The energy requirement for the mare (500kg) from 1 to 3 months of lactation (Mcal DE/day) is v

a) **31.7 to 30.6** b) 28.3 to 27.2

c) 20.3 to 19.2 d) 27.3 to 28.2

Q 29 The energy requirement for the mare (500kg) from 4 to 6 months of lactation (Mcal DE/day) is ________

a) 22.3 to 21.2 b) **28.3 to 27.2**

c) 20.3 to 19.2 d) 27.3 to 28.2

Q 30 A 500 kg mature horse, working at a moderate, one to two hours per day, needs DE about (Mcal /day) ________

a) **23.3** b) 28.3

c) 20.3 d) 27.3

Q 31 Protein accounts for about ______ percent of the fat-free composition of the mature horse.

a) 25 b) 28

c) **22** d) 19

Q 32 The dietary protein requirement of the horse is a function of the __________

a) Needs of the animal

b) Quality of protein available

c) Protein digestibility

d) **All**

Q 33 Average digestible protein/kg of body weight/day required by most of the horses is __________

a) 0.80 b) 0.48

c) 0.42 d) **0.60**

Q 34 A typical horse diet must contain ______ percent lysine.

a) **3.5** b) 1.5

c) 2.5 d) 0.5

Q 35 The first limiting amino acid in the diet of growing foals is __________

a) Leucine b) Methionine

c) **Lysine** d) Threonine

Q 36 The requirement of lysine for weanlings and yearlings are (g/Mcal of DE/day) __________

a) 1.1 and 0.9 b) **2.1 and 1.9**

c) 3.1 and 2.9 d) 4.1 and 3.9

Q 37 To ensure proper growth, the ration to early-weaned or creep-fed foals require crude protein __________

a) **16%** b) 13%

c) 11% d) 10%

Q 38 The ration of weanlings contain crude protein __________

a) 16% b) **13%**

c) 11% d) 10%

Q 39 The ration of yearlings contain crude protein ________

a) 16% b) 13%

c) **11%** d) 10%

Q 40 The ration of a 2 years old horse contain crude protein

a) 16% b) 13%

c) 11% d) **10%**

Q 41 The ration of a 500 kg mare in late gestation (eleventh month) contain crude protein ________

a) **9.5%** b) 13%

c) 8% d) 10%

Q 42 The protein requirement for the mare (500kg) from 1 to 3 months of lactation is ________

a) **14.7 to 15.3%** b) 13.3 to 12.6%

c) 11.3 to 12.2% d) 17.3 to 18.2%

Q 43 The protein requirement for the mare (500kg) from 4 to 6 months of lactation is ________

a) 14.7 to 15.3% b) **13.3 to 12.6%**

c) 11.3 to 12.2% d) 17.3 to 18.2%

Q 44 In horses (500kg), crude protein requirement (g/day) for light work ________

a) 768 b) **699**

c) 862 d) 913

Q 45 In horses (500kg), crude protein requirement (g/day) for moderate work ________

a) **768** b) 699

c) 862 d) 913

Q 46 In horses (500kg), crude protein requirement (g/day) for heavy work ________

a) 768 b) 699

c) **862** d) 913

Q 47 The nutrients requirements of calcium and phosphorus in the diet of mature horse (500kg) at maintenance _____ are ______

a) **0.20 and 0.14%** b) 0.39 and 0.22%

c) 0.36 and 0.26% d) 0.59 and 0.82%

Q 48 The nutrients requirements of calcium and phosphorus in the diet of 3-month old foal are __________

a) 0.20 and 0.14% b) **0.39 and 0.22%**

c) 0.36 and 0.26% d) 0.59 and 0.82%

Q 49 The nutrients requirements of calcium and phosphorus in the diet of Pregnant mares (last 90 days) are __________

a) 0.20 and 0.14% b) 0.39 and 0.22%

c) **0.36 and 0.26%** d) 0.59 and 0.82%

Q 50 The nutrients requirements of calcium and phosphorus in the diet of Lactating mares from foaling to two months are ______

a) 0.20 and 0.14% b) 0.39 and 0.22%

c) 0.36 and 0.26% d) **0.59 and 0.82%**

Q 51 The nutrients requirements of calcium and phosphorus in the diet of mares after three months of lactation are __________

a) 0.20 and 0.14% b) 0.39 and 0.22%

c) **0.37 and 0.23%** d) 0.59 and 0.82%

Q 52 The nutrients requirements of calcium and phosphorus in the diet of hard-working horse (500kg) are __________

a) 0.20 and 0.14% b) 0.39 and 0.22%

c) **0.40 and 0.29%** d) 0.59 and 0.82%

Q 53 The horse diet deficient in selenium results in __________

a) **Muscle degeneration** b) Blindness

c) Paralysis d) None

Q 54 The nutrients requirements of selenium in the diet of horse should be (mg/day) __________

a) 2.0 b) 0.3

c) **1.0** d) 5.0

Q 55 Nutrients requirements (IU/d/horse) of Vitamin A, D and E for all classes of horses (NRC, 2007) __________

a) 25000, 1400 and 1000 b) **15000, 3300 and 500**
c) 1500, 3000 and 400 d) None of above

Q 56 Common grasses used for horse feeding are __________

a) Dub grass b) Anjan grass
c) Angola grass d) **All**

Q 57 Minimum roughage should be offered to horse/day to ensure adequate intake and digestive health (percent of their body weight) __________

a) 2.0 b) 3
c) **1.0** d) 1.5

Q 58 Most popular grain used for feeding of horse is __________

a) **Oats** b) Maize
c) Wheat d) Gram

Q 59 Maize could not be used for horses because of

a) High energy content b) Expensive
c) **Both a and b** d) Wrong statement

Q 60 Broken grams soaked in water are commonly used for indigenous horses in India but racing industry do not use gram in any of their tracks for horses because of __________

a) High protein content b) **Digestive problems**
c) Both a and b d) Wrong statement

Q 61 Silage can be used for horses upto ______ % of roughage portion of their diet.

a) 60% b) 40%
c) 25% d) **50%**

Q 62 Most commonly used protein source in the western countries __________

a) **Soyabean meal** b) Lin seed meal
c) Gram d) Legume seed meal

Q 63 Most of the horse owners in India prefer linseed meal because __________

a) High quality protein
b) High palatability
c) **Improve hair coat condition**
d) All the above

Q 64 Molasses can be used in horse ration during pelleting to improve the palatability upto __________

a) 3% b) 2%
c) **5%** d) 8%

Q 65 At 2 to 4 weeks, foals should provide __________ kg/head/day creep feed along with the mare's milk.

a) **0.5 kg** b) 1.0 kg
c) 1.5 kg d) Not required

Q 66 At 1 to 4 months, horses should provide concentrate mixture __________ kg/100kg of body weight in increasing amounts along with the mare's milk and small quantity of good quality hay.

a) 0.5-0.8 kg b) **1.1-1.6 kg**
c) 2.2-2.8 kg d) Not required

Q 67 At 5 to 6 months, horses should provide concentrate mixture __________ kg/100kg of body weight along with good quality hay.

a) 1.0-1.5 kg b) 0.5-0.8 kg
c) **2.2-2.8 kg** d) Not required

Q 68 For light horses, the concentrate mixture of __________ kg/100kg body weight along with good quality hay is sufficient.

a) **1.0-1.5 kg** b) 0.5-0.8 kg
c) 2.2-2.8 kg d) Not required

Q 69 For weanlings, the concentrate mixture of __________ kg/100kg body weight along with good quality hay is sufficient.

a) 1.0-1.5 kg b) 0.5-0.8 kg
c) **2.2-2.3 kg** d) Not required

Q 70 In general, horse should feed ________ kg of concentrate mixture and ________ kg of hay per 100kg body weight.

a) **2-3 kg and 1-2 kg**
b) 1-2 kg and 2-3 kg
c) 3-4 kg and 2-3 kg
d) 4-5 kg and 3-4 kg

Q 71 The daily ration for working horses should be split into at least three feeds per day, with half the ration fed as the evening feed ________

a) **Correct statement**
b) Incorrect statement
c) Can't say
d) None of the above

Q 72 The disease can occur in working horses that are being fed high grain diets and given one or more days of complete rest with no change in diet ________

a) Monday morning disease
b) Azoturia
c) **Both**
d) None

❑❑❑

Chapter 24

Nutrients Requirements and Feeding of Dog & Cat

Q 1 Latest feeding standard available for Dogs and cats ________

a) **NRC (2006)**
b) NRC (2007)
c) NRC (2001)
d) NRC (2011)

Q 2 Latest Indian feeding standard available for Dogs and cats ___________

a) ICAR (2010)
b) **ICAR (2013)**
c) BIS (1998)
d) ICAR (2006)

Q 3 Which of following is not associated with nutrients requirements of dogs and cats?

a) National Research Council (NRC)
b) Association of American Feed Control Officials (AAFCO)
c) **Bureau of Indian Standards (BIS)**
d) None

Q 4 Standard for practical nutrient profile of dogs and cats based on commonly used feed ingredients __________

a) National Research Council (NRC)
b) **Association of American Feed Control Officials (AAFCO)**
c) Bureau of Indian Standards (BIS)
d) None

Q 5 In adult dogs, the ME for maintenance is (NRC, 2006) _______

a) **130× $BW^{0.75}$**
b) 83× $BW^{0.75}$
c) 110× $BW^{0.75}$
d) 106× $BW^{0.75}$

Q 6 Based on their gastrointestinal system, both dog and cats are __________

a) Omnivores b) Herbivores
c) **Carnivores** d) All

Q 7 The pet which is true carnivores __________

a) **Cat** b) Dog
c) Dog and cat d) None

Q 8 Comparatively more palatable diets are required for __________

a) **Small breeds** b) Medium breeds
c) Large breeds d) All

Q 9 CP requirements for dogs between 4-14 weeks and above 14 weeks (NRC, 2006) __________

a) **22.5 and 17.5%** b) 17.5 and 22.5%
c) 12 and 13% d) 14% each

Q 10 CP requirements for lactating bitches (NRC, 2006) __________

a) **20%** b) 16%
c) 23% d) 13.5%

Q 11 High dietary protein requirements of cats as compared to dog is because of __________

a) Low endogenous N loss b) **High endogenous N loss**
c) High growth rate d) High metabolic rate

Q 12 For growth and reproduction (NRC, 2006), protein requirement of cats is __________

a) 22% b) 13%
c) 17.5% d) **20%**

Q 13 For growth and reproduction (AAFCO, 2008), protein requirement of cats is __________

a) **22%** b) 13%
c) 17.5% d) 20%

Q 14 Crude protein requirement of adult cats for maintenance (NRC, 2006) is __________

a) 8.5% b) 13%
c) **17.5%** d) 20%

Q 15 The amount of metabolizable energy/d (kcal/kg of $BW^{0.75}$) required for pregnancy and lactation of bitches are ________

a) 130 and 148 b) **188 and 470**

c) 470 and 188 d) 148 and 130

Q 16 The requirement of protein in dogs for maintenance and growth (g/kg body weight) is ________

a) **4.8g and 9.6g** b) 9.6g and 4.8g

c) 2.9g and 4.3g d) 4.3g and 2.9g

Q 17 Number of essential amino acids required by pets in their diet ________

a) 7 b) **10**

c) 13 d) 5

Q 18 Calcium and phosphorus requirements (NRC, 2006) for lactating bitches ________

a) 0.5 and 0.8% b) **0.8 and 0.5%**

c) 1.0 and 0.5% d) 2.0 and 1.0 %

Q 19 Calcium requirements (AAFCO, 2008) for dogs for maintenance and growth/reproduction ________

a) **0.6 and 1%** b) 0.8 and 0.5%

c) 1.0 and 0.6% d) 2.0 and 1.0 %

Q 20 Vitamin A and D requirements (NRC, 2006) for dogs (IU/kg) ________

a) 552 and 5050 b) 2050 and 248

c) **5050 and 552** d) 248 and 2050

Q 21 Vitamin A and D requirements (AAFCO, 2008) for dogs (IU/kg) ________

a) 500 and 5000 b) 3050 and 248

c) **5000 and 500** d) 248 and 3050

Q 22 For growth and reproduction (NRC, 2006), dietary fat requirement of dogs is ________

a) **8.5%** b) 5%

c) 12% d) 2.5%

Q 23 On dry matter basis, growing kittens and adult cat diet should contain a minimum fat (AAFCO, 2008) __________

a) 8% b) 5%

c) **9%** d) 2.5%

Q 24 For dogs dietary essential fatty acids __________

a) **Linoleic acid**

b) Arachidonic acid

c) Linoleic acid & Arachidonic acid

d) None

Q 25 For cats dietary essential fatty acids are __________

a) Linoleic acid

b) Arachidonic acid

c) **Linoleic acid & Arachidonic acid**

d) None

Q 26 Cats cannot synthesize Arachidonic acid from linoleic acid due to low activity of __________

a) Δ-3 desaturase b) Δ-9 desaturase

c) Δ-3,6 desaturase **d) Δ-6 desaturase**

Q 27 Dietary requirement of "-lenoleic acid for adult dogs and lactating bitches __________

a) **0.44 and 0.8%** b) 0.8 and 0.44%

c) 0.2 and 0.4% d) 0.4 and 0.2 %

Q 28 Which is not a dog feeding method?

a) Portion-control feeding b) Free choice feeding

c) Timed feeding method d) **None**

Q 29 Dry pet foods contains moisture __________

a) **Less than 14%** b) from 14%to <60%

c) 60% or more d) 2.5%

Q 30 Semi-moist pet foods contains moisture __________

a) Less than 14% b) **From 14% to <60%**

c) 60% or more d) 2.5%

Q 31 Canned pet foods contains moisture ________

a) Less than 14%
b) From 14% to <60%
c) **60% or more**
d) 2.5%

Q 32 Dry pet foods contains linoleic acid (dry matter basis) ______

a) **1%**
b) 2%
c) 3%
d) 0.5%

Q 33 Semi-moist pet foods contains fibre (dry matter basis)

a) 1%
b) 7%
c) **3%**
d) 5%

Q 34 Protein requirement of dog and cat increases with ________

a) Increase in protein quality
b) Improvement in amino acid composition
c) Increase in protein digestibility
d) **Increase in energy density**

Q 35 As a thumb rule, dog should be fed _____ of their body weight.

a) 1%
b) 7%
c) 3%
d) **5%**

Q 36 On dry matter basis, average energy content of dog's food should be ________

a) 2.0-3.0 Mcal/kg
b) **3.0-4.0 Mcal/kg**
c) 1.0-2.0 Mcal/kg
d) 5.0-6.0 Mcal/kg

Q 37 Raw egg should be avoided in the diet of dogs because of presence of anti-vitamin enzyme ________

a) **Avidin**
b) Ovidine
c) Thiaminase
d) Picolinic carboxylase

Q 38 As a thumb rule, a cat needs to consume _____ times the amount of water as its daily intake of food.

a) 5.0
b) **2.5**
c) 1.0
d) 4.0

Q 39 Amino acid required by cats which are only present in animal tissues ________

a) Arginine
b) Tryptophan
c) **Taurine**
d) Lysine

Q 40 Protein suitable for cats must supply minimum _____ mg of taurine/kg diet dry matter.

a) 1000
b) 100
c) 200
d) **500**

Q 41 Unable to synthesize Vit D via dermal photosynthesis due to lack of enzyme 7-dehydrocholesterol.

a) **Cats**
b) Dogs
c) Dogs and cats
d) All carnivores

Q 42 In cats insulin secretion is stimulated by the presence of ______

a) Glucose
b) **Amino acids**
c) Linoleic acid
d) Inulin

Q 43 Cats require dietary source of preformed vitamin A because of the fact that cats cannot convert ß- carotene to vitamin A due to lack of enzyme ________

a) Picolinic carboxylase
b) Glucokinase
c) Carotenase
d) **Dioxygenase**

Q 44 Inadequate dietary level of arginine leads to ________

a) **Hyperammonemia**
b) Niacin deficiency
c) Muscular degeneration
d) Low activity of carboxylase

Q 45 Body condition when waist is visible, ribs can be felt but not seen, abdominal fat pad just detectable indicates ________

a) Thin
b) **Ideal**
c) Overweight
d) Obese

Q 46 In cats absence of dietary carbohydrates will lead to ______

a) Low blood glucose
b) High blood glucose
c) **Not affect blood glucose**
d) Severe energy deficiency

Q 47 In cats, the metabolic requirement for glucose in the cat is derived from ________

a) Alanine b) Glycerol
c) Dietary carbohydrates d) **Alanine and glycerol**

Q 48 In dog and cats, amino acid requirement as a per cent of diet from birth to maturity ________

a) **Decreases**
b) Increases
c) Constant
d) First decreases then increases

Q 49 The difference between dog and cat is that cat cannot synthesize in their body ________

a) Arachidonic acid b) Aminosulfonic acid
c) Taurine d) **All**

Q 50 Number of mice (26g) required by an adult domestic cat weighing 4kg to fulfill their daily needs ________

a) 3-4 b) **9-10**
c) 12-15 d) 5-6

Q 51 Which of the following vitamin is not required by dogs and cats?

a) **Vitamin C** b) Vitamin E
c) Biotin d) Folic acid

Q 52 Animal products do not contain ________

a) **Carotenoids** b) Vitamin A
c) Cobalamin d) Biotin

Q 53 Which teeth in the dogs mouth is more than that of cats mouth?

a) Incisor b) Canine
c) Premolar only d) **Premolar and molars**

Q 54 In Dog and Cat, chemical digestion of food is completed in ________

a) **Small intestine** b) Large intestine
c) Stomach d) Caecum

Q 55 Which of the following factor affect dogs voluntary water consumption?

a) Temperature
b) Type of diet
c) Level of exercise
d) **All the above**

❑❑❑

Chapter 25

Nutrients Requirements and Feeding of Lab Animals

Q 1 Latest feeding standard available for laboratory animals is ____

a) NRC (1992) b) **NRC (1995)**

c) NRC (1994) d) NRC (1998)

Q 2 ME requirement for maintenance of lab rat is __________

a) **114 × $W^{0.75}$ kcal/d** b) 160 × $W^{0.75}$ kcal/d

c) 82 × $W^{0.75}$ kcal/d d) None

Q 3 ME requirement for maintenance of mice is __________

a) 114 × $W^{0.75}$ kcal/d b) **160 × $W^{0.75}$ kcal/d**

c) 82 × $W^{0.75}$ kcal/d d) None

Q 4 The energy requirement (ME, Kcal/Kg) for maintenance, growth and reproduction for Guinea pig per kilogram of diet (NRC, 1995) is __________

a) 3800-4100 b) 1600-1900

c) 2000-2200 d) **2800-3500**

Q 5 The energy requirement (ME, Kcal/Kg) for rat and mice per kilogram of diet (NRC, 1995) is __________

a) **3800-4100** b) 1600-1900

c) 2000-2200 d) 2800-3500

Q 6 The protein requirement for maintenance, growth and reproduction for rats per kilogram of diet (NRC, 1995) are __________

a) **50g, 150g and 150g** b) 180g/kg

c) 60g, 120g and 165g d) 50g

Q 7 The protein requirement for maintenance, growth and reproduction for mouse per kilogram of diet (NRC, 1995) are ___________

a) 50g, 150g and 150g b) **180g**

c) 60g, 120g and 165g d) 50g

Q 8 The protein requirements for maintenance, growth and reproduction for guinea pig per kilogram of diet (NRC, 1995) are ___________

a) 5g, 15g and 15g b) **180g**

c) 6g, 12g and 16g d) 50g

Q 9 The protein requirement for maintenance, growth and reproduction for Guinea pig per kilogram of diet (ICAR, 2013) is ___________

a) 15% b) 18%

c) **20%** d) 14%

Q 10 BIS specifications of crude protein for compound feed for rat and mice is ___________

a) **24%** b) 16%

c) 20% d) 14%

Q 11 BIS specifications of crude fibre for compound feed for rat and mice is ___________

a) 4% b) **6%**

c) 2% d) 9%

Q 12 BIS specifications of total ash for compound feed for rat and mice is ___________

a) 4% b) 6%

c) 5% d) **9%**

Q 13 BIS specifications of vitamin A, D_3 and E per kilogram of diet for rat and mice are ___________

a) **2700 IU, 200 IU and 40mg** b) 1700 IU, 100 IU and 40mg

c) 2500 IU, 200 IU and 40mg d) 2300 IU, 100 IU and 40mg

Q 14 The requirement of fat for rats and mouse per kilogram of diet (NRC, 1995) __________

a) **5%** b) 10%

c) 2.0-3.9% d) 1.33-1.40%

Q 15 About _______ of fat is added per kilogram of diet of guinea pig to avoid essential fatty acid deficiency (NRC, 1995).

a) **5%** b) 10%

c) 2.0-3.9% d) 1.33-1.40%

Q 16 The requirement of essential fatty acids for guinea pig per kilogram of diet (NRC, 1995) __________

a) 50g b) 10g

c) 2.6-6.9g d) **1.33-4.00g**

Q 17 The most limiting amino acid in casein for the growing guinea pig is __________

a) **Arginine** b) Methionine

c) Lysine d) Tryptophan

Q 18 The requirement of arginine, methionine and tryptophan in diet of guinea pig (NRC, 1995) is __________

a) 6g, 6g and 1.8g b) 6g, 3g and 1.8g

c) 10g, 5g and 1.3g d) **12g, 6g and 1.8g**

Q 19 Nutrients requirements of calcium and phosphorus for guinea pig per kilogram of diet (NRC, 1995) are __________

a) **8g and 4g** b) 5g and 3g

c) 5.0-6.3g and 3.0-3.7g d) None

Q 20 Nutrients requirements of calcium and phosphorus for rat per kilogram of diet (NRC, 1995) are __________

a) 8g and 4g b) 5g and 3g

c) **5.0-6.3g and 3.0-3.7g** d) None

Q 21 Nutrients requirements of calcium and phosphorus for mice per kilogram of diet (NRC, 1995) are __________

a) 8g and 4g b) **5g and 3g**

c) 5.0-6.3g and 3.0-3.7g d) None

Q 22 Guinea pigs cannot synthesize vitamin C in their body due to lack the gene to produce the hepatic enzyme __________

a) **l-gulonolactone oxidase** b) l-guloconolactone oxidase
c) l-galactolactone oxidase d) None

Q 23 Vitamin C should be supplied in the diet (mg/kg) of guinea pigs (NRC, 1995: ICAR, 2013) __________

a) 100 b) 150
c) **200** d) 50

Q 24 The raw material which is not commonly used for preparing of lab animal's feed __________

a) Crushed maize b) Whole wheat
c) Barley d) **Broken rice**

Q 25 The animal which is known as "Biological refrigerator" at the farmer's house __________

a) **Rabbit** b) Poultry
c) Guinea pig d) Quail

Q 26 In rabbit, the main site of microbial fermentation of feed is ____

a) Colon b) Fundis
c) **Caecum** d) Small intestine

Q 27 In rabbit, the bacterial ecosystem for fermentation of feed primarily comprised of __________

a) *Fibrobacter spp.* b) ***Bacteriodes spp.***
c) Both a and b d) *Lactobaccillus spp.*

Q 28 Relatively high maintenance energy required for __________

a) Ruminants b) Horse
c) **Rabbit** d) Wrong statement

Q 29 The largest organ in the digestive tract of rabbit is __________

a) Colon b) Stomach
c) **Caecum** d) Food pipe

Q 30 The bacteriocidal fatty acids in milk fat of doe that protect the kids from invasion by detrimental organisms __________

a) **C8 and C10** b) C18 and C20

c) w-3 and w-6 d) None

Q 31 The organisms that develop in the gastrointestinal tract (particularly in the caecum) of rabbit kids towards weaning depends upon the __________

a) Type of carbohydrate b) Protein flow into the caecum

c) **Both a and b** d) None

Q 32 The practice of consumption of faecal pellets directly from the anus by the animal is called __________

a) Coprophagy b) Caecotrophy

c) Refection d) **All the above**

Q 33 During coprophagy, the faecal pellets consumed by rabbits are __________

a) Soft faecal pellets b) Hard faecal pellets

c) **Both a and b** d) None

Q 34 The main nutritional role of coprophagy in rabbits is that it acts, as a source of __________

a) **B complex vitamins**

b) Bacterial protein production

c) Both a and b

d) None

Q 35 Energy requirements (DE Kcal/d) for rabbits for maintenance, growth, gestation and lactation (ICAR, 2013) are ________

a) **2300, 2700, 2700 and 2700** b) 3000, 2900, 2800 and 2700

c) 2300, 2900, 2700 and 2650 d) 3000, 2900, 2800 and 2750

Q 36 Protein requirements (%) for rabbits for maintenance, growth, gestation and lactation (ICAR, 2013) is __________

a) 14, 15, 16 and 18 b) **14, 18, 18 and 19**

c) 14, 18, 19 and 19 d) 14, 14, 18 and 18

Q 37 Minimum fat requirement for rabbits for maintenance, growth, gestation and lactation (ICAR, 2013) is __________

a) 4% b) 5%

c) **2%** d) 1%

Q 38 The nutrient requirement of lysine and arginine for rabbits for maintenance, growth, gestation and lactation (ICAR, 2013) is __________

a) 0.5 and 0.6% b) 0.9 and 0.8%

c) 0.3 and 0.2% d) **0.7 and 0.6%**

Q 39 Maximum fibre (%) requirement for rabbits for maintenance, growth, gestation and lactation rations (ICAR, 2013) is __________

a) **12-14%** b) 8-11%

c) 10% d) 13-16%

Q 40 BIS specifications for energy requirements (ME Kcal/d) for laboratory, meat and wool type rabbits are __________

a) **2500, 2800 and 2600** b) 2600, 2700 and 2700

c) 2500, 2800 and 2900 d) 2500, 2900 and 2700

Q 41 BIS specifications for protein requirements (%) for laboratory, meat and wool type rabbits are __________

a) 13-14, 12-13 and 12-13 b) **15-17, 16-18 and 15-17**

c) 12-13, 16-18 and 12-13 d) 15-17, 16-18 and 19-20

Q 42 Rabbits require high amounts of fibre in their diet to __________

a) Promote intestinal motility

b) Minimize intestinal diseases

c) Provide a substrate for fermentation

d) **All the above**

Q 43 Diets of rabbit, low in fibre increases the incidence of __________

a) **Enterotoxemia** b) Caecal infections

c) Mucoid enteritis d) Both b and c

Q 44 Diets of rabbit, high in fibre increases the incidence of __________

a) Enterotoxemia b) Caecal infections

c) Mucoid enteritis d) **Both b and c**

Q 45 Fibre helps to absorb and eliminate ____________ from the body of rabbit.

a) **Toxins of pathogenic bacteria**

b) Anti-metabolites

c) Excessive digestive juices

d) Both a and c

Q 46 Green leafy vegetables should not be fed to young rabbits because of its ________

a) Low fibre content

b) High anti-nutritional compounds

c) **High water content**

d) Both a and b

Q 47 Daily feed consumption of an adult rabbit is ________

a) 100g b) **150g**

c) 80g d) 300g

Q 48 Rearing of bunnies by another doe for nursing ________

a) Flushing b) Fattening

c) **Fostering** d) Fosterling

Q 49 Chalky white depots in the rabbitry indicated excessive feeding of ________

a) **Calcium** b) Protein

c) Carbonate d) Omega fatty acids

Q 50 Pellet size for rabbit feed is ____________ mm diameter and ____________ mm length.

a) 1-2 mm and 3-4 mm b) **3-4 mm and 6 mm**

c) 4-5 mm and 8-9 mm d) 2 mm and 7 mm

Q 51 Favourite food for guinea pig.

a) **Lettuce** b) Peanuts

c) Oats d) Cucumber

Q 52 Adult guinea pig consumes the diet ______ percent of their body weight.

a) 3% b) 5%

c) **7%** d) 2.5%

Q 53 Daily feed consumption of an adult guinea pig __________

a) 10-30g b) **30-50g**

c) 80-100g d) 5-10g

Q 54 Caecotrophy first starts to function in young rabbits at the age of about __________

a) 5 weeks b) 10 days

c) **3 weeks** d) 8 weeks

Q 55 Daily feed consumption of an adult rat __________

a) 8-0g b) **12-15g**

c) 5-8g d) 20-30g

Q 56 Diets formulated with agricultural products and by-products __________

a) **Natural ingredient diet** b) Purified diet

c) Chemically defined diet d) Compound ration

Q 57 Most commonly used commercial diet for laboratory animals is __________

a) **Natural ingredient diet** b) Purified diet

c) Chemically defined diet d) Compound ration

Q 58 The diet formulated with refined and restricted set of ingredients is designated as __________

a) Natural ingredient diet b) **Purified diet**

c) Chemically defined diet d) Compound ration

Q 59 The diet prepared with elemental ingredients such as individual amino acids, specific sugars, etc. is called __________

a) Natural ingredient diet b) Purified diet

c) **Chemically defined diet** d) Compound ration

Q 60 The diet used for studies in which strict control over nutrient concentrations and specific constituents is essential ________

a) Natural ingredient diet b) Purified diet

c) **Chemically defined diets** d) Compound ration

Q 61 Casein used to prepare __________

a) Natural ingredient diet b) **Purified diet**

c) Chemically defined diet d) Compound ration

Q 62 Chemically extracted form of cellulose used to prepare _______

a) Natural ingredient diet b) **Purified diet**

c) Chemically defined diet d) Compound ration

Q 63 The diet used to study specific nutritional deficiencies or excesses is __________

a) Natural ingredient diet b) **Purified diet**

c) Chemically defined diet d) Compound ration

Q 64 The diet which is expensive and not readily consumed by the laboratory animals __________

a) Natural ingredient diet b) Purified diet

c) Chemically defined diet d) **Both b and c**

Q 65. The diets which are palatable and inexpensive to manufacture __________

a) **Natural ingredient diet** b) Purified diet

c) Chemically defined diet d) Both B and C

Q 66 The sugar above 15% toxic to rats __________

a) **Xylose** b) Sorbose

c) Glycerol d) Glucose

Q 67 The sugar used as primary energy sources in purified diets for guinea pig __________

a) Sucrose b) Lactose

c) Glucose d) **All the above**

Q 68 The best source of carbohydrates in diets of rat __________

a) Glucose b) Glucose precursors

c) **Both a and b** d) None of above

❑❑❑

D. OTHERS

by Dr Jaswinder Singh

Chapter 26

Milk

Q 1 Beestings is the another name of __________

a) **Colostrum**
b) Meconium
c) Whey
d) Immunoglobulin's

Q 2 Which of the following animal's milk has the highest fat content?

a) Cow
b) Buffalo
c) Goat
d) **Sheep**

Q 3 Which of the following animal's milk is more nutritious in terms of nutrient it contain?

a) Cow
b) Goat
c) **Ewe**
d) Mare

Q 4 Tick the wrong statement __________

a) Colostrum is twice as concentrated as milk
b) **Colostrum has high fat, protein and lactose content than milk***
c) Immunity through colostrum is only related to infection which the cow herself has contacted
d) Colostrum has high vitamin A, D and E content than milk

* Lactose is less in colostrums then milk

Q 5 Which of the following condition in the rumen led to milk fat depression?

a) Low acetate combined with propionate and low Vitamin B_{12} synthesis
b) Excess fermentable starch combined with low trans fatty acid production
c) **Partial biohydrogenation of dietary unsaturated lipid combined with low rumen pH.**
d) High saturated fat and high propionate formation

Q 6 On a high grain diet, milk fat depression is caused by _______

a) **Formation of trans fatty acid in the rumen**

b) Lack of vitamin B_{12} production in the rumen

c) Lack of acetate production

d) A hormonal conflict that in essence inhibits fat mobilization

Q 7 Which of the following will lower milk fat?

a) PUFA's b) Low forage diet

c) Low rumen pH d) **All the above**

Q 8 Trans fatty acid have been implicated in milk fat depression, where do trans fatty acid originate from?

a) **Rumen fermentation**

b) Intestinal digestion

c) Liver synthesis

d) Udder breakdown of VLDL

Q 9 Which of the following is not a precursor of milk fat?

a) Acetate b) Butyrate

c) **Propionate** d) Long chain fatty acid

Q 10 As compare to normal milk,which of the following content is low in colostrum?

a) Protein b) Fat

c) Ash d) **Lactose**

Q 11 In newly calved animal, colostral period last for __________

a) **3-7 days** b) 10-15 days

c) 10-15 hours d) 21 days

Q 12 Water content of milk is __________

a) 50% b) 60%

c) **Over 85%** d) 100%

Q 13 Which of the following animal's milk has the highest fat?

a) Cow b) Goat

c) Ewe d) **Sow**

Q 14 Which of the following animal's milk has the higher protein?

a) Cow b) Goat

c) Ewe d) **Sow**

Q 15 Which of the following animal's milk has the higher Ca and P content?

a) Cow b) Goat

c) Ewe d) **Sow**

Q 16 Which of the following protein form the major constituent of the milk protein?

a) **Caseins** b) α-Lactalbumin

c) β-Lactoglobulins d) Immunoglobulins

Q 17 Which of the following sugar constituent the major carbohydrate? in milk

a) **Lactose** b) Glucose

c) Fructose d) Galactose

Q 18 In case someone is allergic to cow milk, which of the following animals milk can be an ideal alternative?

a) Buffalo b) Goat

c) Sow d) **Sheep**

Q 19 Which of the following animal has comparatively higher amount of vitamin C in her milk?

a) Cow b) Buffalo

c) Goat d) **She camel**

Q 20 Yellow colour of cow milk is due to presence of __________

a) **Carotene** b) Vitamin A

c) Casein d) Calcium

Q 21 White colour of buffalo milk is due to presence of __________

a) **Fat globules & casein** b) Carotene

c) Vitamin A d) Riboflavin

Q 22 The light blue colour of whey is due to presence of ________

a) **Riboflavin** b) Vitamin A

c) Casein d) Carotene

Q 23 Which of the following content is higher amount in milk in late lactation stage of a buffalo?

a) Lactose b) **Fat**

c) Quantity of milk d) None of the above

Q 24 In milk of mastitic animal, which of the following change occur?

a) Lactose content decreased

b) Potassium content decreased

c) Na & Cl content increased

d) **All the above**

Q 25 Which of the following cow has quality milk?

a) **Jersey** b) H.F

c) Cross bred cow d) All have the same

Q 26 Which of the following does not show an increasing trend in the later stage of lactation?

a) Fat b) Crude protein

c) **Lactose** d) SNF

Q 27 The production of low fat milk may be associated with ______

a) **Lack/low roughage diet** b) High grain content

c) High cake content d) None of the above

Q 28 For production of 1Kg of MILK of 4% fat, DCP required is ___

a) **45 g** b) 35 g

c) 25 g d) 70 g

Q 29 Metabolic energy required for production of 1Kg milk of 4% fat ________

a) **1.13 Mcal** b) 1.80 Mcal

c) 2.13 Mcal d) 2.80 Mcal

Q 30 Calcium required for producing of 1Kg milk of 4% fat ______

a) **2.7 g** b) 3.7 g

c) 4.7 g d) 5.7 g

Q 31 Phosphorus required for producing of 1Kg milk of 4% fat ______

a) **2.0 g** b) 3.0 g

c) 4.0 g d) 5.0 g

Q 32 The digestible nitrogen required per 100g milk nitrogen in HF cow is ______

a) **156.4 g** b) 110 g

c) 100 g d) 210.5 g

Q 33 Digestible nitrogen required for 100g of milk nitrogen is ______

a) **132 g** b) 122 g

c) 182 g d) 192 g

Q 34 To calculate milk protein, milk nitrogen is multiplied by which of the following factor?

a) 6.25 b) **6.38***

c) 6.50 d) 6.10

* Because milk protein contained 15.87% nitrogen as compared to 16% nitrogen of normal protein.

Q 35 Lactose in cow milk is around ______

a) 5.2-5.6% b) **4.6- 4.8%**

c) 7.6-8.2% d) 1.0-2.5%

Q 36 Butyric acid and citric acid generally used in milk replacer help in ______

a) Faeces expulsion

b) **Development of rumen papillae**

c) Early eruption of teeth

d) All the above

Q 37 Generally how much quantity of standard milk replacer is equivalent to 1 kg milk ______

a) **175 gm** b) 50 gm

c) 200 gm d) 500 gm

Q 38 Cow milk is generally richer than buffalo milk in what?

a) Fat
b) **Carotene**
c) Minerals
d) Protein

Q 39 Casein constitute about how much percent of total milk protein present in milk?

a) **80**
b) 90
c) 60
d) 30

Q 40 The castor oil is added in artificial colostrums, because it has __________

a) **Laxative effect**
b) Immuno protective effect
c) Good protein content
d) All the above

Q 41 A standard colostrometer is placed in a cylinder containing colostrums and allowed to float freely. The upper level of colostrums is at green level. Then, the colostrums contain __________

a) <20 mg/ ml of Ig
b) 20 to 50 mg/ ml of Ig
c) **> 50 mg/ ml of Ig**
d) 1 mg/ ml of Ig

Q 42 If the upper level is at yellow. Then, the colostrums contain __________

a) <20 mg/ml of IgG
b) **20 to 50 mg/ ml of Ig G**
c) > 50 mg/ml of IgG
d) 1 mg/ml of IgG

Q 43 If the upper level is at red. Then, the colostrums contain __________

a) **<20 mg/ ml of Ig G**
b) 20 to 50 mg/ml of Ig G
c) > 50 mg/ml of IgG
d) >100 mg/ml of IgG

Q 44 The optimum level of IgG in colostrums to consider it as high quality is __________

a) 20 mg/ml of IgG
b) 30 mg/ml of IgG
c) 10 mg/ml of IgG
d) **>50 mg/ ml of IgG**

Q 45 Cow have ________ streak canal/teat.

a) **1**
b) 2
c) 3
d) 4

Q 46 The rear quarter produce __________ % of the daily milk yield.

a) 20% b) 40%

c) **60%** d) 80%

Q 47 Normally, in fat corrected milk, fat percentage is adjusted at __________

a) **4 %** b) 5%

c) 6% d) 7%

Q 48 The formula used for fat corrected milk (4%) is __________

a) **FCM (kg)= 0.4 (kg milk) + 15 (kg fat)**

b) FCM (kg) = 4 (kg Milk) + 1.5 (kg Fat)

c) FCM (kg) = 15 (kg milk) + 0.4 (kg fat)

d) FCM (kg) = 1.5 (kg Milk) + 4 (kg Fat)

Q 49 The net energy content of 1 kg of Fat corrected milk is ________

a) 650 Kcal b) **750 Kcal**

c) 850 Kcal d) 950 Kcal

Q 50 On a high grain diet, the milk fat depression is caused by _____

a) **Formation of trans fatty acid in the rumen**

b) Lack of vitamin B_{12} in the rumen

c) Low acetate production

d) All the above

Q 51 Which of the following condition will lower the milk fat?

a) PUFA's supplementation b) Low forage diet

c) Increased trans fatty acid d) Low rumen pH

e) **All the above**

Q 52 Which of the following conditions in the rumen leads to milk fat depression?

a) Low acetate combined with propionate and low vitamin B_{12} synthesis

b) Excess fermentable starch combined with low trans fatty acid production

c) **Partial biohydrogenation of dietary unsaturated lipid combined with low rumen pH**

d) High saturated fat and high propionate formation

Q 53 Trans fatty acid have been implicated in milk fat depression, where do trans fatty acid originate from?

a) **Rumen fermentation**

b) Intestinal digestion

c) Liver synthesis

d) Udder breakdown of VLDL

Q 54 Milk fat depression is due to what ?

a) **Incomplete rumen biohydrogenation of polyunsaturated fat**

b) Change in VFA pattern

c) Lack of fat in the diet

d) All the above

Q 55 What per cent of milk is water?

a) 82 per cent b) **87 per cent**

c) 93 per cent d) 50 per cent

Q 56 What pathway in young calves directs milk into the abomasum, bypassing the rumen, reticulum, and omasum?

a) Rumen bypass groove b) Masticulas passinomis

c) **Esophageal groove** d) Rumen passinomis

Q 57 When is the best time to feed anionic salts to dairy cows?

a) The day before calving

b) **Two weeks prior to calving**

c) While the cow is calving

d) Immediately after calving

Q 58 As a rule of thumb when milk production ________, the milk fat content ________.

a) **Decreases, increases** b) Decreases, decreases

c) Increases, increases d) Stops, increases

Q 59 When you fed your mid to late lactating cow 100 calories, how many calories do you get back in the form of milk?

a) 10-15 b) **20-25**

c) 40-50 d) 60-70

Q 60 NRC 2001 recommended that amount of IgG provided to calf should be at least __________

a) 50 mg
b) 100 mg
c) **100 g**
d) 200g

Q 61 Compared to whole milk, most milk replacer contain ________

a) **Less energy**
b) Less fat
c) More energy
d) Less protein

Q 62 Which of the following immunoglobulins constitute the major portion of immunoglobulin in colostrum?

a) **IgG**
b) IgA
c) IgM
d) Can be any

Q 63 Which of the following immunoglobulins present in colostrum has the higher half life?

a) **IgG**
b) IgA
c) IgM
d) All have equal

Q 64 Half life of immunoglobulin G (IgG) in calf blood is _______

a) 4 days
b) 1 days
c) **21 days**
d) 2 days

Q 65 Half life of immunoglobulin M (IgM) is __________

a) 1 days
b) **4 days**
c) 2 days
d) 21 days

Q 66 Half life of immunoglobulin A (IgA) is __________

a) 1 days
b) 4 days
c) **2 days**
d) 10 days

Q 67 Antibody(immunoglobulins) content of colostrum is lowest in __________

a) **First calving**
b) Second calving
c) Third calving
d) Fourth calving

Q 68 Which of the following breeds of cows has lowest level of antibodies in colostrum?

a) Jersey
b) **Holstein**
c) Sahiwal
d) All have equal

Q 69 Which of the following factor affects the antibodies (IgG) concentration in colostrum?

a) Length of dry period
b) Breed
c) Volume of colostrum
d) **All the above**

Q 70 The major determinant of milk volume is __________

a) **Lactose**
b) Protein
c) Water
d) Minerals

Q 71 Which of the following sugar is only made by mammals?

a) Glucose
b) Sucrose
c) Fructose
d) **Lactose**

Q 72 Which of the following constitute form the major part(97-98%) of milk fat?

a) **Triglycerides**
b) Phospholipids
c) Free fatty acid
d) Cholesterol

Q 73 "Sunlight flavour" in milk occur due to degradation of _______

a) **Methionine**
b) Fat
c) Lactose
d) Calcium

❑❑❑

Chapter 27

Miscellaneous

A. Horse

Q 1 The prehensile organ of the horse is ________

a) Tongue
b) **Upper lip**
c) Lower lip
d) Teeth

Q2 The average saliva secreted in a horse fed normally is ______

a) 100-150 litre
b) **10-15 litre**
c) 40-50 litre
d) 50-75 litre

Q3 In which part of the equine digestive system, protein and soluble carbohydrate are mainly digested?

a) Caecum
b) Stomach
c) Large intestine
d) **Small intestine**

Q4 In horse, which of the following mineral is lost in greater amount in sweat?

a) Na
b) K
c) **Cl**
d) Ca

Q 5 Which of the following animal is less efficient in digesting forages?

a) Cow
b) Buffalo
c) Goat
d) **Horse**

Q 6 "Margo plicatus" structure is found in which animal?

a) Dog
b) Cow
c) Pig
d) **Horse**

Q 7 The junction between glandular and non-glandular stomach of horse is known as ________

a) Saccus caecus b) **Margo plicatus**

c) Saccus entericus d) None of the above

Q 8 The largest gland in horse body is ________

a) **Liver** b) Pancreas

c) Margo plicatus d) Brunner gland

Q 9 Which of the following is not a macromolecule in living organism?

a) Protein b) Nucleic acid

c) Polysaccharide d) **Amino acid**

Q 10 Protein constitute about ______ of the horse body.

a) 10% b) **18%**

c) 40% d) 2%

Q 11 Number of essential amino acids required for foal is ________

a) **10** b) 12

c) 13 d) 7

Q 12 Equine motor neuron disease (EMND) occur due to deficiency of ________

a) Vitamin A b) **Vitamin E**

c) Vitamin C d) Vitamin D

Q 13 Equine degenerative myeloencephalopathy (EDM) occur due to deficiency of ________

a) Vitamin A b) **Vitamin E**

c) Vitamin C d) Vitamin D

Q 14 The ideal Ca: P ratio for horse is ________

a) 1:1 b) **1.5:1**

c) 3:1 d) 1:2

Q 15 A deficiency or excess of which mineral leads to similar symptoms ________

a) Se b) Fe

c) **I** d) Zn

Q 16 The latest NRC edition for horse nutrient requirement was __________

a) **NRC (2007)** b) NRC (2010)
c) NRC (2001) d) NRC (1992)

Q 17 Horse caecum has a capacity of __________

a) **25-35 litre** b) 10-15 litre
c) 100-150 litre d) 80-100 litre

Q 18 Crushed or cracked feed that has been cooked prior to the extrusion process is known as __________

a) **Kibbling** b) Quidding
c) Crumbling d) Middlings

Q 19 Byproduct of the flour milling process that is graded according to the proportion of bran, germ and endosperm is known as __________

a) Kibbling b) Quidding
c) Crumbling d) **Middlings**

Q 20 The dropping of small amount of feed from the horse mouth during chewing (Most often as a result of sharp teeth or damage to mouth or tongue) is known as __________

a) **Quidding** b) Kibbling
c) Crib bitting d) Voiding

Q 21 Gall bladder is absent in __________

a) Dog b) Pig
c) Cat d) **Horse**

Q 22 The most popular grain for horse is __________

a) **Oat** b) Corn
c) Sorghum d) Wheat

Q 23 The most common protein supplement for horse is __________

a) **Soyabean meal** b) Cottonseed meal
c) Peanut meal d) Maize gluten meal

Q 24 Which is the longest part of the horse digestive system?

a) Large intestine b) Caecum
c) **Small intestine** d) Oesophagus

Q 25 Which of the following nutrient is a concentrated form of energy and is used in small quantity to increase the energy density of the diet?

a) **Fat** b) Starch

c) Protein d) Minerals

Q 26 Compared to other farm animals, stomach of a horse is________ in size.

a) Large b) **Smaller**

c) Relatively same d) Can be larger or smaller

Q 27 The stomach of the horse make up ________ % of the entire digestive tract.

a) **10** b) 40

c) 30 d) 60

Q 28 Small intestine of the horse make up ____________% of the entire digestive tract.

a) 10 b) 60

c) **30** d) 75

Q 29 In the horse, ________________ is the primary site for water absorption.

a) Stomach b) **Caecum**

c) Small intestine d) Rectum

Q 30 Nutritional secondary hyperparathyroidism (NSH) in equine is also known as __________

a) Bran disease b) Millers disease

c) Fibrous osteodystrophy d) **All the above**

Q 31 Excessive feeding of bran coupled with high oxalate content in the feed of horse can lead to __________

a) Tying up b) Laminitis

c) **Big head disease** d) None of these

Q 32 Which of the following animal has more lactose in her milk?

a) Cow b) Goat

c) Sheep d) **Mare**

Q 33 Which of the following is not an example of fructans?

a) Inulins b) Levans

c) Graminan d) **Galactans**

Q 34 Which of the following straw is generally used for horse feeding?

a) Wheat straw b) **Oat straw**

c) Rice straw d) Rye straw

Q 35 The most palatable of all the straw is __________

a) Wheat straw b) **Oat straw**

c) Rice straw d) Rye straw

Q 36 Foregut in horse does not include __________

a) Mouth b) Stomach

c) Small intestine d) **Caecum**

Q 37 Tick the wrong statement __________

a) Caecum is fully functional in horse at about 2 years of age

b) **Crude fibre is more digestible in horse as compared to ruminants**

c) Gall bladder is absent in horse

d) Caecal fermentation is not as efficient as rumen fermentation

Q 38 The water required per Kg of DMI in horse is __________

a) 5-10 litre b) 0.5-1.0 litre

c) **2-4 litre** d) 10-15 litre

Q 39 The most expensive nutrient in horse ration is __________

a) **Protein** b) Carbohydrate

c) Fat d) Minerals

B. Poultry / Swine

Q 1 Feed required by commercial broilers to produce 1 kg of broiler meat is __________

a) 3-4 kg b) 4-5 kg

c) 0.5- 1.0 kg d) **1.8- 2.0 kg**

Q 2 Feed required by laying pullet to produce 1 kg of eggs is ______

a) 1-1.5 kg
b) **2.5- 3.0 kg**
c) 0.5-1 kg
d) 4-5.5 kg

Q 3 Which state is known as egg basket of India?

a) Punjab
b) Haryana
c) **A.P**
d) Maharashtra

Q 4 Drum sticks are common name of chicken __________

a) **Legs**
b) Ribs
c) Both legs and ribs
d) Claws

Q 5 Crude protein content of dried swine excreta __________

a) 35%
b) 43.88%
c) **18%**
d) 5%

Q 6 Crude protein content in poultry manure (dried poultry dropping) is __________

a) 15%
b) 10%
c) 45%
d) **24%**

Q 7 Which of the following intestinal parameter can not be related with better performance of birds?

a) High villus height (VH)
b) **Larger crypt depth**
c) Thin intestinal wall
d) High villus height: crypt depth ratio

Q 8 Generally, maize constitutes _________ percentage of broiler/ layer feed.

a) **50-60%**
b) 30-35%
c) 20-30%
d) 70-80%

Q 9 Which of the following is an example of protective food*?

a) Milk
b) Eggs
c) Fruits
d) **All the above**

* Protective food are so called because of their ability to balance diets commonly over rich in starch, sugars and fat and all too frequently lacking in balanced protein, minerals and vitamins

Q 10 Egg is deficient in ________

a) Vitamin A b) Vitamin D

c) Riboflavin d) **Vitamin C**

Q 11 Practically all the Fe content in the egg is localized in ______

a) Albumin b) **Yolk**

c) Equally distributed d) Egg don't have any Fe in it

Q 12 Tick the right statement ________

a) **There is no air cell in an egg at the moment it is laid**

b) Air cell is usually at pointed end

c) Air cell size remain the same from laying to until it is broken

d) Air cell is formed from the expired air of chick embryo

Q 13 Which of the following is not a part of egg shell?

a) Mammillary layer b) Spongy layer

c) Pores d) **Air cell**

Q 14 Germ spot is present in ________

a) **Every egg** b) Fertile egg only

c) Brown egg only d) Albumin of the egg

Q 15 The mean percentage of shell and edible content of the egg is?

a) 57 & 32 b) **11 & 89**

c) 60 & 40 d) 29 & 71

Q 16 The average percentage of shell, albumin and yolk in normal egg is ________

a) **11,57 & 32** b) 57,11 & 32

c) 32,11 & 57 d) 57,32 & 11

Q 17 The average percentage of protein in whole egg is ______

a) 5% b) **12%**

c) 22% d) 32%

Q 18 The average per cent fat content in whole egg is ________

a) 5% b) 20%

c) **10%** d) 17%

Q 19 The per cent water content in whole egg is ________

a) 25.5% b) 35.5%

c) 55.5% d) **65.5%**

Q 20 Which of the following egg part contain higher per cent protein content?

a) Egg white b) **Egg yolk**

c) Both have equal d) Egg shell

Q 21 Which of the following egg part contain higher fat percentage?

a) Shell membrane b) Shell

c) Egg white d) **Egg yolk**

Q 22 Peewee size of the egg refers to ________

a) Extra large size b) Large egg

c) Medium egg d) **Smaller egg**

Q 23 Haugh unit values ranges from ________

a) 0-50 b) **0-110**

c) 0-100 d) 0-140

Q 24 Barley can be added to poultry ration upto ________

a) 40 b) 35

c) **15** d) 50

Q 25 Oat should not constitute more than ______ % of the poultry ration.

a) 40 b) 50

c) **20** d) 60

Q 26 Maize can be incorporated in poultry ration upto ________

a) 20% b) 30%

c) 40% d) **60%**

Q 27 Fletcher scale is used to determine the ________

a) **Yolk colour** b) Yolk quantity

c) Yolk thickness d) All the above

Q 28 Freshly laid egg has a pH of ________

a) **7.6** b) 6.0

c) 5.4 d) 4.5

Q 29 Storing the egg for long time makes its content ________

a) **More alkaline**

b) More acidic

c) Neutral

d) Depends upon composition of egg

Q 30 Storage of egg for longer period leads to ________

a) **Increase in yolk size** b) Decrease in yolk size

c) No change in yolk sac d) Can increase or decrease

Q 31 Dried poultry litter can be included in the ration of layer at a level of ________

a) **5-10%** b) 20-25%

c) 12-18% d) 26-28%

Q 32 Rice Polish in poultry ration can be used upto ________ %.

a) 10 b) 20

c) 30 d) **50**

Q 33 Which of the following is not a very palatable feed stuff for poultry?

a) Maize b) Rice

c) **Barley** d) Wheat

Q 34 Ground nut meal can be incorporated into poultry ration upto ________ extent.

a) 10% b) 15%

c) 25% d) **35%**

Q 35 The maximum level of mustard meal to be used in poultry ration is ________

a) 20 b) **10**

c) 25 d) 35

Q 36 Blood meal is deficient in ________

a) Arginine b) Lysine

c) **Methionine** d) All the above

Q 37 Phosphorus content of the meat meal should be less than _____

a) 10%
b) **4.4 % ***
c) 15%
d) 20 %

* If phosphorus content is more than 4.4,then this meat meal should be classed as meat and bone scrap.

Q 38 Blood meal can be incorporated in the poultry ration upto __________

a) 20%
b) 25%
c) **10%**
d) 35%

Q 39 Magnesium content in limestone should be less than ________

a) 10%
b) 15%
c) **5%***
d) 20%

* Limestone's that contain more amount of magnesium are known as Dolomites.

Q 40 One pound is equal to _________

a) **454 gm**
b) 28.35 gm
c) 353 gm
d) 284 gm

Q 41 One ounce is equal to _________

a) 454 gm
b) **28.35 gm**
c) 353 gm
d) 284 gm

Q 42 In broiler farming, total feed consumed/total body weight gives the _________

a) Feed efficiency
b) Feed conversion efficiency
c) Feed conversion ratio
d) **All the above**

Q 43 Formula for protein efficiency ratio is _________

a) Feed intake (g)/ body weight gain (g)
b) **Body weight gain (g)/ total protein consumed (g)**
c) Total protein consumed (g)/ body weight gain (g)
d) Total protein intake (g)/ feed efficiency

Q 44 Tick the wrong statement __________

a) **Higher value of FCR (>2) is desirable**

b) Higher value of BCR(>1) indicates profitability

c) Lower value of FCR indicate better feed efficiency

d) If BCR =1, it indicates no profit no loss

Q 45 Major site of action of pepsinogen in poultry is __________

a) Crop b) **Proventriculus**

c) Gizzard d) Caeca

Q 46 Laboratory analysis of a feed ingredient show 13% protein, 13% fat and 13 % fibre, which of the following ingredient it is?

a) Wheat bran b) **Rice bran**

c) Broken rice d) Millet

Q 47 Soybean meal is deficient in __________

a) Lysine b) Tryptophan

c) Threonine d) **Methionine**

Q 48 In NaCl, the percentage of Na and Cl is __________

a) **39** and **60%** b) 60 and 39%

c) 70 and 30% d) 80 and 20%

Q 49 The word "pullet" is used for female of __________

a) **Chicken** b) Turkey

c) Duck d) Quail

Q 50 The calcium content in the plasma of laying hens is around __________

a) 80-120 mg/l b) 150-200 mg/l

c) **300-400 mg/l** d) 50-80 mg/l

Q 51 In egg, which of the trace minerals is present in greater amount than the others?

a) **Iron** b) Copper

c) Zinc d) Iodine

Q 52 In birds, the main end product of protein metabolism are __________

a) Urea b) **Uric acid**

c) Allantoin d) Creatinine

Q 53 Non-ruminant, omnivorous, animal having a complex foregut and a reletively simple intestine tract is __________

a) Pig b) **Poultry**

c) Cow d) Rabbit

Q 54 An oesophageal out pocketing present in most of the birds is __________

a) **Crop** b) Gizzard

c) Proventriculus d) Pancreas

❑❑❑

Chapter 28

Test Your Knowledge

Q 1 The exceptionally sweet taste of honey is due to _ ( )

a) Glucose b) Sucrose

c) Fructose d) Galactose

Q 2 Which of the following alcohol is produced from reduction of glucose? ( )

a) Sorbitol b) Dulcitol

c) Mannitol d) All the above

Q 3 The second most abundant mineral in animal body _ ( )

a) Ca b) P

c) Mg d) k

Q 4 The most prevalent mineral deficiency in grazing livestock across the world is of _ ( )

a) Ca b) P

c) Se d) S

Q 5 Mucosal block theory involved in absorption of which mineral? ( )

a) Cu b) Zu

c) Fe d) Se

Q 6 In full fat soyabean, the percentage of fat is around _ ( )

a) 5% b) 10%

c) 18% d) 28%

Q 7 The most abundant nutrient in the body is _ ( )

a) Water b) Mineral

c) Carbohydrate d) Protein

Q 8 The "Vitamin H" term is used for _ ( )

a) Biotin b) Folic acid

c) Niacin d) Pantothenic acid

Q 9 Which of the following vitamin has most complex structure of all the vitamin? ( )

a) Vit B_{12} b) Vit B_2

c) Vit B_6 d) Vit B_5

Q 10 Pink colour discolouration of egg albumin may occur, when layer are fed on _ ( )

a) Cotton seed cake b) Mustard cake

c) Soyabean Cake d) Groundnut cake

Q 11 Anti-nutritional factor present in castor cake in _ ( )

a) Ricin b) Strychnine

c) Dicumoral d) Linamarin

Q 12 Which of the following is k/a muscular stomach in birds? ( )

a) Crop b) Proventriculus

c) Gizzard d) None of the above

Q 13 The enzyme 'Ptyalin is abrent in the saliva of _ ( )

a) Ruminants b) Poultry

c) Pig d) All of the above

Q 14 The foremost part of ruminant stomach is _ ( )

a) Rumen b) Reticulum

c) Omasum d) Abomasum

Q 15 Rumination is also known as _ ( )

a) Cud chewing b) Reverse peristalsis

c) Controlled vomiting d) All of the above

Q 16 Principle of organ of prehension in pig is _ ( )

a) Upper lip b) Lower lip

c) Tongue d) Incisor

Q 17 For effective microbial protein synthesis in urea supplemented diet the optimum ration of N:S ratio is _ ( )

a) 10:1 b) 1:10

c) 5:10 d) 10:5

Q 18 The term "Defaunation" generally pertain to removal of which microorganism from the rumen? ( )

a) Fungi b) Protozoa

c) Archea b) Bacteriophage

Q 19 Who reported the presence of Fungi in the rumen for the first time? ( )

a) Orpin b) Gruby & Delafond

c) Parker d) Vansoest

Q 20 Metabolic water formed when one gram fat oxidized is _ ( )

a) 0.56g b) 0.40g

c) 1.07g d) 0.88g

Q 21 Which of the following Amino acid is bitter in taste? ( )

a) Glycine b) Alanine

c) Serine d) Arginine

Q 22 Broadly, the enzymes are divided into how many groups? ( )

a) 6 b) 5

c) 4 d) 3

Q 23 Which of the following is not an example of internal indicator? ( )

a) Lignin b) Acid insoluble ash

c) Silica d) Carminered

Q 24 Sample size to bag surface area ratio and be around Insacco technique _ ( )

a) 10-20 mg/cm^2 b) 20-50 mg/cm^2

c) 50-70 mg/cm^2 d) 70-100 mg/cm^2

Q 25 Apparent digestibility of feed is _______ than the true digestibility. ( )

a) Less b) Equal

c) Higher d) May be on any side

Q 26 Among the VFAs, which one has the highest GE value? ( )

a) Acetic acid b) Propionic acid

c) Butyric acid d) All have the same

Q 27 Pteroylglutamic acid is the chemical name of which vitamin? ( )

a) Folacin b) Niacin

c) Pantothenic acid d) Riboflavin

Q 28 Pearl Millet is commonly k/a _ ( )

a) Bajra b) Jowar

c) Javi d) Soybean

Q 29 BIS specifications of minerals mixture for cattle are of following type _ ( )

a) Two b) Three

c) Four d) One

Q 30 Copra meal is synonymous for _ ( )

a) Kranz meal b) Coconut meal

c) Soyabean meal d) Flax seed meal

Q 31 The optimum pH for good quality silage is _ ( )

a) 2 b) 4

c) 6 d) 8

Q 32 The solvent extracted cake generally contain this much oils( )

a) Less than 1% b) Less than 5%

c) More than 5% d) Nearly 5-10%

Q 33 Conversion of lypsinogen to trypsin in done by _ ( )

a) Hcl b) Pepsin

c) Enterokinase d) Gastrin

Q 34 Niacin deficiency in poultry birds lead to a condition _ ( )

a) Black tongue b) Black leg

c) Toe paralysis d) None of the above

Q 35 Following animal is prone to iodine toxicity _ ( )

a) Cattle b) Swine

c) Poultry d) Horse

Q 36 Which of the following is not a leguminous fodder? ( )

a) Senji b) Guar

c) Lucerne d) Teosinte

Q 37 Father of nutrition is _ ( )

a) Antony Lavosier b) Hippocrates

c) Van Holvant d) None of those

Q 38 Percentage of metabolizable protein formed from dietary protein in ruminant animal is _ ( )

a) 60% b) 55%

c) 75% d) 95%

Haylage is forage conserved at higher moisture content than hay but lower than silage or Haylage is drier than silage but less drier than hay

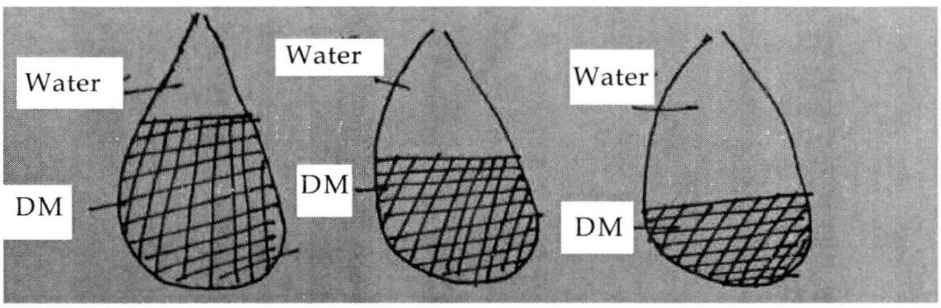

Water = 20 %	Water = 50 %	Water = 70 %
DM = 20 %	DM = 50 %	DM = 30 %
Hay	Haylage	Silage

Q 39 An estrogenic substance namely "Genistein" is found in _ ( )

a) Soyabean seed b) Neem seem meal

c) Linseed meal d) Rape seed

Q 40 Sulphur atoms present in "cystine" are _ ( )

a) 1 b) 2

c) 3 d) 4

Q 41 Which mineral is present in enzyme "Xanthine oxidase"? ( )

a) Mn b) Mg

b) Mo d) Zn

Q 42 Recommended calorie: protein ration for broiler starter is _( )

a) 135:1 b) 155:1

c) 140:1 d) 180:1

Q 43 Fat content in double tonned milk is _ ( )

a) 1.5% b) 2.5%

c) 2% d) 3%

Q 44 One Kcal is equal to _ ( )

a) 2.205 KJ b) 6.25 KJ

c) 3.185 KJ d) 4.185 KJ

Q 45 "Steaming up" is the practice of feeding extra concentrate_ ( )

a) After calving b) Last 6-8 wk of pregnancy

c) During transition period d) After conception

Q 46 Nitrogen present in 6.25gm protein is _ ( )

a) 1 gm b) 2 gm

c) 3 gm d) 4 gm

Q 47 Van Soest method of feed analysis was proposed in _ ( )

a) 1966 b) 1977

c) 1982 d) 1952

Q48 Mixture of ingredients including water which is consumed by animal on a particular time is known as _ ( )

a) Ration b) Feed

c) Diet d) Food

Q49 The term "Specific Dynamic Effect" was corned by _ ( )

a) Rubner b) Atwater

c) Kellener d) Lavoisier

Q 50 Physiological fuel value for protein is _ ( )

a) 4.0 kcal/g b) 9.0 kcal/g

c) 9.4 kcal/g d) 4.9 kcal/g

Q 51 Percentage of absorbed nitrogen retained by the body is known as _ ( )

a) Biological value b) Gross protein value

c) Net protein retention d) Protein efficiency ratio

Q 52 Essential Amino Acid India (EAAI) for measuring protein quality for monogastric was proposed by _ ( )

a) Black & Mitchell b) Laplace & Lavoisier

c) Oser d) Atwater

Q 53 The part of leaf, twig, growth of shrubs, wooding vines & tree available for animal for animal consumption is known as _( )

a) Herbage b) Cover

c) Browse d) Forage

Q 54 Minimum number of animals required for metabolic profile test for significant interpretation are _ ( )

a) 2 b) 5

c) 7 d) 10

Q 55 The optimum range of milk urea nitrogen (MUN) in _ ( )

a) 12mg/150ml b) 12-18mg/100ml

c) 18-25mg/100ml d) 25-30mg/100ml

Q 56 Which of the following in also known as "Anti-infective vitamin"? ( )

a) Vitamin A b) Vitamin E

c) Biotin d) Vitamin C

Q 57 Which of the toxic mineral is also used as growth promoters in poultry birds? ( )

a) Cadmium b) Arsenic

c) Murcury d) Lead

Q 58 Under Anaerobic condition glycolysis yield how many moles of ATP? ( )

a) 2 b) 4

c) 6 d) 8

Q 59 The net energy content of 1kg fat corrected milk is _ ( )

a) 650 kcal b) 750 kcal

c) 850 kcal d) 950 kcal

Q 60 Which of the following animals milk have the highest fat content _ ( )

a) Cow b) Goat

c) Ewe d) Sow

Q 61 The light blue colour of whey is due to presence of _ ( )

a) Riboflavin b) Vitamin A

c) Casein d) Carotine

Q 62 Calcium required for producing 1 kg of milk with 4% fat is _ ( )

a) 2.7g b) 3.7g

c) 4.7g d) 5.7g

Q 63 Ipil-pil is another name of _ ( )

a) Subabul b) Tamarind

c) Acacia d) Khejri

Q 64 Falling disease in ruminant occur due to deficiency of _ ( )

a) Fe b) Ca

c) Cu d) Pb

Q 65 In India, the first feed mill was established at _ ( )

a) Ludhiana b) Karnal

c) Hyderabad d) Odisha

Q 66 Shearing is the combination of _ ( )

a) Cutting & grinding b) Cutting & crushing

c) Soaking & crumbing b) Cutting and steaming

Q 67 IGFRI (Indian Garassl and & Fodder Research Institute) is located at _ ( )

a) Jhansi (UP) b) Makhdoom (UP)

c) Bikaner (Rajasthan) d) Chandigarh (Punjab)

Q 68 The unit of bulk density is _ ( )

a) Kg/cft b) Cm/m^3

c) Kg/m^2 d) Kg/m

Q 69 The term "Nutraceutical" was coined by _ ( )

a) Stephen Defelice b) Hippocrates

c) Mccollum d) Loosli

Q 70 Number of proximate principles in Weende system of feed analysis is _ ( )

a) 5 b) 6

c) 3 d) 10

Q 71 PPM (Part per million) is _ ( )

a) g per kg b) mg/kg

c) μg/kg d) ng/kg

Q 72 Which of the following fraction is not included in ADF (Acid detergent fibre)? ( )

a) Hemi-cellulose b) Cellulose

c) Lignin d) Silica

Q 73 Nature of ruminant saliva is _ ( )

a) Highly acidic b) Slightly acidic

c) Slightly alkaline d) Distinctly alkaline

Q 74 'Degnaladesease" in ruminant occur due to excess of _ ( )

a) K b) Se

c) Mg d) F

Q 75 DCP of wheat straw is _ ( )

a) 3.0 b) 4.0

c) 0.0 d) 5.0

Q 76 Feeding of beneficial microbes is _ ( )

a) Probiotic b) Prebiotic

c) Synbiotic d) Xenobiotic

Q 77 The term "Animal Starch is used for _ ( )

a) Glucose b) Galactose

c) Glycogen d) Fructose

Q 78 The term 'Transition period' is generally complied to _ ( )

a) 3 week before & after parturition

b) 3 week before calving

c) 3 week after calving

d) 3 week before & after conception

Q 79 In ruminant eructation, which gas is in higher percentage _ ( )

a) CO_2 b) CH_4

c) H_2S d) NO_2

Q 80 The maximum crude fibre in swine diet is _ ( )

a) 20% b) 10%

c) 15% d) 25%

Q 81 The term "Draff" is used for _ ( )

a) Brewer's grain b) Spent hops

c) Spent yeast d) Wort

Q 82 The effect of one nutrient on the other in the digestive system is known as _ ( )

a) Allosteric effect b) Associative effect

c) Specific dynamic effect d) Cholinergic effect

Q 83 NRC system of feeding standard belongs to _ ( )

a) USA b) UK

c) Australia d) South Africa

Q 84 Which of the following is an example of "Holotricks"? ( )

a) Entodinium b) Epidinium

c) Ophroscolex d) Dasytricha

Q 85 'Post Parturient Dyspepsis' in cattle is also k/a _ ( )

a) Milk Fever b) Hypocacemia

c) Post Parturient Paresis d) Ketosis

Q 86 Toluene distillation technique is used for measuring _ ( )

a) Dry matter content of silage

b) VFA production in rumen

c) Ammonia production in rumen

d) Acid content of silage

Q 87 Major acid produced in ensiling process which helps in preservation of fodder _ ( )

a) Lactic acid b) Butyric acid

c) Acetic acid d) Valeric acid

Q 88 The concept of hay equivalence was used in which feeding standard? ( )

a) Savage b) Morrison

c) Scandinavian d) Thaer

Q 89 Kasni (Cichroiumin intybus) is a used generally found with _ ( )

a) Bajra b) Barseem

c) Maize d) Jowar

Q 90 Tube silage is making silage in _ ( )

a) Tunnel b) Trench

c) Polythene d) Tower

Q 91 Which of the following is known as Epsom salt? ( )

a) $MgSo_4$ b) $Cuso_4$

c) $MnSo_4$ d) $ZnSo_4$

Q 92 In Northern India, lean period comprises of _ ( )

a) Jan-Feb b) Aug-Sep

c) May-June d) Dec-Jan

Q 93 The term used for freshly cut green forage fed to animal is_( )

a) Stillage b) Soilage

c) Haylage d) Ensilage

Q 94 The RQ value for fat is _ ( )

a) 0.7 b) O.9

c) 1.0 d) 1.5

Q 95 B-Hydroxy butyrate and aceto acetic are used as source of energy preferably by _ ( )

a) Skeletal muscle b) Liver

c) Spleen d) Kidney

Q 96 Loss of nutrient due to rain is known as _ ( )

a) Leaching b) Bleaching

c) Seepage d) Effluent loss

Q 97 The recommended level of urea in concentrate for ruminants animals in _ ( )

a) 2% b) 3%

c) 1% d) 2.5%

Q 98 Press mud is the byproduct of which industry? ( )

a) Rice milling b) Fruit juice making

c) Beverge industry d) Sugar industry

Q 99 Calf starter contain how much CP _ ( )

a) 22-23% b) 15-16%

c) 10-15% d) 35-40%

Q 100 Gossypol in cotton seed can cause the deficiency of _ ( )

a) Cu b) Co

c) Fe d) I

Q 101 Feeding of Antibiotic as growth promoters was banned in which country ? ( )

a) Europe Union b) India

c) Pakistan d) Malaysia

Q 102 HOT process technology for UMMB making was developed by _ ( )

a) NDDB, Anand b) NDRI, Karnal

c) IVRI, Izatnagar d) PAU, Ludhiana

Q 103 Encephalomalacia in poultry birds occur due to deficiency of _ ( )

a) Vit A b) Vit E

c) Vit B_6 d) Vit B_2

Q 104 Extra feeding sow before breeding is known as _ ( )

a) Flushing b) Sleaming up

c) Challenge feeding d) Creep ration

Q 105 Feed conversion efficiency in broiler is _ ( )

a) 1.8:1 b) 2.5:1

c) 3:1 d) 4:1

Q 106 The main component of endogenous urinary nitrogen (EUN) in mammal is _ ( )

a) Uric acid b) Urea

c) Amino acid d) Amines

Q 107 How many caeca are present in poultry digestive system? ( )

a) 1 b) 2

c) 3 d) 4

Q 108 Which of the following animal practiced coprophagy? ( )

a) Cow b) Horse

c) Rabbit d) Goat

Q 109 Which of the following VFA is glucogenic in nature? ( )

a) Acetic acid b) Prepronic acid

c) Butyric acid d) Isovaleric acid

Q 110 Carbon in protein is present to the extent of _ ( )

a) 23% b) 16%

c) 50% d) 7%

Q 111 Which of the following is also K/a animal protein factor? ( )

a) Vit B1 b) Vit. B6
c) Vit B2 d) Vit B12

Q 112 Which part of stomach is fully developed incalf of 4 week of age? ( )

a) Raticulum b) Rumen
c) Omasum d) Abomasum

Q 113 Water content in calf at birth is_ ( )

a) 75-80% b) 50-60%
c) 30-50% d) 10-20%

Q 114 Which of the following is a kharif crop? ( )

a) Berseem b) Oats
c) Mustard d) Cowpea

Q 115 The term treacle can also be used for _ ( )

a) Molasses b) Table scrap
c) Teosinte d) Bran

Q 116 AOAC (Association of Official Agricultural Chemists) found _ ( )

a) USA b) Canada
c) UK d) Australia

Q 117 Formation of glucose from non carbohydrate sources in known as _ ( )

a) Glucogenesis b) Glycogenesis
c) Glycogenolysis d) Glycolysis

Q 118 Salt sickness is occurs due to _ ( )

a) Deficiency of Cu b) Excess of Cu
c) Deficiency of salt d) Excess of salt

Q 119 Thumps in piglet occur due to deficiency of _ ( )

a) Fe b) I
c) Zn d) Cu

Q 120 Highest quality of milk is produced by _ ( )

a) Jersey b) HF

c) Ayrchice d) None of the above

Q 121 Alsi is common name for _ ( )

a) Flaxseed b) Salseed

c) Seasam d) Lin seed

Q 122 Which of the follow nutrient effect the milk fat percentage? ( )

a) Fibre b) Protein

c) Fat d) Mineral

Q 123 Which of the following is involved in quality in animal feed? ( )

a) BIS b) Codex alimentarius

c) HACCP d) All the above

Q 124 Limiting amino acid in soyabean is _ ( )

a) Lysine b) Methionine

c) Arginine d) Leucine

Q 125 Milk coagulation enzyme of calf is _ ( )

a) Renin b) Pepsin

c) Erepsin d) Steapsin

Q 126 Tankage is _ ( )

a) Bone meal b) Feather meal

c) Blood meal d) Meat meal

Q 127 Calcium salt of fatty acid is a _ ( )

a) Soap b) Bypass protein

c) Inert fat d) Degradable fat

Q 128 Which of the following is not the essential fatty acids? ( )

a) Linoleic acid b) Linolenic acid

c) Oleic acid d) Arachidonic acid

Q 129 Parakeralosis occur due to deficiency of _ ( )

a) Zn b) Mn

c) Mg d) S

Q 130 Gees blade is absent in which of the following? ( )

a) Cattle b) Horse

c) Dog d) Pig

Q 131 Excessive ammonia produced in rumen is converted into urea by the _ ( )

a) Rumen microbes b) Rumen wall

c) Liver d) Spreen

Q 132 Which of the following is not hind gut fermenter? ( )

a) Horse b) Rabbit

c) Pig d) Goat

Q 133 The word "Bunk" in Bunk management pertain to _ ( )

a) Manger b) Shed

c) Surrounding d) All the above

Q 134 The average weight of newly born buffalo calf is _ ( )

a) 25-30kg b) 15-20kg

c) 35-50kg d) 50-60kg

Q 135 Lactose, the milk consists of _ ( )

a) One molecule of glucose & molecule of glutose

b) One molecule of glucose & molecule of fructose

c) One molecule of glucose & molecule of sucrose

d) One molecule of glucose & molecule of maltose

Q 136 Which of the following is cyclic amino acid ? ( )

a) Lysine b) Tyrosine

c) Threonine d) Glutamic aid

Q 137 Which of the following is not a hexose sugar? ( )

a) Glucose b) Fructose

c) Mannose d) Arabinose

Q 138 Fat is present in milk as _ ( )

a) Colloidal srespension b) Emulsion

c) True solvent d) Homogenised

Q 139 Formation of ketone bodies from bulyric acid of rumen occur in _ ( )

a) Liver b) Extra hepatic tissue

c) Blood d) Rumen epithelium

Q 140 The average egg weight is _ ( )

a) 57gm b) 50gm

c) 62gm d) 45gm

Q 141 The thumb rule of feeding the green fodder to the ruminant is_ ( )

a) 10% of the body wt b) 5% g body wt

c) 40% of the body wt d) 2.5% of body wt

Q 142 Inculation of rumen microbes from one species to animal of another speciesis k/a _ ( )

a) Transfaunation b) Transferation

c) Tramslocation d) Transduction

Q 143 The water conduct in succulent fodder is _ ( )

a) 10-20% b) 20-35%

c) 40-45% d) 60-90%

Q 144 Which mineral is required for the production of Vit B_{12} _ ( )

a) Ca b) Co

c) S d) I

Q 145 Excessive feeding of paddy straw canlead to deficiency of_( )

a) Co b) Ca

c) I d) Fe

Q 146 Which of the following is not a Non Protein Nitrogen source forruminant? ( )

a) Urea b) Polypeptide

c) Biuret d) Amino acid

Q 147 Weende System of proximate analysis was given by _ ( )

a) Hennberg and Stohmann b) Laplace and Lavorsice

c) Vansoest d) None of these

Q 148 The term Pashu chocolate is generally used for _ ( )

a) Bheli feed b) Black salt

c) Straw bale d) Uromin lick

Q 149 The surface area law i.e.heat given of bywarmblooded animals is directly proportional to their body surface was given by_( )

a) Rubner b) Atwater

c) Kellener d) Loosely

Q 150 The hormone Gastrin was secreted by _ ( )

a) Gastric mucose b) Pancreases

c) Small intestine d) Both a & b

Q 151 The amount of food energy required to keep the animal at a constant body weight and composition is called _ ( )

a) Maintenance energy b) Net energy

c) Gross energy d) Heat increment

Q 152 Nutrient requirement of animals are related to _ ( )

a) Body weight b) Stage of maturity

c) Both d) None

Q 153 Metabolic body weight is defined as body weight raised to the power _ ( )

a) 0.78 b) 0.75

c) 0.72 d) 0.70

Q 154 Activity increment for birds kept in cages is _ ( )

a) 37% b) 50%

c) 25% d) None

Q 155 The heat production at specified time after the last feeding is_ ( )

a) Fasting metabolism b) Fasting catabolism

c) Basal metabolism d) All the above

Q 156 Estimation of protein requirement for maintenance & growth in pig & poultry is done by _ ( )

a) Factorial method b) N-balance method

c) Feeding trial method d) All the above

Q 157 "Rachitic Rosasy" occur due to deficiency of _ ( )

a) Vit A b) Vit D

c) Vit E d) All the above

Q 158 CNCP system was proposed by _ ( )

a) Chalupa and Sniffen b) Vansoest and Sniffer

c) Preston and Leng d) None of these

Q 159 Which is the best biomarker for assessing the status of ketosis? ( )

a) Glucose b) Cholesterol

c) Non-esterified fatty acid d) All the above

Q 160 National Institute of Animal Nutrition & Physiology is located at _ ( )

a) Bangalore b) Hydrabad

c) Izatnagar d) New Delhi

Q 161 The study of effect of nutrient on gone expression is known as_ ( )

a) Nutrigenomic b) Nutraceuticals

c) Nutrient dynamic d) All the above

Q 162 The major drug detoxification organ in the body is _ ( )

a) Liver b) Kedney

c) Spleen d) All the above

Q 163 Which is the major protein of feather? ( )

a) Collagen b) Elastin

c) Keratin d) Chromoprotein

Q 164 Heated product of urea is known as _ ( )

a) Urea b) Biuret

c) Uric acid d) Allantoions

Q 165 The nature of enzyme is _ ( )

a) Protein b) Fat

c) Carbohydrate d) Mixture of all

Q 166 SF_6 tracer technique is used for the estimation of _ ( )

a) CH_4 production in rumen b) VFA in silage

c) Proximate principle d) None of the above

Q 167 In UMMB (Urea-mineral-molasses block), the ratio of urea to molasses is generally _ ( )

a) 1:1 b) 1:2

c) 1:3 d) 1:10

Q 168 'D' value of the food is related with _ ( )

a) Percentage digestible organic matter in the dry matter

b) Percentage digestible protein in the dry matter

c) Percentage digestible fiber in the dry matter

d) Percentage digestible fat in the dry matter

Q169 Sweet clover disease is associated with which vitamin? ( )

a) Vit A b) Vit D

c) Vit C d) Vit K

Q 170 Which of the following cannot be used as silage additive? ( )

a) Sugar rich material

b) Clostridium containing inoculants

c) Enzymes

d) Formalin

Q 171 The mineral required by enzyme cytochrome oxidase is _ ( )

a) Cu b) Fe

c) Zn d) Se

Q 172 Vitamin involved in flavoprotein is _ ( )

a) Thiamine b) Riboflavin

c) Biotin d) Niacin

Q 173 Which vitamin supplementation can entrance the iron absorption? ( )

a) Vit A b) Thiamin

c) Vit C d) All the above

Q 174 Vitamin needed for Coenzyme (COA) formation _ ( )

a) Pantothenic acid b) Biotin

c) Riboflavin d) Thiamin

Q 175 "Oat hay poisoning" occurs due to high content of _ ( )

a) Nitrate b) Cyanide

c) Glucosinolate d) Tannin

Q 176 Which of the following is not a carbohydrate? ( )

a) Hemicellulose b) Pectin

c) Lignin d) Chondroitin

Q 177 Glycoside present in bitter almond is _ ( )

a) Amygdalin b) Linamarin

c) Dhurin d) Vicianin

Q 178 In ruminant, majority of energy needed for maintenance is provided by _ ( )

a) VFA b) Glucose

c) Fat d) All the above

Q 179 "In situ" method of determine the digestibility of feed stuff is synonymous with _ ( )

a) In vitro b) In sacco

c) In vivo d) In laboratory

Q 180 Supplementation of oligosaccarides in ruminant animals is also known as _ ( )

a) Antibiotic b) Prebiotic

c) Synbiotic d) Xenobiotic

Q 181 How frequently should an average cow freshen? ( )

a) Once every 24 months b) Once every 12 months

c) Once every 20 months d) Only once in her lifetime

Q 182 In nutrition, NPN stands for _ ( )

a) Non Protein Nitrogen
b) Normal Protein Nitrogen
c) Neutral Protein Nitrogen
d) Natural Protein Nitrogen

Q 183 Colostrum has approximately __________ calcium, as does regular milk. ( )

a) Two times
b) Three times
c) Four times
d) Same as of regular milk

Q 184 Fats are broken down by a dairy cow in what part of her body? ( )

a) Rumen
b) Pancreas
c) Small intestine
d) Large intestine

Q 185 Which of the following Vitamin is not colourless? ( )

a) B_6
b) Pyridoxine
c) Choline
d) B_{12}

Answers

1. c 2. a 3. b 4. b 5. c 6. c 7. a 8. a 9. a 10. a
11. a 12. a 13. a 14. b 15. d 16. b 17. a 18. b 19. a 20. c
21. d 22. a 23. d 24. a 25. a 26. c 27. a 28. a 29. a 30. b
31. b 32. a 33. c 34. a 35. d 36. d 37. a 38. c 39. a 40. b
41. b 42. a 43. a 44. d 45. b 46. a 47. b 48. b 49. a 50. a
51. c 52. a 53. c 54. c 55. b 56. a 57. b 58. a 59. b 60. b
61. a 62. a 63. a 64. b 65. a 66. b 67. a 68. a 69. a 70. b
71. b 72. a 73. d 74. b 75. c 76. a 77. c 78. a 79. a 80. b
81. a 82. b 83. a 84. d 85. d 86. a 87. a 88. a 89. a 90. c
91. a 92. c 93. b 94. a 95. a 96. a 97. c 98. d 99. a 100. c
101. a 102. a 103. a 104. a 105. a 106. b 107. b 108. c 109. b 110. d
111. d 112. d 113. a 114. d 115. a 116. a 117. a 118. a 119. a 120. a
121. a 122. a 123. d 124. b 125. a 126. d 127. c 128. c 129. a 130. b
131. c 132. d 133. a 134. a 135. a 136. b 137. d 138. b 139. d 140. a
141. a 142. a 143. d 144. b 145. b 146. b 147. a 148. d 149. d 150. d
151. a 152. c 153. b 154. a 155. a 156. d 157. b 158. a 159. c 160. a
161. a 162. a 163. c 164. b 165. a 166. a 167. c 168. a 169. d 170. b
171. a 172. b 173. c 174. a 175. a 176. c 177. a 178. a 179. b 180. b
181. b 182. a 183. a 184. c 185. d

Chapter 29

Questions: Animal Nutritionist Ought to Know

Q 1. What is the difference between animal nutrition, biochemistry and physiology?

Though there is no clear cut demarcation between these three. Animal nutrition is a branch which deals with what to fed, how much nutrients and anti-nutritional factor a feed have. Once the feed ingested, then came the physiology. How feed eaten is digested by enzymes in various part of GIT comes under the physiology. When feed is completely broken into their last absorbable form and it is absorbed in small intestine. After absorption what happened to these absorbable forms of nutrient, it comes under the biochemistry.

Q 2. Why cattle milk/milk fat is yellowish in colour but that of buffalo is white in colour ?

It is carotene (yellowish pigment) rather than vitamin A, which is present in plants. In majority of animals, this carotene is converted into Vitamin A, which is then absorbed. In species like rat, pig, goat, sheep, rabbit, buffalo and dog almost all the carotene is cleaved in the intestine but in human, cattle, horses significant amount of carotene can be absorbed, which is then stored in liver, fatty tissue and give yellowish colour to body weight and milk fat. Whereas, animal that does not absorb carotene have white fat/white milk.

Q 3. Why there is gaps in true series of B-complex vitamin?

Many substances have been referred as vitamin, as they are once believed to be vitamin. But now they are no longer considered as such and the numbers that are assigned to them, now form the gaps in true series of vitamin B series.

B_4	Adenine
B_8	Adenosine monophosphate
B_{10}	Para amino benzoic acid
B_{11}	Pteryl-hepta-glutamic acid
B_{13}	Orotic acid

Q 4. Why urine become neon yellow on taking vitamin B-complex?

B- Series of vitamin is water soluble and excess of vitamin B series vitamins are excreted in urine. Riboflavin, Folic acid and vitamin B_{12} are having orange yellowish and red tinge, so they impart dark yellow (Neon) colour to urine.

Q 5. What is the difference between rapeseed and canola?

Canola is developed through conventional plant breeding from rapeseed, an oilseed plant already used in ancient civilization as a fuel. The word "rape" in rapeseed comes from the Latin word *rapum* meaning turnip. Canola was bred naturally from rapeseed at the University of Manitoba, Canada, by Keith Downey and Baldur R. Stefansson in the early 1970s, and had a different nutritional profile, in addition to much less erucic acid. In the international community, canola is generally referred to as rapeseed 00 or double zero rapeseed to denote both low glucosinolates and low erucic acid

Q 6. Why prolong boiling of egg sometimes leads to development of greenish black colour in yolk?

When eggs are subjected to prolong boiling, the high temperature some breakdown in the cysteine present in the egg albumin. This release hydrogen sulphide gas, which penetrate the yolk membrane and react with iron of the yolk, producing a greenish black iron sulphide discolouration, which most people find objectionable. Reducing the boiling time to minimum needed to produce hard boiled egg and cooling the egg immediately in cold water largely prevents the development of the discolouration.

Q 5. If a pig is fed a diet with mainly saturated fatty acid, its body fat will be saturated, if it is fed unsaturated fatty acid, its body fat will be unsaturated. But in ruminant carcass fat is more of saturated type irrespective of the diet. Why?

Pig is a simple stomach animal while ruminant animals have compound stomach. In rumen, the microorganism presents causes the biohyrogenation of unsaturated fatty acid of the diet. So, in ruminant animal much of the body fat is synthesized from absorbed acetate produced from biohydrogenation of the fat.

Q 6. What is trans- fat or fatty acid, How it is related with health of the consumer?

The presence of double bond in a fatty acid molecule mean that the fatty acid can exist in two forms, depending upon the spatial arrangement of the hydrogen atoms attached to the carbon atoms of the double bond. When the hydrogen atom lie on the same side of the double bond, the acid is said to be in cis- form and if hydrogen atoms lies on opposite side, it is known as trans form. Generally, all the naturally occurring fatty acid have cis-configuration, naturally occurring trans fatty acids arise from bacterial synthesis. During hydrogenation some of trans fatty acids are formed along with saturated fatty acid. Digestion, absorption and metabolism of the trans fatty acid are comparable with their cis counterpart. As compared with the consumption of an equal number of calories from saturated or cis –unsaturated fatty acid, the consumption of trans fatty acid raises level of LDL cholesterol, reduces HDL cholesterol, promotes inflammation that can cause endothelial dysfunction and increases plasma TAG's, thereby increases the chances of atherosclerosis and coronary heart disease. Trans- fatty acid have extended half life, flavour stability and have higher melting point than their cis analogues.

Q 7. Why sheep and goat meat has a typical smell?

The odour and flavour are due to medium length branched chain fatty acid like 4 methyloctanoic, 4 methyl nonanoic and 4 ethyl analogues. They are formed from methyl melonate, which is produced from propionate. The concentration of branched chain fatty acid in body fat is higher in grain fed than in pasture raised animals because of the higher propionate production with higher concentration diet.

Q 8. Why canola and olive oils are considered to be healthier than other vegetable oils?

Both these oils are having high concentration of monounsaturated fatty acids (MUFA). In canola, about 59% of total fatty acids is MUFA and in olive oil, it is 74% of the total fatty acid. Both MUFA and PUFA have serum cholesterol lowering properties in humans. However unsaturated fatty acids are susceptible to peroxidation and MUFA are, therefore, lesser susceptible for auto-oxidation.

Q 9. Why the rice bran gets quickly rancid?

In whole rice, the fat and lipase enzymes are distributed in aleurone and testa layers respectively. So, as long as the bran surface is uninjured and protected by the husk, the enzymes remain dormant. But as the bran surface is ruptured and separated from the brown rice, the enzyme lipase gets activated and it comes in contact with fat and causes its hydrolysis into free fatty acids. These free fatty acids rancidification is the main cause of rice bran rancidity. But now by heating or extrusion technology, rice bran is heated >100°C to inactivate the lipase, which prolong the life of rice bran.

Q 10. Why very small and very large herbivores are not usually ruminants?

Gut volume among herbivores varies directly with body weight, whereas metabolic rate varies with a fractional power of body weight. Thus, small herbivores have a high metabolic requirement for energy and they must consume high quality diet to meet their energy requirement. So, for this reason smallest ruminants are concentrate selectors. Small non-ruminant's herbivores are better able to utilize forage than small ruminants because of direct digestion without fermentation. As the body size of ruminant decreases, fermentation of forages can no longer meet the increasing energy requirements. With very large ruminants, however, insufficient fibrous feed can be ingested to meet the energy requirements of a large body mass through fermentation by products. Large animals in the wild generally are not able to select sufficient amounts of the rapidly digested foods used by smaller concentrate selectors because the foods are comparatively rare. Thus, large body size favour non-ruminants' herbivores, such as elephant or rhino.

Q 11. Why butyric acid in a silage is considered as bad although it is one of the volatile fatty acid present in the rumen of cow?

Butyric acid is a normal end product of carbohydrate fermentation in the rumen. On the other hand high butyric acid in silage indicates that the silage has undergone clostridial fermentation, which is one of the poorest fermentation. Silage high in butyric acid has poor nutritive value (higher ADF and NDF value) because many of the soluble nutrients have been degraded. This type of silage may have high soluble protein content and may contain amines, which can adversely affect the performance of the animal. High level of butyric acid in silage some time induced ketosis in lactating cow because low energy level of silage and higher level of butyric acid in the blood of cow.

Q 12. Why beauty pageants are reluctant to eat oily things or fried snacks?

Oil particularly, PUFA when heated in iron or copper pan under goes auto-oxidation. UV rays also stimulate the auto-oxidation, which leads to generation of free radicals. Free radicals are harmful for the skin and it may causes wrinkles beside other side effects. So, that is why most beauty pageants are reluctant to eat such things. High calories intake is another reason.

Q 13. Why DL-methionine is used as a feed additive instead of L-methionine?

Only L - amino acids are used in protein synthesis. In some case, animal can convert the d-isomer to the L - isomer form (Methionine), whereas, in other case (Lysine) they can not. So, DL Methionine is used as a feed additive but lysine is available only as L-lysine.

Q 14. Why new born calves are more sensitive to cold than older calves or cow?

New born calves have a greater surface area/pound of body weight as compared with older animals. The amount of heat production by an animal at maintenance is proportional to body weight, but the amount of heat dissipated is proportional to body surface area.

Q 15. All animals are monogastric. Justify.

Animal scientists have categorised autoenzymatic digester as monogastric or non-ruminants. These terms are unsatisfactory. All animals are monogastric i.e. have one gastric stomach. Many animals like ruminants have a complex compartmentalized stomach but technical, they are monogastric.

Q 16. Why do cats have high dietary requirement for niacin?

Niacin is synthesized from tryptophan with numerous intermediates. There are species differences in activities of enzymes involved in niacin biosynthesis. In cat, picolinic acid is formed rather than niacin. Thus, cat has a high dietary requirement for niacin. In other species dietary, tryptophan has a sparing effect on the niacin requirement.

Q 17. What is the difference between slug feeding, target feeding, challenge feeding, flat rate feeding transitional feeding and phase feeding?

Slug feeding - It is faulty feeding to animals. Slug feeding is when cows are fed a large amount of grain or molasses at one time or sudden change of diet i.e. grain type to another or from low energy/high NDF diet to high energy/low NDF diet. It negatively affects the rumen health, digestion and reduces milk production.

Flat rate feeding - Feeding a constant amount of concentrate through out the entire lactation. It is not recommended as during early lactation concentration fed is insufficient, while during late lactation it will be too much.

Targets concentrate feeding - If due to financial constraints, it is not possible to fed as much concentrate as would be ideal, then it is best to feed all the concentrate available during early lactation. During early lactation cow need plenty of nutrients to cater body need than that required during late lactation.

Challenge feeding/Lead feeding - This method of concentrate feeding is practised in lactating animals. Begins with a low level of concentrates and gradually increases the amount of concentrate fed each day until the point is reached, when adding concentrate does not result in an increase in the next day milk production. This is also known as lead feeding. Continue with this level of feeding for the first 12 weeks of the lactation. After 12 weeks, the amount of concentrate fed should depend upon the milk production.

Transitional feeding - Transition period is 3 weeks prior and 3 weeks after the calving. Feeding during this phase is very critical and requires proper attention to get the maximum output from animals.

Phase feeding - Phase feeding is a concept introduced in the early 1980 and is centred around diet modification based on the relationship among milk production, feed intake and body weight change occurring through out the lactation cycle.

Q 18. Why green fodder should be cut in the evening?

Forages will have low sugar content early in the morning because the plant cellular respiration will have been utilizing sugar all night. By the afternoon, photosynthesis should have produced a lot of sugars. A cold night will reduce the rate of respiration, so the following morning the forage should have higher sugar content than normal.

Q 19. What is the difference between essential, non-essential, critical and limiting amino acids?

Some amino acids are not synthesized in the body or if so, they are not adequate. So, they must be provided in the diet. Such amino acids are known as essential amino acids or indispensible amino acids. Amino acids required but synthesized in the body adequately are known as non-essential amino acids or dispensible amino acids.

Among the essential amino acids, certain amino acids are likely to be low in feeds. These are known as critical amino acids.

Among critical amino acids lysine, methionine are the most deficient amino acid and are known as limiting amino acids.

Q 20. What are the advantages of hind gut fermentation in horse over the rumen fermentation in ruminants?

Soluble carbohydrates, such as glycogen, are available to the animal before they are available to the microbes. Therefore, the brain, which can only utilise glucose, receives a good, constant supply with relatively less time and energy utilised than in the ruminant. The ability to process food more rapidly than foregut fermenters gives hindgut fermenters an advantage at very large body size, as they are able to accommodate significantly larger food intakes.

Q 21. Why fat, such as pig lard, beef and mutton, tallow is firm and hard, where as fat from fish and plant oils are softer and oily in nature?

Fat from plant and marine oils especially of fish are more highly unsaturated than those of mammalian origin. This is because of the presence of varying amount of linolenic acid (18:2), linolenic acid (18:3) and oleic acid (18:1). In fish oil (fat) significant concentration of highly unsaturated fatty acid C20 and C22 are also present. In mammalian depot fat, the proportion of high molecular weight saturated acid like palmitic acid (16:1), stearic acid (C18) are present along with smaller but significant contribution from lauric (C12) and myristic acids (C14). So, due to this reason, there fat is firm and hard.

Q 22. Why elderly people always suggest to drink the milk before going to bed for a good sleep?

Milk is good source of biological active peptides. The enzymatic hydrolysis of the milk protein casein releases opioid peptides, which have pharmacological activities, such as analgesia and sleep inducing effects. Both of these activities can lead to a good sleep.

Q 23. Why pig did not suffer from gout?

Gout is caused by crystal of insoluble uric acid precipitating in soft tissue and joint and causing pain. Pigs do not get gout because they convert uric acid to water soluble allantoin.

Q 24. Why does goat meat or beef fat contains odd chain and branch chain fatty acid but poultry fat does not?

Goat meat fat or beef fat contain odd and branched chain fatty acid because of microbial metabolism of lipid in the rumen, which produce various VFA i.e. propionic acid, valeric acid and isobutyric acid.

Q 25. Vitamin D is a hormone. Justify.

Vitamin D is a steroid and is a hormone because it is produced in a gland i.e. kidney and transport by the blood to the target tissue (intestine). Its formation and secretion are controlled by a feedback mechanism i.e. blood calcium concentrate.

Q 26. Why do cows excrete cow pies while sheep excrete pellets?

As the relative size of fore-stomach increases, there is a decrease in the abdominal space available for colon which tends to decrease in relative size. Decrease length of the colon, reduces the capacity for water absorption. Sheep has comparatively less voluminous rumen and greater colon space for water absorption. So, due to more water absorption, it excretes pellets.

Q 27. Explain why DCAD is expressed as milliequivalent per 100 gram DM rather than a per cent of ration DM?

The DCAD is used to create mild metabolic acidosis i.e. when the ration has a negative DCAD. Mechanism by which DCAD helps prevent milk fever and hypocalcemia is related to the physiological need to maintain electrical neutrality of the blood. Na, K, Cl and S are four elements used for DCAD calculation. Each ion exerts its effect according to its valence or electric charge rather than in proportion to its weight.

Q 28. Explain how the negative DCAD in late lactation reduces the chances of hypocalcemia and milk fever?

Feeding of negatively charged mineral like ammonium chloride in late lactation causes a drop in blood pH and thereby produces a mild state of metabolic acidosis. In order to maintain the blood pH in normal physiological range of 7.0-7.4, the body will mobilize the calcium carbonate from the bone. The carbonate in acidic blood is converted to bicarbonate that neutralized the high concentration of H^+. In this process, the calcium and some phosphorus are released incidentally from the bones. This will result in higher Ca concentrations in the blood. This higher blood calcium lowers the chances of hypocalcemia and milk fever in the freshly calved animals.

Q 29. Which egg-cooked or raw should be fed to dogs?

Feeding of raw egg, sometimes leads to vomiting and diarrhoea. Research revealed that raw egg white started leaving the stomach almost as soon as swallowed. As early as an hour and half after swallowing, the egg white was well along in small intestine. In contrast boiled egg white remained in the stomach for 2-3 hours until well digested. Raw egg white fed to dogs was often found in stools. Raw egg white feeding can lead to deficiency of biotin due to presence of avidin. Dog could utilize only 50-60% of raw egg white and cooked was found to be 90% utilized.

Q 30. What is the difference between foregut and hindgut fermentation?

The difference between them is the site of fermentation and the organ used for fermentation. Other attributes of the fermentation chamber remain the same, like - **anaerobic environment**, plenty of fluid, regulated pH, steady nitrogen supply and the correct temperature.

- Foregut Fermentation – Foregut fermenters animals includes cow, buffalo, sheep, goat, ox and deer, camels, llamas, they ferment their food before it reaches the 'true' stomach. The stomach of a ruminant exists as four chambers which are the **rumen, reticulum, omasum** and **abomasum** (true stomach). Ruminants digest food more efficiently than hindgut fermenters, as they are able to consume food into the rumen – the site of fermentation, allow microbial digestion and then regurgitate the 'cud' and chew it some more. This means by the time the ingested food reaches the abomasum, all the extractable nutrients have been metabolised (some microflora from the rumen may also be digested in the abomasum, which increases nutrient intake).
- Hindgut Fermentation – Hindgut fermenters (e.g. elephant, horse, guinea pig, rabbit, herbivorous reptiles, e.g. tortoise and herbivorous birds) have a digestive system very similar to carnivores, except due to the large amounts of fibre and other difficult-to-digest components of the diet, the complete digestive tract is much longer. Hindgut fermenters also have a working, enlarged caecum which is the site of bacterial fermentation. The process of fermentation is the same as that of foregut fermenters, however, as the caecum is located after the stomach and small intestine, the majority of food reaches the caecum undigested. Bacterial fermentation occurs in the caecum and colon allowing some volatile fatty acids to be absorbed, but then the digested food is excreted (along with the microflora). This is why some hindgut fermenters are seen eating their faeces – the food making

up the faeces has been digested by the microflora making it of nutritional value. The ingestion of the faeces allows the restoration of the microflora population.

Q 31. Why the epithelium of small intestine allow passage of intact immunoglobulin's (large protein molecule present in colostrums) during the first 24 hours of calf life?

Exact reason is not known, but various theories have been put forward to explain this :

1. Low acidity in the abomasums, due to under development of the parietal cells of the abomasums (that produce HCl) up to 24 hours after birth.
2. Absence of enzyme that would normally degrade the protein.
3. Presence of anti-tryptic enzyme in colostrums.
4. Presence of a non-heat coagulable protein in colostrums that may act in manner analogous to that of a surface active agent.
5. Thickening of the intestinal wall as a result of bacterial flora becoming established.
6. Hormonal balance of the calf.

Q 32. Why egg is used in artificial colostrums?

The scientific basis for this lies in that egg white has marked anti-bacterial action on at least certain strains of *E.Coli*, the causative agent of calf diarrhoea. It has also been observed that egg albumin like the globulins of colostrums can pass unchanged into the blood stream of the calf during the first 24 hours of life. This entry into the blood stream via lymphatic system is possibly helped by the large amount of the emulsifying agent, lecithin in egg yolk. It is also a good source of vitamin A.

Q 33. What are the advantages and disadvantages of suckling colostrums over bucket feeding?

Advantages

1. Immunoglobulin's tend to be greater in calves obtaining colostrums by suckling their dams than in those given by colostrums by bucket.

2. Suckling promotes early expulsion of meconium as compared to bucket feeding.
3. Milk letdown is facilitated for zebu cattle, which do not readily release their milk unless a calf is present.

Disadvantages

1. Extension of the postpartum interval to rebreeding. The extent depends upon the amount of suckling. Adlib suckling may cause complete lactational anoestrous. This reproductive delay is due to reduced LH output of pituitary gland when calf suckles.
2. Exact amount of milk production can not be measured.
3. If calf allows suckling at last of milking, then this milk contain more fat. So, overall fat content of the remaining milk decreased.
4. Sometimes due to death of calf, dam is reluctant to release the milk.
5. Suckling delays the onset of oestrous after calving.

Q 34. What is the difference between feed supplement and feed additive?

Feed supplement : It refer, to feed stuffs that are used to improve the value of basal feeds. They can be used in large quantity like protein supplement or in very small quantity like vitamins or trace mineral supplements.

Feed additive : They can be of nutritive and non nutritive type and are usually added in small quantity to obtain the desired effect like improvement of performance, or feed utilization.

Q 35. Why colostrums get coagulated on heating but milk does not?

Colostrums contain higher amount of albumin and globulins. So, when colostrums are heated, these proteins get coagulated. But in milk, these albumin and globulin are in much amount, so it does not get coagulated.

Q 36. Do the rumen fluid always have the same colour?

Normally, rumen liquor colour is olive green to greenish brown. However, it can vary and partially resemble the composition of diet.

Grass fed/green fodder fed animals: Grey to Olive green

Maize silage/ straw fed: Grey brown or yellowish brown

Blackish green: Feeding of charcoal/ rumen purification

Dark Brown: Simple inactivity of rumen biota

Reddish Discolouration: Bleeding die to rumenocentesis/feeding of beetroot

These feed stuffs contain carotene, xanthophyll, chlorophyll and phaeophytin, etc. type of pigment which directly or indirectly give the characteristic colour to rumen fluid.

Q 37. Feeding of sodium bicarbonate in dairy ration is best management practice in early lactation but a worst management practice during the transition period (before calving). Explain, why?

Sodium bicarbonate is a buffer which prevents the occurrence of acidosis, which can otherwise, leads to reduced feed intake, anorexia, bloat, and reduced milk production depending upon the extent of acidity. Sodium bicarbonate by preventing rumen acidosis stimulate dry matter intake. It plays a crucial role in buffering the increased amount of volatile fatty acid produced in the rumen after calving due to high DMI and increased proportion of concentrate in the diet especially in the diet of high yielder.

On the contrary in transition period before calving, recommendation is of negative DCAD to lower the incidence of milk fever and hypocalcemia. Four elements Na, K, Cl and S are used for DCAD calculation. So, feeding of sodium bicarbonate at this stage increases the level of sodium and there by making the DCAD positive. This prone the animal for milk fever and hypocalcemia post calving.

Q 38. What is the difference between silage, shredlage, haylage, earlage and snaplage?

Silage: Green fodder preserved under anaerobic condition is known as silage

Shredlage: In this method, before ensiling fodder crops are shredded longitudinally, while simultaneously chopped. This silage will provide more peNDF and have more readily available starch and sugar as compared to normal silage.

Hay lage: It is ensiled corn grain, cobs and in some cases, husks and a portion of the stalk. It is higher in energy than normal corn silage.

Snaplage: This term pertain to ensiled corn grain, cobs and husks typically harvested with a forage harvester equipped with a corn snapper header so that only the ear and a portion of the ear shank is removed, chopped and ensiled.

Q 39. Can the adult dairy animal ration or lactation ration can be given to the calf as a starter ration?

No, adult dairy animal ration or lactation ration can't be given to newly born calf as a starter ration because this type of ration have lesser protein, more fibre content, no B-complex vitamins, no coccidiostat, no antibiotic, no yeast and sometimes no molasses. In adult animal, rumen bugs can synthesize vitamin B complex, so no need to supplement these from externally but in calves' rumen is not developed; so, they need them in their feed. Similarly, coccidiostat and antibiotic are added in calf starter to prevent the incidence of diarrohea and to promote the growth by preventing the growth of pathogen in GI Tract.

Q 40. Why it is not a good practice to feed a well balanced early lactation diet as transitional diet to the cow in the last three weeks of pregnancy?

In transitional phase, low sodium and potassium diet is desirable so as to reduce the incidence of milk fever. But they are high in lactation diet as buffer and molasses are added in this diet to maximize the productivity. These two elements increase the DCAD in the diet. This can increase the chances of milk fever post calving.

On the other hand, it takes almost three weeks for the rumen bugs to develop as per new diet. So, the lactation diet can be started 3-4 days before calving in a gradual manner. Use of anionic salts is helpful to lower the DCAD before calving.

Q 41. What is the difference between plain, fortified and chelated mineral mixture?

Plain mineral mixture is the mixture, in which inorganic salts of various minerals are mixed in a proper amount and ratio so that it will be able to meet the requirement of the animals. It costs less and has nominal charges.

In fortified mineral mixture, some herbs, vitamins etc are added and mixed in the plain mineral mixture. Main aim is to overcome the deficiencies improved the absorption of minerals and performance of the animals. It cost, more than the plain mineral mixture.

In chelated mineral mixture, mineral (s) are attached with certain organic moiety known as ligand through a coordinate covalent bond. Ligand may be certain amino acid, certain organic acid or may be polysaccharide. This requires a proper technique. This type of mineral mixture is costly than the above two mineral mixture and is recommended for high yielding animals.

Q 42. Why oat is preferred over maize for horse feeding?

In stomach of horse, good population of lactobacilli exist, which produces gas from fermenting sugar and starch. Since maize is a good source of energy, it can lead to lacto acidosis and stomach damage. On the other hand, oat has lower energy level and high fibre content, so it is preferred because it causes less trouble in stomach of horse.

Q 43. Why chicken soup of feet's and legs is recommended by elderly people in case of bone fracture?

Skin of legs and feet of the chicken contain about eight times as much 7-dehydrocholesterol (Provitamin D_3) as the body skin. So, it helps in bone formation through promoting absorption of calcium in small intestine.

Q 44.Why is it that milk fat percentage is so easily influenced in a given species, whereas the lactose percentage is fairly constant?

The milk fat content is determined by the acetic and butyric acid production from rumen fermentation, constituting 50% to 60% and 12% to 18% respectively of the total VFAs. Diet and the status of the microbes in the rumen greatly influence the proportion of VFAs. Only 40% of milk fatty acids are produced directly out of carbohydrate degradation in the rumen and remaining 60% of the milk fat is produced over metabolomics synthase from VFA's of the digestive tract and free non-esterified fatty acids from body fat degradation. Both milk fat content and composition are, therefore, influenced by the feedstuffs like fiber, carbohydrates, fats. Propionic acid through glucose is precursor the milk lactose content. Lactose is formed in the mammary gland from glucose. Studies suggest that the rate of lactose synthesis appears to be dependent upon the α - LA to GT ratio. β 1,4 Galactosyl transferase (GT) is the enzymatic subunit of lactose synthase. α -Lact albumin (α-LA) a milk when protein is necessary for the synthesis of lactose. α-LA is only expressed in the mammary gland, lactose synthesis only occurs in the mammary gland. In addition, expression of the α-lact albumin gene is closely regulated by hormones and lactose synthesis only occurs during the lactating state of the tissue. So, the content of lactose in the milk is nearly stable.

Q 45. Why fat has greater gross energy value/gram as compared with carbohydrate?

Relative composition of protein, fat and carbohydrate in per cent is as :

	C	H	O	N
Fat	77	12	11	–
Protein	52	6	22	16
Carbohydrate	44	6	50	–

In carbohydrate, there is enough oxygen present in the molecule to take care of all the hydrogen present, thus heat arises only from the oxidation of the carbon. In case of fat, however, there is relatively much less oxygen present and relatively more oxygen atoms are required from outside and combustion involves the oxidation of hydrogen as well as carbon. The burning of 1g H2 produces over four times as much heat (34.5Kcal/g) as compared to the case of carbon (8 Kcal/g). So, this is the reason why Fat has higher gross energy as compared to fat.

Q 46. Why meat from older animal is tough on cooking?

Collagen content increases with aging of the animal. Collagen has characteristic of shrinkage on heating because of its high proline and hydroxyproline content. So, this shrinkage of collagen gives the toughness to the meat of older animal.

Q 47. What is the difference between Nutraceuticals, Nutrigenomic and Nutrigenetics?

Nutraceuticals : Nutraceutical (Nutrient + Pharmaceuticals) is defined as any food/feed or ingredient having some health benefit including disease treatment and prevention. This term was coined by " Stephen Defelice". Sarah 2003 reported that Nutraceuticals, when fed to the birds/animals must improve the performance effectively & economically, with little therapeutic use, without causing cross resistance to other antibiotic at actual use level, without involving with transferable (infectious) drug resistance, without causing deleterious disturbance to the normal gut flora, Without creating environmental pollution and must be nontoxic to the animals and its handlers. Booth (1997) defined the term "Veterinary Neutraceutical" as a non-drug substance that is produced in purified or extracted form and administered orally to provide agents required for normal body structure and function with the intent of improving health and well-being of animals.

Nutrigenomic: It is the study of effect of feed or feed constituents on gene expression. It is a molecular level study involving interaction between nutrients and other dietary bioactive with the genome. Or it is defined as response of gene to dietary nutrients.

Nutrigenetics: It studies the effect of different gene changes on nutrient metabolism or it is the study of molecular relationship between genes, their response to specific nutrients and how those response can impact animal health and performance.

Q 48. What is Precision Animal Nutrition?

It is defined as providing the animal (in question) with the feed that precisely meet its nutrients requirements for optimum production, reproduction, health for producing wholesome animal products without having any negative effect on environment. Basic deriving force behind this is to improve profitability and social milieu.

Objectives of Precision Animal Nutrition

1. To provide the feed to animal which precisely match their requirements.
2. To improve the profitability or gross return by ensuring the better feed efficiency.

3. To maintain the cleaner environment by lowering a) the excretion of N, P, K etc in excreta b) methane production in rumen.
4. Effective use of available feed resource (conventional and unconventional) to match the animal nutrients requirement.
5. To make the future of mankind bright by preserving feed resource and environment besides, providing the quality animal food.

Q 49. How many eggs are produced by a hen in a day?

A *hen* requires about 24 to 26 hours to produce an *egg*. After the *egg* is laid, the *hen* starts all over again about 30 minutes later. So, a hen will give one egg per day and will have some days, when it does not lay an egg at all.

Q 50. What are the cost and benefits of rumen digestion?

Benefits

1. Because of rumen microbes present in reticulo-rumen complex, animal can use fibrous feed which is otherwise too fibrous for non-ruminants.
2. Can use cellulose- the most abundant carbohydrate present as a major nutrient.
3. Rumen microbes are able to synthesise all components of vitamin B Complex provide the adequate Co for vitamin B_{12} synthesis.
4. Rumen microbes can synthesis high quality microbial protein from low quality protein, non-protein nitrogen and recycled nitrogenous end products.
5. Unconventional fibrous feed can be used easily.

Costs

1. Spend a large part of their life (1/3 rd) on chewing. On an average 8 hours/day.
2. Contrary to monogastric, in ruminant animal what they fed is not reached in the true stomach in same proportion and amount.
3. Feeding of high quality protein can be converted to lower quality protein.

4. Need complicated mechanism to keep the fermentation vat working efficiently like a) regular addition of large quantities of alkaline saliva, b) powerful mixing movements in the forestomach c) mechanism for the elimination of the gases of fermentation.
5. Almost 8-9 % energy is lost as methane.

Q 51. Explain Cu-Mo-S interactions.

This interaction of Cu-Mo-S was first reported by Dick and Bull in 1945.

1. Teart – England & wales- Pasture- Mo very high - Cause rapid scoring though Copper content is in normal range.
2. Peat Score – Newzealand - Moderate High Mo- but pasture Copper is below normal range- copper depletion- Scour
   - High sulphate or grazing in a minning area rich in "S" leads to production of rumen sulphide, which reduces Cu absorption through the formation of insoluble copper sulphide.
   - Chronic Copper poisoning can occur in sheep with moderate Copper intake but very low level of Mo and Sulphate.
   - Conversely the depletion of animal Copper reserve or copper deficiency can arise on normal copper but high Mo and sulphate intakes. So, Mo and sulphate can either increase or decrease the copper status of the animal.
   - Under the influence of Mo and SO_4- absorption of Cu decreased, rate of accumulation of copper in liver decrease.
   - According to one theory- these anions restrict copper utilization in sheep by depressing copper solubility in GIT through the precipitation of insoluble cupric sulphide.
   - The present theory says that Mo exerts its limiting effect on copper retention in the animal only in the presence of S. Sulphide is formed in rumen by microorganism, which in turn combine with copper to form an insoluble copper thiomolybdate ($CuMoS_4$) thereby limiting the absorption of dietary copper. Thiomolybdate if formed in excess- absorbed and exert a systemic effect on copper metabolism in animal. Tri and tetrathiomolybdate complexes responsible for reducing copper absorption, while di and tri thiomolybdate effects the copper metabolism in the body.

- Formation of thiomolybdate also effects the kinetics of S-metabolism by affecting sulphide formation and absorption. Thiomolybdates rapidly react with particulate matter and protein to form complex that bind Cu strongly, reducing its solubility, decreasing the H_2S concentration.
- Rain increases the Mo content - thereby reduced the copper level.

Q 52. Explain Vitamin E and Se relationship.

There is a close working relationship between vitamin E and Se. Se has a sparing effect on vitamin E and sulphur amino acids particularly protect against or delay onset of several form of Se deficiency syndromes. Tissue breakdown occurs in most species receiving diet deficient in both vitamin E and Se.

Peroxides and hydroperoxide are highly distructive to tissue integrity and lead to disease development.

1. Vitamin E in cellular and subcellular membranes is the first line of defence against peroxidation of vital phospholipids but even with adequate vitamin E some peroxides are formed. Se as a part of enzyme glutathione peroxidise is a second line of defence that destroy these peroxides before have an opportunity to cause damage to membranes. Therefore, Se, Vitamin E and S containing amino acids through different biochemical mechanism are capable of preventing some of the same nutritional diseases. Vitamin E prevents fatty acid hydroperoxide formation, S amino acids are precursors of glutathione peroxidise and Se is a component of glutathione peroxidise.
2. To some extent, vitamin E and Se are mutually replaceable but there are lower limits below which substitution is in effective. In diet severely deficient in Se, vitamin E does not prevent or cure exudative diathesis, whereas addition of little Se completely prevent this disease.
3. Both vitamin E and Se provide protection against toxicity with three class of heavy metals :

   i) Ist class consists of metal like Cadium and Mercury- In which Se is highly effective in altering toxicities but vitamin E has little influence.

ii) Second class includes silver and arsenic- Vitamin E is highly effective and selenium is also effective but only at relatively high level.

iii) Third class include Lead- Vitamin E is effective but Se has little effect.

4. Both Vitamin E and Se play an important role in protecting leukocytes and macrophages during phagocytosis- the mechanism whereby mammals immunologically kills invading bacteria. Both Vitamin E and Se may help these cells to survive the toxic product that are produced in order to effectively kill ingested bacteria.

5. Requirements of both Vitamin E and Se are greatly dependent on the dietary concentration of each other. Vitamin E is known to reduce the selenium requirement in at least two ways i) By maintaining body Se in an active form or preventing loss from body. ii) By preventing destruction of membrane lipids within membrane thereby inhibiting the production of hydroperoxides and reducing the amount of glutathione peroxidise needed to destroy peroxide in the cell.

   Se is known to spare vitamin E in at least three ways :

   i) It is required to preserve the integrity of the pancreas, which allow normal fat digestion thus normal vitamin E absorption.

   ii) It reduces the amount of vitamin E required to maintain the integrity of lipid membranes via glutathione peroxidise.

   iii) It aids in some unknown ways in retention of vitamin E in blood plasma.

6. Adult cows with a Se/Vitamin E deficiency may be more likely to suffer from retention of placenta, abnormal calving, metritis, cystic ovaries and higher risk of infertility.

Q 53. Why roaster crow but hens do not?

Syrinx is the voice box in the chicken. The chicken voice is produced by air pressure on a sound valve and modified by muscle tension. Both roaster and hens are able to crow. The reason hens don't normally crow is because they 'don't feel like it' due to female hormone effects and the absence of sufficient levels of the male hormone. When the ovaries become diseased and the level of female hormones decrease, many hens will start to show male characteristics including crowing.

Q 54. Why molasses based diet is not recommended to the animal approaching calving? or Is potassium beneficial or detrimental in a prefresh diet?

Feed anionic salts as part of the pre calving feeding program prevents milk fever and retained placentas. Anionic salts provide anions (chloride and sulphate) to counteract the cations (potassium and sodium) in the diet. This will help to lower body pH, stimulate calcium release from the bones, stimulate calcium absorption from the gut, prevent milk fever and retained placenta at calving. However, diets high in cations do the reverse and lead to milk fever or sub clinical hypocalcaemia. High cationic concentration reduces the sensitivity of bone toward PTH hormone and limit the release of Calcium. So, avoid or minimise feeds in the diet that have a high sodium (buffers: sodium bicarbonate), potassium (molasses, sorghum, ryegrass) or calcium (lucerne) content, as they increase the risk of milk fever and retained placentas. Balance the diet for a low calcium content to increase the mobilisation of calcium from the bones and reduce the risk of milk fever and retained placenta.

Note: Anionic slats (ammonium chloride (*Nishader*), calcium chloride) are quite unpalatable and may further depress DM and energy intake. To determine whether the anionic salts are working, test the urine with pH test strips. Target a urine pH of less than 6.5.

Q 55. How urinary pH testing can be helpful in monitoring the status of transition cow especially in relation to prevention of hypocalcaemia?

Feeding of anionic salt is advocated as a preventive measure to reduce the risk of post calving hypocalcaemia. The optimum pH should be between 6.0-6.5. If diet is over acidified with excess of anionic salt, urine pH fall below 6.0 and if not enough anionic salts are being fed, then urinary pH remain close to neutral (pH of 7.0).

Q 56. Name the anionic salts which can be used in transition cow feed to prevent milk fever.

- Magnesium sulphate
- Calcium sulphate
- Calcium chloride
- Ammonium Chloride (Nishader)
- Magnesium chloride

Q 57. What are the similarities and differences between silage fermentation and rumen fermentation?

Similarities

- Anaerobic fermentation
- Lactic acid bacteria are required.

Differences

- Yeast are undesirable in silage but required in rumen fermentation.
- Acetic acid bacteria are undesirable in silage fermentation but required in rumen fermentation.
- Butyric acid is undesirable product in Silage but is one of the volatile fatty acid in rumen.
- Rumen fermentation is a continuous process but in silage, fermentation is a limited process and restricted to phase 2 or to a lesser extent in phase 3.
- If everything normal, rumen microflora continuous flourish but due to acidic pH in optimum silage, bacterial population decrease in stable phase.
- Acetic acid is predominant acid (50-60%) in rumen fermentation but it should be less than 2% in stable silage. In silage, Lactic acid is predominant acid.
- Rumen pH 6.8-7.2 and in silage, it is 3.8-4.2.

Q 58. Why cattle need fibre?

- For rumen fill.
- Maintaining normal rumen fermentation through optimum rumination.
- Maintain Normal milk fat percentage.
- Protecting post calving disorder.

Q 59. Why sheep is less susceptible to nitrate toxicity than the cattle?

In rumen, Nitrate is reduced to nitrite by the rumen bugs, which when absorbed and oxidized the ferrous iron of haemoglobin to ferric ion, which is known as methaemoglobin which can not carry oxygen to body tissue. The susceptibility of any ruminant species depends upon its ability to reduce methaemoglobin. The rate of methaemoblin reduction in erythrocyte is the highest in sheep and lowest in cattle. So, sheep is less susceptible to nitrate toxicity.

Q 60. Why Neutral Detergent Fibre (NDF) is generally higher than crude fibre (CF)?

Crude fibre consists of hemi-cellulose, cellulose and lignin, however, during CF estimation part of hemicellulose and lignin are reflected in Nitrogen free extract (NFE). NDF consist of hemicellulose, cellulose, lignin, silica and some pectin.

Q 61. How big should a heifer be at breeding and at calving?

Stage	Puberty	Breeding	1st calving'	2nd calving	3rd calving
% Mature body size	45-50%	55%	82%	92%	100%

A puberty calf should be around 45-50% of is expected mature body size, at breeding it should be 55% of mature body size, at first calving 82%, at 2nd calving 92% and by 3rd calving at 100%.

Q 62. Difference between rumen fermentation in cattle and caecum fermentation in horse?

First and foremost is position of fermentation chamber (rumen in cattle and caecum in horse) in relation to small intestine. In rumen fermentation, it is cranial to small intestine, so all the products coming from this chamber has to go through small intestine, where in horse it is caudal to small intestine. In ruminant microbial protein is utilized as a source of protein, whereas in horse it is almost lost.

Q 63. Peculiar difference between dog and cat digestive physiology?

- Cat lack the enzyme deoxygenase necessary to cleave beta carotene hence it required preformed vitamin A as compared to dog which can cleave the beta carotene.

- Cat need an additional essential amino acid (beta amino sulphonic acid), which most other mammals are able to synthesize taurine from sulphur containing amino acid. The cat's ability to snthesize is very limited.
- Cat has a higher requirement for dietary protein than the dog.
- Cat is an obligate carnivore where as dog is omnivore.
- Cat can not synthesize nicotinic acid from tryptophan.
- Cat can not convert sufficient linoleic acid to meet its requirement for arachidonic acid. Similarly, cat can not synthesize eicosapentaenoic acid from alpha - linolenic acid due to lack of enzyme delta-6-desaturase.
- Dentition of the dog include molars for crushing plant material, where as cat lack these teeth.
- Cat's small intestine is shorter than dogs (even when corrected to overall body length).
- Cat's have even fewer taste buds than dogs.
- Cats are unable to meet their metabolic needs for vitamin D via dermal photosynthesis because they lack 7-dehydrocholesterol, which is required for synthesis.

Q 64. Difference between Finishing and Flushing?

Finishing: the process of bringing meat animals to a desired state of body condition prior to slaughter is known as finishing. In broiler, it represents the last one third of life, for pig it start from around 50-55 kg to slaughter.

Flushing : A feeding strategies consisting of an increasing plane of nutrition in animal usually applied before mating. Practiced in sheep and pig to have more numbers of offsprings.

Q 65. Why churning of milk cream leads to butter formation?

Milk fat is secreted from the mammary epithelial cells as fat globules and it consists of a mixture of compounds including triacylglycerols, diacylglycerols, monoacylglycerols, phospholipids, cerebrosides, gangliosides, sterols and sterol esters and derivatives, carotenoids, tocopherol, vitamins A, D, E, C, B1, and B2 and free fatty acids. They are not soluble in water, or aqueous liquids. The milk fat globule is encapsulated by a lipid bilayer membrane made up of proteins, phospholipids, lipoproteins, cerebrosides, nucleic acids, enzymes, trace elements, and bound water. The FGM (fat globule membrane) provides stabilization for the fat globule in the aqueous environment of the milk serum. During churning, the FGM membrane get ruptured, the fat globules join together into a solid mass of fat known as butter.

Q 66. Why green colour of fodder is converted into yellowish/brownish/golden colour in silage?

This is due to action of organic acids on the chlorophyll, which converts the chlorophyll into a brown magnesium free pigment, phaeophytin. This pigment gives the brownish/ golden colour to the silage.

Q 67. Why threobromine toxicity is a significant risk for pet dogs but not for pet cat?

Dogs are sensitive to and show preference for sweet foods like chocolate, which can lead to threobromine toxicity but cat donot prefer the food so does not consume the chocolate or other sweet foods. Conversely, cats but not dogs are attracted to flavours that are even bitter.

Q 68. Why plants contain ANF?

It is natural mechanism through which many members of plants kingdom save themselves from the other living organism. These plants synthesize certain unique chemical compounds for defense mechanism. Many of these compounds can be detrimental or fatal, if ingested by man or animal. So, these compounds are given the name as antinutritional factor (ANF). Plants contain thousand of compound which depending upon the situation, can have beneficial or deleterious effects on organism consuming them. These compounds with the exception of nutrients are referred as allelochemicals. ANFs may be regarded as a class of these compounds. Being an ANFs is not an intrinsic characteristic of a compound but depend upon the digestive process of the ingesting animals. For example, trypsin inhibitors, which are ANF's for monogastric animals, do not exert adverse effects in ruminants because they are degraded in rumen.

Q 69. Why lactation feed can not be fed to calves?

Lactation complete feed do not contain sufficient energy to support good calf growth.

They may also contain in appropriate amount of protein and minerals.

Also, lactation feed may contain added fat ,animal byproducts or other additives that reduces the palatability.

Lactation complete feed do not contain B-vitamin and coccidiostat.

More percentage of fibre in lactation feed.

Comparatively less palatble.

❑❑❑

Chapter 30

Going for Interview: Fill This Form

1. The cost of green fodder Rs.........per Kg or Rs................../tonn
2. Cost of wheat straw Rs.................../kg
3. Cost of concentrate Rs............../kg or Rs............../50kg Bag.
4. Cost of wheat grains Rs............../kg or Rs..................../tonn.
5. Cost of maize Rs.............../kg or Rs.................../tonn.
6. Cost of rice Rs................/kg or Rs................../tonn.
7. Cost of ricebran Rs................./kg or Rs................../tonn.
8. Cost of rice polish Rs................./kg or Rs................./tonn.
9. Cost of mustard cake Rs................../kg or Rs................./tonn.
10. Cost of cottonseed cake Rs................../kg or Rs................./tonn.
11. Cost of mineral mixture Rs................../kg
12. Cost of fish meal Rs............................/tonn
13. Cost of DCP Rs..
14. Cost of LSP Rs..
15. Cost of adult cow with 10 litre milk Rs ....
16. Cost of 1kg broiler - Rs..
17. Cost of 30 egg/tray Rs..

18. Space requirement for animals

Animals	Floor space requirement		Feeding space requirement
	Open	Covered	
Cows	–	–	–
Buffaloes	–	–	–
Bull	–	–	–
Calves	–	–	–
Doe	–	–	–
Buck	–	–	–
Kid	–	–	–
Sow	–	–	–
Boar	–	–	–

Some Important Books

1. Animal Nutrition by P Mcdonald, RA Edward, JFD Greenhalgh, CA Morgan, A Sinclair, G. Wilkinsin.
2. Matching Ruminants Production System with Available Resource in the Tropic and Subtropic by T R Preston and R A Lang.
3. Animal Nutrition in the tropic by S K Ranjan.
4. Vitamin in Animal Nutrition by Lee Rusell Mcdowell.
5. Minerals in Animal and Human Nutrition by Lee Rusell Mcdowell.
6. Comparative Animal Nutrition and Metabolism by P R Cheeke and E S Dierenfeld.
7. Animal Nutrition by Maynard and Loosli.
8. Feeds and Principals of Animal Nutrition By G C Banerjee.
9. Animal Feed Technology by SK Kundu, SK Mahanta, Sultan Singh and PS Pathak.
10. Principle and Practice Animal Nutrition By Jagdish Prasad.
11. Basic of Animal Nutrition by J S Hundal, Udaybir Singh and Jaswinder Singh.

❑❑❑